# Pain Free 1-2-3!

## A Proven Program to Get YOU Pain Free Now!

JACOB TEITELBAUM, M.D.

*Disclaimer*

Every effort has been made to ensure that the information contained in this book is complete and accurate. However, neither the publisher nor the author is engaged in rendering professional advice or services to the individual reader. The ideas, treatments, medications, procedures, and other suggestions contained in this book are not intended as a substitute for consulting with your physician. All matters regarding your physical health require medical supervision. Neither the author nor the publisher shall be liable or responsible for any loss, injury, or damage allegedly arising from any information or suggestion in this book.

*Pain Free 1-2-3!* and other Deva Press books are available at special quantity discounts.

For information contact:
Cheryl@endfatigue.com or call 410-573-5389

**Other books by Jacob Teitelbaum MD** (available at www.vitality101.com) **include:**

***From Fatigued to Fantastic! A Manual for Moving beyond Chronic Fatigue Syndrome and Fibromyalgia,*** and

***Three Steps to Happiness – Healing through Joy!***



ISBN 0-9647599-1-8
Library of Congress Cataloging-in-Publication Data

Printed in the United States of America

*To Laurie, my wife,*
*my special lady and the*
*love of my life;*
*my children, David, Amy, Shannon,*
*Brittany, and Kelly;*
*my mother, Sabina, and father, David,*
*whose unconditional love made this*
*book possible.*
*Drs. Janet Travell, Billie Crook,*
*and David Simons who laid the*
*foundation for this work,*
*and to my patients, who have taught*
*me more than I can ever hope to*
*teach them.*

# Acknowledgments

So many special people helped make this book possible that I cannot possibly list them all. In truth, I have created nothing new; I have simply synthesized the wonderful work done by an army of hard-working and courageous physicians and healers.

I would like to extend my sincerest thanks to:

First and foremost, my staff. Their hard work, compassion, and dedication (and, I must admit, patience with me) are what made my work possible.

My wonderful research partner Birdie (Barbara Bird). Her dedication to quality shows in every facet of her work. My office manager and "right hand person" Cheryl Alberto (the real boss), who makes sure that everything works as it should—no matter how much chaos I create. Amy Podd, Mary Groom, Angela Borlik, and Angela Bearden who make everything run smoothly. Bren Jacobson and Alan Weiss, who love me enough to call me on my "stuff" and keep me intellectually honest. The Anne Arundel Medical Center librarian, Joyce Miller. Over the last twenty years, I have often wondered when she would politely tell me to stop asking for so many studies. So far, she has not. In fact, she always smiles when I ask her for more.

My many teachers, the real heroes and heroines in their fields, whose names could fill this book. They include William Crook, Max Boverman, Brugh Joy, Janet Travell, David Simons, Jerry and Esther Hicks and the Abraham team, Hal Blatman, William Jefferies, Jay Goldstein, Leonard Jason, Michael Rosenbaum, Murray Susser, Charles Lapp, and Alan Gaby. I would like to thank my formatter, Doug Judy and my editor, Mary Zeilbeck, for her help and patience with me in the face of all my changes. I would also like to thank Doug Judy for his superb job of formatting and cover design. And I would especially like to thank my loving wife for her incredible and devoted dedication and help in making sure this book was the best possible guide it could be for helping people get their lives back.

I would also like to thank the many chronic pain, chronic fatigue syndrome and fibromyalgia support groups. These are easily the best patient support groups I have ever seen.

And finally, God and the universe, for the guidance and infinite blessings I have been given and for using me lovingly as an instrument for healing. ■

# Table of Contents

# Introduction—From Pain to Pain Free!

1975 was a very difficult year. After having several very stressful years that made medical school look easy, I came down with fibromyalgia, myofascial pain syndrome, and chronic fatigue syndrome (CFS). This gave me first-hand experience with widespread muscle pain and what it was like. It also gave me an enormous incentive to learn how to overcome these problems. Having widespread achiness was difficult, but taught me an enormous amount. In watching my body, I learned how a tight muscular knot (trigger point) in one area could cause pain and tenderness elsewhere in the body. I also found that tight muscles could cause other apparently unrelated symptoms like nausea and diarrhea. It was quite an education!

Several other experiences broadened my "pain horizon" dramatically. During my medical residency in 1979, I was working in the outpatient clinic. We would all cringe when one of the patients, an ornery, hunched-over elderly woman, came in. She was always in severe back pain and no one could help her. During one of her visits, she told me that when she pushed on a lump that was about a foot away from her discomfort it triggered her back pain. I mentioned this to my instructor, Dr. John Stuckey, and his eyes lit up. He said, "watch this," and with a smile he injected the lump with a little lidocaine (Novocain®). The woman was able to stand up straight, pain free for the first time in years. Without the chronic pain, she was the sweetest person you could imagine! At that time I had no idea why this had worked, but I rapidly learned about doing trigger point injections. Several years later, after reviewing thousands of research studies and attempting many experiments to ease my own discomfort, I had developed an effective metabolic approach to treating muscle pain. Despite being an internist I had, by default, become the pain specialist in town.

I was soon to find that other doctors had also discovered similar principles of pain management. Two of these spectacular physicians, Dr. Janet Travell and Dr. David Simons, had written a book, which a patient of mine gave me, called *The Trigger Point Manual*. In it, the authors had long before documented the concepts that I had "discovered." Dr. Travell was a professor at George Washington Medical School and the White House physician for Presidents Kennedy and Johnson. She has since passed on. Dr. Travell and Dr. Simons are the "grandparents" of modern pain management. Their book expanded the understanding of treatment dramatically for pain specialists. They also laid the foundation for your getting well!

### *Am I Alone with My Pain?*

Chronic pain is a very common problem affecting millions of Americans. In a 1999 American Pain Society survey, nine percent of the American adult population was found to suffer from moderate to severe non-cancer related chronic pain. 56 percent of these had suffered for over five years. When the researchers reviewed 805 chronic pain patients, they found that over half of them had changed doctors because their physicians were unwilling or unable to adequately and appropriately treat their pain.[1]

### *I Know How Pain Affects Me, but What Are the Costs to Society?*

In addition to the ways in which it devastates people's lives, chronic pain is one of the most expensive medical conditions in the United States. The price tag, including loss of productivity, loss of income, and medical costs, exceeds $100 billion annually.[2] Over $61 billion is lost in productive work time because of pain, even if the person is able to work.[3] Our track record for treating cancer-related pain is also devastating. The American Cancer Society estimates that an enormous number of advanced cancer patients suffer from inadequately treated chronic pain.[4]

The financial costs pale compared to the suffering and loss of personal relationships, functional ability, and even length of life, as well as the depression and anxiety caused by the chronic pain. **The good news is that most chronic pain now can be effectively treated.** Unfortunately, most doctors have not yet been trained in proper pain management. This does not, however, mean that you have to wait to get relief. This book has been written to give you and your physician the information you need so that you can be pain-free and get your life back.

### *How Does Traditional "Pharmaceutical" Medicine Handle Pain?*

I can summarize most of what I was taught about pain in medical school in one paragraph. Use Tylenol® and/or Advil® family medications. If the patient has cancer, you can use narcotics if you have to.

Were I a surgeon, surgical options might be added. I was given the impression that chiropractors, and anyone else who offered something that wasn't taught in medical school, were quacks trying to steal people's money and that physicians needed to protect gullible patients from them.

Although this may seem like a sad assessment, I suspect that most of you who have chronic pain will agree with it. Many physicians reading this book will also find that this mirrors their experience. The good news is that you don't have to be in pain anymore!

## *What Happens When Physicians Combine Natural and Allopathic Medicine?*

The use of both natural and allopathic (prescription) medicine dramatically increases our ability to help you get well. Although both allopathic and natural medicines have their weaknesses, when you combine them almost all pain can be effectively treated. It's the difference between having only one tool—say a hammer, which is like allopathic medicine—or a whole tool kit that includes the dozens of other healing arts available in natural medicine. A hammer can be a very useful tool, but unfortunately when all you have is a hammer, everything starts to look like a nail! It's much easier to get the job done safely and effectively when you are using all the tools available to you.

Doctors are usually better at treating acute, short-lasting pain (e.g. injuries, surgery, etc.) because they are better able to find the source and are more comfortable using available treatments on a short-term basis. Treating chronic pain problems—such as fibromyalgia and myofascial/muscle pain, cancer pain, arthritis, headaches, back pain, and nerve pain—is more of a challenge for physicians.

## *How Can I Bridge the Split between the Two Systems?*

There seems to be much confusion and conflict over whether natural or prescription medicines are the best. On one hand, there are those who claim that pharmaceuticals are the new panacea and a cure-all for everything, while natural remedies are unregulated, unproven, ineffective forms of snake oil. On the other hand, there are those who say that surgery and prescription medications are highly toxic and too expensive. They claim that we should only use natural medicines and point out their safety record. How are we to make sense of all this confusion?

I choose to keep the best of both systems. Over the decades, I've often had to struggle with the perceived conflict between these two wonderful and powerful branches of the healing arts. When we examine these systems closely, however, there is no conflict between them. So-called CAM, Complementary and Alternative Medicine, i.e. natural, therapies offer the vast variety and power that nature brings to healing through herbs, nutrition, touch, love, and energy/spirit. Using a mix of intuition, experience, and science, it is a more feminine "motherly love" kind of approach. Although CAM factors in what science has to say, like a mother taking care of her child, it is most interested simply in what works and what is safe. This often results in it being very open-minded and accounts for its current rapid growth. Allopathic medicine focuses largely on that which is patentable. It mainly deals with prescriptions, and can sometimes use the powerful tools of science to develop effective new remedies. Scientific debate within the medical community can be very useful for sorting out what works and dealing with things that the scientists believe in (i.e. prescriptions). Allopathic medicine, however, is much too biased to be objective when it comes to evaluating natural remedies. For example, if given the power to regulate natural medicines, the FDA would likely regulate them out of existence. Because of this, Congress appropriately protects natural products.

Although natural therapies have their strengths, they also have their shortcomings. One of these is quality control. Where an allopathic medication has to go through stringent testing for potency and purity, natural remedies are viewed as foods and do not have adequate regulation. Because of this, many products have little or none of the potency they claim to have and therefore, although cheap, do nothing (if someone offers you something that costs a dollar to make for only 50 cents, be suspicious!). Because this is a major problem, I am very picky about which products and companies I recommend. For example, two natural products companies, Enzymatic Therapy and Integrative Therapeutics/ITI, have voluntarily registered with the FDA as pharmaceutical companies, which means their products have the same quality control as prescriptions. In time, Congress will recognize that quality control regulation is needed for all natural products, but hopefully will put it in the hands of people who are knowledgeable and open-minded about natural products.

I simply propose that you use the best of both systems. To make this easier for you, and to maintain objectivity, I have a policy of not taking money from any companies (natural or pharmaceutical) whose products I recommend. In addition, for the products I make, 100 percent of my royalties go to charity. There's nothing wrong with money. I simply don't want it to get in the way of your getting well!

### *So Effective Treatment for Most Pain Exists, but Doctors Are Not Aware of the Research?*

Exactly! In this book, I will teach you how to recognize the cause of your pain, and teach you both natural and prescription approaches that can help the pain go away. To help your doctor become more comfortable with these treatments, I have included information from a large number of research studies, which are listed at the end of the book. You do not need to know the technical stuff to learn how to get well. Some of you would like more detail, and others simply want the "bottom line." Because of this, I have written the book using two different color backgrounds. As you read along, feel free to skip anything in a "gray background," which is the more technical information. In addition, Appendix A summarizes how to use the treatments in the book that will take you step-by-step to being Pain Free.

I can tell you first hand that pain is treatable. My pain is gone! ■

**Important Points**

1. Just because medical schools have not yet effectively taught physicians about pain management does not mean that effective treatment is unavailable. On the contrary, most pain can be effectively treated.
2. The conflict between prescription and natural medicine is based more on belief systems and money than on science. Both can be useful tools. I recommend that you use the best of both systems.
3. **I am very picky about what treatments I use. To maintain objectivity and credibility, I have a policy of not taking money from any companies, natural or pharmaceutical, whose products I recommend. In addition, for products that I make, 100 percent of my royalties go to charity.**
4. Throughout this book, I will review how to determine the cause of your pain, and how to make it go away.

***The tribal wisdom of the Lakota People, passed on from generation to generation, says:***

*"When you discover you are riding a dead horse, the best strategy is to dismount."*

***However, in government, medicine, and in corporate America, more "advanced" strategies are often employed, such as:***

1. Buy a stronger whip.
2. Appoint a committee to study the horse.
3. Lower the standards so that dead horses can be included.
4. Reclassify the dead horse as living-impaired.
5. Harness several dead horses together to increase speed.
6. Declare that as the dead horse does not have to be fed, it is less costly, carries lower overhead and therefore contributes substantially more to the bottom line of the economy than do some other horses.
7. Promote the dead horse to a supervisory position.

# Section 1

# *General Principles of Pain Relief— Giving Your Body What It Needs to Heal and Eliminate Pain*

A number of general principles apply to pain relief and pain management. I will give a detailed overview of these in this section and provide specific details in later chapters when they apply to specific types of pain. In addition, to simplify things, Appendix A contains a summary (like "Cliff Notes") and flowcharts to help quickly evaluate your pain and determine how to treat it.

### *The two main principles of pain relief are:*

1. Supply your body with what it needs for healing and tissue repair. This includes optimum nutrition (often well beyond RDA levels), 8 to 9 hours of deep sleep each night, and optimal hormonal levels (simply having a hormonal blood test be "normal" may not be adequate). Each of these three areas is critical. Pain often will not go away until each area is adequately handled—regardless of the cause of the pain.

*Continued on next page*

2. Treat or eliminate things that stress your body and cause pain. These include infections; toxins (e.g. chemical and heavy metal) and inflammation; mechanical stresses on the body; excessive situational, psychological or physical stresses; and abnormal tissue compression (e.g. cancers). All need to be considered and treated. For example, it may surprise you to know that nutritional and hormonal deficiencies and/or fungal infections (usually secondary to antibiotic use) can aggravate neuropathic or back pain. Because of this, it is a good idea for you to read this entire section, at the end of which I outline a simplified approach for making sure the key principles for treating your pain are addressed. I also provide tools you can use to make the pain relief treatment much easier. ■

# Chapter 1
# *Getting Started—Why We Have Pain*

I know that you are tired of being in pain and are ready to have the pain go away. Many of you have received little relief from current medical approaches. In fact, many of you do not even know what is causing your pain.

*Pain Free 1-2-3!* is a workbook that will teach you how to determine the cause of your pain, and how to make it go away. Although, an enormous amount of new research is emerging on the complex biochemistry of pain—and this information helps when creating new approaches for pain relief—dazzling you with this difficult biochemistry is not my goal. My purpose is to give you the information you need to determine the cause of your pain, give your body what it needs so the pain can go away, and help you move forward so you can get a life that you love. This book will do that for you.

I will begin by briefly reviewing the purpose of pain and general principles of pain relief. I will then discuss the different types of pain. By knowing the type of pain that you have—nerve, muscle/ligament/tendon, bone/arthritic, inflammatory/infectious, etc.—you can tailor your treatment approach to make it more effective. Once you understand the different types of pain and how to treat them, your ability to make the pain go away increases dramatically. Mind-body issues will also be reviewed, as will other problems—sexual dysfunction, fatigue, insomnia, weight gain, and depression—that can be associated with and caused by pain. I will also discuss the pros and cons of both holistic and prescription approaches, enabling you to make the best use of all available treatments.

After giving you an overview of pain types and therapies, I will discuss the most common causes of pain—headache, back pain, arthritis, etc.—and how to effectively treat them. For some of you, the pain is widespread. For others, it is localized. For most kinds of pain there are general principles that are helpful for healing. These are especially important for myofascial (muscle, tendon, etc.) pain, but are important for most other pain conditions as well.

In some sections of the book, I've structured a "Question and Answer" approach. In other sections I give a step-by-step outline. While I won't give all of the thousands of research studies and reports that this book is based on, I will give the references that I think your doctor (or those of you with a scientific interest) will find helpful. The more technical information that you can skip over is shaded in light gray. For now, let's start with the basics.

## *What Is Pain?*

The International Association for the Study of Pain defines pain as "an unpleasant sensory and emotional experience associated with actual or potential tissue damage or described in terms of such damage." Fortunately, most of you don't need such a complex definition. You know pain when you feel it.

It is useful to categorize pain. Let's start with two basic categories:

1. Acute pain, which usually results from tissue injury, inflammation, or illness. It often occurs suddenly after surgery or injury. Usually doctors can figure out what caused it, and it goes away on its own or with treatment.
2. Chronic pain can last for many years and is poorly treated medically, which is why it lasts for years. Chronic pain is the main focus of this book, although acute pain also will be addressed.

## *Pain Is Horrible! Why Do We Have Pain?*

Although chronic pain can be devastating, it serves a critical function. For example, there is a horrible genetic disease that is uniformly fatal and leaves people horribly deformed and disabled. People who suffer from this disease are born without a pain system, and therefore without any ability to feel pain. You may think this would be wonderful. It is not. As a child, if a sufferer of this disease falls off a roof and breaks a leg, he or she has no pain and still tries to walk, causing further damage. If his hand is on a hot stove or in a fire, he does not know it until he smells something burning. Pain is a critical warning system for your body. It tells you when you need to avoid something so that you do not cause damage to yourself. In addition, pain tells you when your body is not getting what it needs (e.g. sleep, nutrients, oxygen, etc.).

Pain is not the enemy; it is an important warning system. But when pain goes out of balance and becomes chronic, it may end up causing more harm than good. **In addition to teaching you how to turn off the pain signal, I will also help you understand what pain is trying to tell you about what your body needs.**

## *How Do I Turn Off the Pain Signal?*

You turn off the pain by giving your body what it needs and by eliminating what is damaging or toxic to your body. For example, one of the most common types of pain is myofascial or muscle pain. The medical profession very poorly understands this type of pain. Although we might think that muscles will go limp if they do not have what they need, consider rigor mortis. When someone dies and the muscles are not getting what they need, they do not become loose—in fact they become stiff as a board. As noted above, if your muscles do not have adequate nutrients, optimal hormone levels, or enough sleep for tissue repair, they will get stuck in the shortened position and cause pain. Underlying infections can also cause your muscles to get stuck in the shortened position. Pain is your body's way of saying that these problems need to be addressed. You'll be amazed at how pain that has lasted decades can go away quickly when these problems are taken care of. We will discuss this in depth in Section 1 and also in the chapter on myofascial pain.

Often, finding the right medication for pain is like trying on different shoes to see which pair fits best. In the current "medical shoe store" there are one or two pairs to try on. If the shoes don't fit, you are out of luck. Fortunately, there are dozens of treatments to try, and when one doesn't fit another often will.

In addition, pain management is a perfect place to combine traditional and complementary therapies. The difficulty that patients have in finding doctors that can effectively treat their pain is driving them to alternative healers in droves. In fact, according to the *Journal of the American Medical Association*, pain is the number one reason why people use alternative medicine,[1] which includes Chiropractic, Naturopathic Medicine, Acupuncture, Biofeedback, Massage, Reiki, Meditation, and other techniques. Often, it is difficult to treat chronic pain with a single "magic bullet." It takes a practitioner who is both knowledgeable about many treatment modalities and who is also a compassionate listener. ■

***For those of you who watch what you eat, here's the final word on nutrition and health. It's a relief to know the truth after all those conflicting medical studies:***

1. The Japanese eat very little fat and drink very little red wine, and they suffer fewer heart attacks than the Americans.
2. The Mexicans eat a lot of fat and drink lots of Tequila, and they suffer fewer heart attacks than the Americans.
3. The French eat lots of fatty cheese and rich food and drink lots of wine, and they suffer fewer heart attacks than the Americans.
4. The Italians drink excessive amounts of red wine and eat lots of carbohydrate-rich pasta, and they suffer fewer heart attacks than the Americans.
5. The Germans drink a lot of beer and eat lots of sausages and fats, and they suffer fewer heart attacks than the Americans.

***Conclusion:***

*Eat and drink what you like. Speaking English is apparently what kills you.*

CHAPTER 2

# Optimizing Nutritional Support Easily

The American diet is awful. In fact, it is often called the Standard American Diet (S.A.D.) and the initials are appropriate. Let's look at why this occurs.

## Food Processing

The average American's diet includes 150 pounds of added sugar per year, accounting for approximately 18 percent of your caloric intake. Since a healthy diet without added sugar may have only a 10 percent margin of safety for supplying optimum amounts of nutrients, the added sugar alone makes the average American diet a disaster.[1]

Sugar also suppresses your immune system, encouraging the growth of yeast in your bowel and stimulating yeast overgrowth. Yeast grows by fermenting sugar and the yeast says thank you by making billions of baby yeasts.

Another dietary stress is white flour. Vitamins were discovered by a settler who went on sailing expeditions with Dutch explorers. He found that the colonists were becoming ill, and the colony's chickens were looking unusually healthy. Finding this to be curious, he began feeding the chickens' food to the people. Over a period of several weeks, the people became stronger and healthier. He (incorrectly) named the chicken feed "vital amines," meaning "vital proteins," and began selling it. The name was later shortened to "vitamins."

Today, scientists understand what happened to those colonists. Polishing off the brown outer coat, or bran, from rice had become fashionable. The rice bran was then used as chicken feed. The bran, however, contains most of the vitamins and minerals that are present in rice. The colonists therefore quickly became nutritionally deficient, while the chickens flourished.

In the U.S., approximately 18 percent of calories come from white flour. However, white flour, just like white rice, has had the bran removed and therefore is also significantly depleted of vitamins and minerals.[2]

As you can see, from just the use of white flour and added sugar, Americans often reduce their vitamin and mineral intake by around 35 percent. Adding to this problem are the nutrients that are lost in the canning of vegetables and in the processing of foods, which can cause vitamin losses of up to 80 percent.[3]

As Dr. S. B. Eaton noted in his study in the prestigious *New England Journal of Medicine,* "Physicians and nutritionists are increasingly convinced that the dietary habits adopted by Western society over the past one hundred years make an important etiologic [causative] contribution to coronary heart diseases [angina], hypertension, diabetes, and some types of cancer.[4] This is the same conclusion that was reached by the authors of *Western Diseases: Their Emergence and Prevention* by the Harvard University Press. [5]

Just as nutritional deficiencies can cause these medical problems, not having adequate nutrients can cause pain and keep the pain from going away. The late Dr. Janet Travell, White House physician for Presidents John F. Kennedy and Lyndon B. Johnson and professor emeritus of internal medicine at George Washington University, co-wrote *Myofascial Pain and Dysfunction: The Trigger Point Manual,* which is acknowledged as the authoritative work on muscle pain. In one chapter alone, Dr. Travell and coauthor Dr. David Simons referenced 317 studies showing that problems such as hormonal, vitamin, and mineral deficiencies can contribute to muscle disorders.[6] Dr. Travell strongly encouraged me in my work and my landmark study on effective pain management was dedicated to her memory.

Numerous other studies have shown that adequate amounts of vitamins and minerals, especially folic acid, zinc (found to be very low in people with FMS), and selenium, are critical for proper immune function—that is, for defense against infections. Vitamin A, beta-carotene, vitamin B6, vitamin C, vitamin E, iron, and many other nutrients also have been found to be very important in keeping your body's defenses strong.[7 – 12]

I sometimes hear doctors express skepticism about the importance of nutritional supplements. A typical comment is: "Five hundred years ago, there were no vitamin tablets, and people seemed to do just fine." These doctors forget that 500 years ago sugar was expensive and not readily available. The king of England might have sprinkled a teaspoon of sugar on his food as a sign of power, but when he wanted sugar and had none left, he had to send someone to the West Indies to get it!

The argument about people not needing vitamin tablets 500 years ago simply does not apply to the average modern American. One study that was reported in the *American Journal of Clinical Nutrition* showed that fewer than 5 percent of the study participants consumed the recommended daily amounts (RDAs) of all their needed vitamins and minerals.[13] What is frightening is that this study was conducted in Beltsville, Maryland, on employees of the U.S. Department of Agriculture (USDA) research center.

Despite this, some cynics still like to say that the vitamins go out in your urine, so all you're doing by taking vitamin supplements is making expensive urine. Using this line of reasoning, these cynics can stop drinking water (it just goes out in their urine). That way, they'll soon stop annoying people who are in the process of getting themselves well.

## Vitamin and Mineral Supplementation

Every vitamin and nutritional mineral, amino acid, and nutritional cofactor is **very** important in some way to health. The body depends on receiving vitamins and minerals from the diet because it cannot make them itself. **If you are low in vitamins, minerals, and other nutrients, your pain simply will not go away**. Because of this, an excellent nutritional supplement is critical to your becoming pain free.

For example, inositol, vitamins B1, B6 and B12, zinc and antioxidants are critical for healing neuropathies (nerve pain). For muscle pain, magnesium, B vitamins, antioxidants, zinc, iodine, selenium, and malic acid are critical. In fact, each kind of pain has different nutrients that are important for pain relief.

As there are literally dozens of different nutrients that are critical for tissue repair, and it would take at least 35 supplement tablets a day to replace them all, I recommend that you use a powdered nutritional supplement called the Energy Revitalization System® by Enzymatic Therapy. I developed this product so that my patients could easily get the nutritional support they need without taking handfuls of tablets. As noted above, 100 percent of my royalties go to charity, and the product is available in most health food stores (or at www.Vitality101.com ). One good tasting drink and one capsule replace over 35 tablets of supplements a day. The Energy Revitalization System contains 50 nutrients (almost all in optimal forms and amounts) and can supply outstanding nutritional support for almost everyone. It contains almost all the key nutrients that you need to get from your diet except for iron (which is toxic to take unless you are iron deficient), calcium (which blocks thyroid hormone absorption and should be taken at nighttime), and essential fatty acids (oil and water don't mix). Many people find that simply taking this product for optimal nutritional support can help them to feel much better while decreasing and sometimes eliminating their pain (after 6 weeks). It can replace the multi-vitamin and almost all of the nutritional supplements that most people take. (To make it easy, when I recommend specific nutrients I will often note whether or not they are in the vitamin powder and B-complex. Alternatively, the individual nutrients I recommend can be obtained separately or in other forms.)

Some people will develop diarrhea from magnesium containing products. Most people, however, find that it simply makes them wonderfully regular. If diarrhea is a problem, one can cut the dose of the powder in half or take it with milk, and this will usually take care of it. In addition, any supplement containing B vitamins can turn your urine bright yellow. This is normal.

Although many excellent physicians use them, I do not recommend using tests for checking blood levels for most nutrients because the tests are often inaccurate, expensive, and/or unnecessary. I feel it is better and less expensive to simply use the vitamin powder. The exceptions would be iron and vitamin B12 levels. Let's discuss some key nutrients in a bit more depth.

## *Iron*

Iron is important because an iron level that is too high or too low can cause pain, fatigue, poor immune function, cold intolerance, decreased thyroid function, and poor memory.[14 - 19]

I routinely recommend that all my chronic pain patients have their iron level, total iron binding capacity (TIBC), and ferritin levels checked. Although only checking an iron level is not useful by itself, dividing the iron level by the TIBC gives you a *percent saturation,* which is a useful measure. The ferritin blood level will often discover iron deficiency earlier, but is not reliable if inflammation is present. Combining these three tests is the best way to measure iron status. Some insurance companies balk at paying for all three tests, but they are worth doing. Even if a person's iron percent saturation is low but still normal, that person will often feel fatigued and in pain, despite not being anemic. Significant iron deficiency can often occur in the absence of anemia.

As an example, a study reported in the British medical journal *The Lancet* showed that infertile females whose ferritin levels were between 20 and 40—a ferritin level over 9 is technically normal—were often able to become pregnant when they took supplemental iron.[20] Other research shows that low-normal iron levels cause poor mental functioning and poor immune function. This suggests that levels considered sufficient to prevent anemia are often inadequate for other body functions. Because of this, anyone whose ferritin level is below 40, **or** whose percent saturation is less than 22 percent, should be given a trial treatment of iron therapy. In addition, a surprisingly large number of people display early hemochromatosis on their iron studies. Hemochromatosis is a disease of excess iron. Early in the disease, pain and arthritis are often the only symptoms. If caught early, hemochromatosis is remarkably easy to treat. If caught late, however, it is disabling and even life-threatening. This is an additional reason to check the iron level carefully.

## Vitamin B12

Vitamin B12 is another key nutrient. Technically, the B12 level is normal if it is over 208 picograms per deciliter (pg/dL) of blood. However, studies have shown that people can suffer severe and sometimes long-term nerve and brain dysfunction from B12 deficiency, even if their levels are as high as 300 pg/dL. Why are the "normal" levels set so low? In part, the normal values were initially set according to what prevents anemia. But the needs of brains and nervous systems for vitamin B12 are often much higher than those of the bone marrow. Also, as much as I hate to admit it, medical schools have greatly enjoyed poking fun at the old-time doctors who gave vitamin B12 shots for fatigue. The use of B12 shots, despite "normal" blood levels, is considered almost a symbol of unscientific, archaic medicine. As noted in an editorial in *The New England Journal of Medicine,* however, current findings suggest that those old-time doctors may have been right.[21] In addition, a recent study using the respected Framingham database showed that metabolic signs of B12 deficiency occur even with levels over 500 pg/dL.[22] I suspect, though, that the modern medical establishment will be a little slow to eat crow.

It is no surprise, then, when their other problems are also treated, many people respond dramatically to B12 injections. In addition to fatigue, it can be very helpful for nerve pain, migraines, and other problems. If a patient's B12 level is under 540 pg/mL, I treat that person with a 1-cc (1,000 to 3,000 microgram) injection of Vitamin B12, 1 to 5 times a week, for 15 injections. These shots are very safe and fairly inexpensive. Although most regular pharmacies carry only the 1,000-microgram-per-cc strength, holistic pharmacies (Cape Apothecary is an excellent one that can mail prescriptions worldwide—see Appendix C: Resources) can make up injectable vitamin B12 that contains 3,000 to 5,000 micrograms per cc. Usually, if a patient is going to benefit from the shots, I see improvement by 10 weeks. I usually stop after 10 to 15 shots. If a patient feels worse when the injections are stopped, I resume giving the shots, usually giving 1 every 1 to 5 weeks (but as often as 3 to 4 times a week in some cases) for an extended period of time. Most people, however, can maintain excellent B12 levels by taking at least 500 micrograms of B12 daily by mouth (see Appendix C: Resources).

## *Other B Vitamins*

Vitamins B1, B2, B6, and B12 have been found to be clinically effective in helping a number of chronic pain conditions, including low back pain, migraines, sciatica, trigeminal neuralgia, and diabetic neuropathy (see references in the chapters on these problems). Now researchers at the Parker Institute in Dallas have conducted a study suggesting that these vitamins may also help treat painful sprains, old fractures, burns, and bruises. The study suggests that B vitamins may possess the ability to block a certain type of pain receptor, especially in patients with neuropathic pain. [23]

## *Magnesium*

Magnesium is probably the single most important nutrient for pain relief. It is involved in hundreds of different functions and is routinely low in the American diet as a result of food processing. The average American diet supplies less than 300 mg of magnesium per day, while the average Asian diet supplies over 600 mg per day.[24, 25] I generally recommend taking 900 mg of malic acid and 150 to 200 mg of magnesium glycinate a day. If diarrhea and cramps are not a problem, you can take up to 500 mg of magnesium daily. If you get uncomfortable diarrhea from the magnesium, cut the dosage back and then slowly increase the dose as is comfortable.

If your body's magnesium stores are low, your muscles will stay in spasm and your pain will not resolve. This is one of the reasons that taking magnesium is so critical. In addition, magnesium is important for your muscle and body strength and energy. Most of your magnesium is inside your cells and the blood tests only measure the magnesium in your blood, making blood tests an unreliable measure. **Everyone** with pain should take magnesium. An exception is if you have kidney failure with a blood test creatinine level over 1.7 mg per deciliter (mg/dL), which is rare in chronic pain patients. If your creatinine is 1.5 to 1.6 mg/dL, take just 150 mg of magnesium a day for 2 to 3 months and discuss your dosage and regimen with your physician.

Magnesium absorption is very difficult, which is why I like to use the glycinate form. Plain magnesium oxide is also available and is the most inexpensive form of magnesium, but your body may not absorb it well. If you choose to take magnesium oxide, take 500 mg per day.

In addition to helping muscle pain when taken by mouth or intravenously, intravenous (and often oral) magnesium has other benefits as well. Two grams of intravenous magnesium given over a few minutes will routinely knock out an acute migraine. In addition, it is very good for esophageal spasms when given twice a week for about a month. For those with spasm of the fingertips (Raynaud's phenomenon—if your fingers turn white and painful when you put them in the freezer), muscle cramps, decreased circulation in the legs with pain, and walking and/or kidney stone pain, magnesium can also be very helpful. As one example, research suggests that oral magnesium and Vitamin B6 decrease the frequency of recurrent calcium kidney stones by 90 percent.[26]

## Vitamin C

In a study of 324 patients with arthritis of the knee, those taking over 200 mg a day of vitamin C had less pain than those taking smaller amounts. One epidemiologic study also suggested vitamin C may prevent the development of pain and worsening of the arthritis on X ray.[27]

## Calcium

Most people do not need calcium supplementation, and (as is the case with iron) taking it at the same time as a thyroid hormone will block the thyroid hormone's absorption. Some people's pain improves with taking calcium and others get worse. In addition, calcium is best taken at night as it helps sleep.

Most calcium tablets are made of calcium carbonate (chalk) and often will not dissolve in the stomach. They then go out in the stool, having done no good along the way. It is better to use chewable calcium or other forms of calcium such as calcium citrate or chelates, taking 500 to 600 mg at bedtime and perhaps the same amount at dinner. This is most important, however, in women over 40 years old. Although calcium gets much attention in the treatment of osteoporosis, other nutrients are as, or more, important. In fact, countries with the highest calcium intakes often have the highest rates of osteoporosis.

## Vitamin D

Unfortunately, Americans have been misled into thinking that sunshine is bad for them. Most of the skin cancers that are caused by excess sun exposure are not especially dangerous and are easy to treat. Some doctors also think that the rise in dangerous skin cancers (melanomas) is also associated with excess sun exposure. I do not believe this is the case, as most melanomas occur in clothed areas that are not exposed to the sun. As time goes on, I think we'll find that the increase in this single type of dangerous skin cancer is caused by other factors besides sunshine. Unfortunately, humans tend to get most of their vitamin D from exposure to sunlight. Dr. Michael Holick, director of the Vitamin D research lab at Boston University Medical Center, thinks that "the current message that all unprotected sun exposure is bad for you is too extreme... the original message was that people should limit their sun exposure, not that they should avoid the sun entirely. I do believe that some unprotected exposure to the sun is important for health." This is supported by evidence that vitamin D **deficiency** can contribute to many cancers including prostate, colon, and breast cancer. Dr. Holick feels that vitamin D may also help protect against heart disease, autoimmune disease, and even type 1 diabetes. For example, multiple sclerosis is mostly seen in northern latitudes where people get less sunshine. Now we are also finding that vitamin D deficiency may contribute to unexplained muscle and bone pain. In a study of 150 children and adults with unexplained muscle and bone pain, almost all were found to be vitamin D deficient—with many being severely deficient with very low vitamin D levels.

Researchers noted that it was a big surprise that the worst vitamin D deficiencies occurred in young people—especially women of childbearing age. In addition, all the African Americans, Hispanics, and Native Americans who participated in one pain study were vitamin D deficient, as were all of the patients under the age of 30. Dr. Plotnikoff notes that "the message here is that unexplained pain may very well be linked to vitamin D deficiency. My hope is that patients with unexplained pain will be tested for vitamin D status and treated if necessary." [28] I prefer to simply recommend 600 units of vitamin D instead of spending several hundred dollars on blood testing.

Although the RDA (which I feel is often **inadequate**) for vitamin D is 200 to 400 IU/day for most people, Dr. Holick believes that most people need approximately 1000 IU of vitamin D daily. It is not easy to get this from food alone. For example, one glass of fortified milk or orange juice has approximately 100 units of vitamin D and most multivitamins have 400 units or less.

To put it in perspective, a light skinned person wearing a swimsuit at the beach will get about 20,000 units of vitamin D in the time it takes his or her skin to get lightly pink. It is difficult during the winter for people living in northern climates to get the vitamin D that they need from the sun. During the summer at the beach however, you can get what you need in five minutes.[29] Another fringe benefit is that in one study, those taking over 400 units of vitamin D a day had a 40 percent lower risk of developing multiple sclerosis than those who were not taking supplementation.[30]

## Copper

This nutrient is "a double-edged sword." Because it is pro-inflammatory, it can aggravate arthritis and many other inflammatory and autoimmune processes. On the other hand, copper deficiency can contribute to deficiencies of a critical antioxidant called superoxide dismutase. The bottom line is that it's good to get just a tiny bit of copper. To be on the safe side, I recommend approximately 1/2 mg a day.

## Essential Fatty Acids

Although we get excessive fat in the American diet, most of it is not the type that our bodies need. Your body needs specific fats for proper hormonal (e.g. prostaglandin) and cell function. For example, fish oils are anti-inflammatory and can be helpful in rheumatoid arthritis and other types of pain. I had a patient who came to see me while on chronic high dose morphine. His pain went away when he took fish oil supplementation. As a fringe benefit, high intakes of fish oil are associated with a decreased risk of Alzheimer's disease and cognitive impairment.[31]

I do not routinely recommend essential fatty acid supplementation for everyone. If you have dry eyes or dry mouth, however, this suggests fish oil deficiency. For years I would only use flaxseed oil (which is poorly converted to the type of oil found in fish) because most fish oils contain toxins such as mercury and lead and are also rancid. Fortunately, there are now a few brands of fish oil that have no toxins and are not rancid. One brand I recommend is Eskimo 3 Fish Oil®, 1 to 3 tsp a day for 9 months. if you have dry eyes or dry mouth symptoms that are suggestive of this deficiency (see Appendix C: Resources).

Although I strongly recommend taking nutritional supplements to ensure obtaining the necessary nutrients, I also want to stress that eating a good healthy diet is important. Eat a lot of whole grains, fresh fruits (whole fruit, not fruit juice), and fresh vegetables. Many raw vegetables have enzymes that improve digestion and help to decrease pain. You do not have to cut out all foods that might be "bad" or eat a diet that is impossible to follow. All you need to do is eat a diet that is reasonably healthy and low in added sugar. When I tell people to cut out sugar, I like to add the three magic words "Except for Chocolate!" I consider chocolate to be a healthy food. To have your cake and eat it too (so to speak), consider sugar free chocolates. Some are awful but others are spectacular. Russell Stover® has a whole line of sugar free chocolates that are outstanding. There are many healthy sugar substitutes. Stevia is excellent, healthy, and easy to use. The best tasting brands of stevia I've found are from Body Ecology® and Stevita® (see Appendix C: Resources). Many others are bitter. Inositol (which helps anxiety and nerve pain) and xylitol (which decreases osteoporosis) look and taste just like sugar. Saccharin (which comes in the pink packets) is also OK. I do not recommend aspartame (NutraSweet®). Some sugar substitutes can cause gas or diarrhea.

In addition, most Americans are chronically dehydrated and this can make you feel worse as well. I do not recommend that you count glasses of water; this is an annoying way to spend a day. Simply check in with your mouth and lips every so often. If they are dry, you are dehydrated and need to drink more water. Many people are appropriately concerned about the quality of tap water. An excellent filter is made by Multi Pure® (see Appendix C: Resources).

The more unprocessed your diet is, the healthier you will be. On the other hand, **things that give you pleasure and make you feel good are generally good for you (contrary to popular belief)**. Your body will tell you what's good for you by making you **feel good**. (Note: All nutrients recommended in this chapter except for iron, calcium, and essential fatty acids/fish oils are in the vitamin powder/B-complex—see Appendix C: Resources). ■

### Important Points

1. Remove sugar and other sweets from your diet (except for chocolate). Stevia, a sweet-tasting herb, and saccharin taste good and are acceptable sugar substitutes.
2. Most Americans are dehydrated. If your mouth or lips are dry you are thirsty. Drink more water.
3. Use the Energy Revitalization System vitamin powder and B-complex for excellent overall daily nutritional support. It replaces over 35 supplement tablets a day with one good tasting drink and one capsule (see Appendix C: Resources).
4. If you have dry eyes or mouth, use fish oil (1/3 to 1 Tbsp daily for 6 to 9 months). If you have low iron on blood testing, take iron. Consider calcium at dinner and bedtime if you are at risk for osteoporosis.
5. Except for sugar, eat what makes you feel good (which may or may not be what you crave).

# CHAPTER 3 Getting 8 to 9 Hours of Sleep a Night—The Foundation of Pain Relief

To eliminate muscle and many other sources of pain, it is critical to get 8 to 9 hours of solid, deep sleep each night on a regular basis. Disordered sleep is, in my opinion, a major underlying process that perpetuates pain.

Inadequate sleep can occur for a number of reasons. Many Americans simply do not make enough time for adequate sleep. One hundred years ago, the average American was getting 9 hours of sleep a night. Anthropologists tell us that 5000 years ago, the average night's sleep was 11 to 12 hours a night. When the sun went down, it was dark, boring, and dangerous outside, so people went to bed. When the sun came up, they woke up. The average time from sunset to sunrise is 12 hours. The use of candles initially shortened sleep time. Then light bulbs were developed followed by radio, TV, computers, etc. We are now down to an average of 6 ½ to 7 hours of sleep a night, and this is simply not adequate to allow proper tissue repair.

Some people get inadequate sleep because of poor sleep hygiene, often occurring because pain keeps them awake. Others have insomnia because the sleep center in the brain (called the hypothalamus) is suppressed by the same process that is causing the pain.

A 2001 poll conducted by the National Sleep Foundation found that 58 percent of Americans had sleep difficulties. This had increased from 51 percent the year before. Fifteen percent of Americans use a prescription or over-the-counter sleep aid. In addition, those who slept less than six hours a night felt more stressed, angry, sad and tired than the people who got more sleep. The survey of over 1000 adults also found that only 30 percent of people reported getting the recommended 8 hours of sleep a night, down from 38 percent the year before. The average amount of sleep also decreased to under seven hours.[1]

In animal studies conducted by Carol Everson, Ph.D. at the University of Tennessee, sleep deprivation resulted in immune suppression, resulting in multiple infections (including yeast overgrowth in the gut).[2] Many other abnormalities also occurred because of the sleep disorder. These same processes seem to occur in people with fibromyalgia pain.[3]

Sleep has a distinct architecture with five key stages. Stages 1 and 2 sleep are fairly light, while stages 3 and 4 (or delta wave) sleep are the deeper stages of sleep. My experience, and that of many other clinicians, suggests that what is deficient in fibromyalgia and likely in many pain patients are the deeper, restorative stages of sleep (stages 3 and 4). These are the stages where you produce growth hormone, which results in tissue repair and healing. Unfortunately, most sleeping pills in common use keep people in light stage 2 sleep, which can actually make their problem worse. The good news is that there are a number of exceptions.

Several studies have shown that if you continually wake up people whenever they go into deep sleep, or even shake them lightly so that they go from deep sleep into light sleep, they will develop pain within one to two weeks and often within one night.[4, 5]

In fact, inadequate sleep has repeatedly been shown to contribute to pain. In one study of fibromyalgia patients, it was found that increased pain sensitivity is associated with greater sleep disturbance[6]. Another study of female office employees in one large company showed that women who suffer from frequent muscle pain also have insufficient sleep.[7] Another study by Dr. Moldofsky, a respected researcher on sleep in fibromyalgia, found that things that disrupted deep sleep resulted in normally healthy people waking feeling unrefreshed, with widespread muscle pain, tenderness, and fatigue. He concluded that "there is a reciprocal relationship between sleep quality and pain."[8] In another study of 105 fibromyalgia patients, it was also found that sleep quality was important in mediating pain and fatigue.[9]

I find that when my patients get 8 to 9 hours of solid sleep regularly each night for 6 to 9 months, their pain and, interestingly, their inability to fall asleep both resolve. They are then able to markedly reduce the amount of sleep and pain medication that they need. It is because of this that breaking the cycle of poor sleep and maintaining quality sleep for at least 6 to 9 months is critical to breaking the cycle of pain.

Eight to nine hours of solid sleep each night, without waking or hangover is the goal and, hard as this may be to believe, it is very attainable using the suggestions that I will give you in this chapter.

## *How Can I Get 8 Hours of Deep Sleep Each Night if I Have Insomnia?*

In general, I think it is a good idea to begin with natural remedies and good sleep hygiene. Many of you, however, will have a problem with your sleep center (the hypothalamus) not working or with the pain simply keeping you awake at night. Because of this, in light of how critical it is that you get 8 to 9 hours of solid sleep a night, I would strongly encourage you to add prescription therapies if the natural approaches are not adequate. This will make a big difference in making your pain go away, and you can usually come off the prescriptions about six months after you are feeling better.

## Natural Sleep Remedies

Most of the natural sleep remedies discussed here are not sedating, yet they will help you fall asleep and stay in deep sleep. Some are available in combination formulas as well. I recommend the following natural sleep aids:

1. Begin with the Revitalizing Sleep Formula®, which I helped to formulate (see Appendix C: Resources). This contains a mix of six excellent sleep herbals in a single capsule. In addition, these herbals can be helpful in alleviating both pain and anxiety. Take 1 to 4 capsules at bedtime if you have trouble **staying** asleep, or take the same dosage 30 to 90 minutes before bedtime if you have trouble **falling** asleep. You'll see the effect of a given dose on sleep the first night you take it, although the effectiveness increases with continued use. It can also be taken during the day to relieve pain and anxiety. If you're still not getting 8 to 9 hours of sleep a night, add in the natural remedies below. The Revitalizing Sleep Formula herbal contains:
   - Wild lettuce extract 28 mg—one of the most powerful sleep herbals available
   - Jamaican dogwood extract 12 mg—helps with sleep and is a muscle relaxant
   - Hops extract 30 mg
   - Passionflower extract 90 mg—helps both sleep and in alleviating anxiety
   - Valerian extract 200 mg
   - Theanine 50 mg (from green tea)—helps sleep and strengthens immune function

2. Magnesium, 75 to 250 mg. Calcium, 600 mg at bedtime, also helps sleep.

3. Hydroxy L-tryptophan (5-HTP). Take 200 to 400 mg at night. When used for 6 weeks, a 300 to 400 mg dose has been shown to decrease fibromyalgia pain and often helps people to lose weight. 5-HTP is what your body uses to make serotonin, a neurotransmitter that helps improve the quality of sleep and can decrease levels of substance P, your body's pain messenger. The one caution I give is that if you are taking other treatments that increase serotonin

(these include anti-depressants like Prozac®, St. John's Wort, Ultram®, Desyrel®, etc.), limit the 5-HTP to 200 mg at night. It takes 6 to 12 weeks to see the full effect of 5-HTP, and it is more expensive than the other remedies. Nonetheless, it may be worthwhile in treating chronic pain.

4. Melatonin. This is a hormone produced by the pineal gland. Although it is natural and available over the counter, this does not mean that it is without risk. My concern with any hormone is that although it might be quite safe when used within the body's normal range, I worry about toxicity when people take more than the body would normally make. For most people, all it takes to restore melatonin to normal levels is ½ mg. The usual dose you find in stores, however, is 3 mg, which is 6 to 10 times the dose that most people need. Except for a small subset of people, who likely have trouble absorbing it properly, the ½ mg dose is every bit as effective for sleep as higher doses. I would use a dose higher than ½ mg only if it **clearly** helps you sleep better than the lower dose.[10]
5. Delta wave sleep-inducing compact disks or cassettes. To fall asleep, you can play deep sleep-inducing tapes or CDs. If you wake up during the night, you can push your sound system's replay button. Better yet, get a CD or tape player that can replay continuously throughout the night. These tapes and CDs are available on my web site at www.Vitality101.com.

## Good Sleep Hygiene

These are some important things to consider that enhance good sleep hygiene:

- Do not consume alcohol near bedtime.
- Do not consume any caffeine after 4:00 P.M.
- Do not use your bed for problem solving or doing work.
- Take a hot bath before bed.
- Keep your bedroom cool.
- If your partner snores, sleep in a separate bedroom (after tucking in or being tucked in by your partner) or get a good pair of earplugs and use them. The wax plugs that mold to the shape of the ear are often the best ones.
- If you frequently wake up to urinate during the night, do not drink a lot of fluids near bedtime. Most pain patients wake during the night because their sleep center is not working properly or because of the pain. Because they also have a full bladder, they think they are waking up because they have to urinate. This is not the case.

They are waking up because of their pain syndrome. There is a simple way to remedy this problem. If and when you wake up during the night and you notice your bladder is full, just talk to it (in your mind, so your spouse doesn't think you're nuts) and tell it, "Nighttime is for sleeping. We will go to the bathroom in the morning when it is time to wake up." Then roll over and go back to sleep. If you still have to urinate five minutes later, go to the bathroom. Most of you will find that your bladder will happily go back to sleep, and when you wake up in the morning, you won't even have to urinate as badly as you did when you woke up in the middle of the night.

- Put the bedroom clock out of arm's reach and facing away from you so you can't see it. Looking at the clock frequently aggravates sleep problems and is frustrating.
- Have a light snack before bedtime. Hunger and hypoglycemia cause insomnia in all animals, and humans are no exception. For your snack, eat foods high in the amino acid tryptophan, such as milk and turkey, which contributes to sleep.

## Sleep Medications

Although I much prefer natural remedies to prescription medications, the sleep disorder in some pain patients may be too severe to be dealt with by natural remedies alone. However, even if you are someone who needs prescription sleep aids, adding natural remedies can be very helpful and usually decreases the amount of medication that you will need, resulting in fewer side effects. In addition, once you come off the sleep medications (usually after 9 to 18 months, although they can be used indefinitely if needed) you may find that all you require are the natural remedies. Whatever treatments you use, though, it is important that they not only increase the duration of sleep but also maintain or improve the deep stages (stages 3 and 4) of sleep. Unfortunately, most sleeping pills in common use (for example, Dalmane®, Halcion®, and Valium®) may actually worsen the quality of sleep by increasing the amount of light stage (especially stage 2) sleep and decreasing the deep stages of sleep even further. You want to be certain that the treatments and medications you use leave you feeling better the next day, not worse.

There are several approaches to sleep when treating pain patients. Some doctors prefer to use a single medication or treatment and push it up to its maximum level. If that works, great; if not, they stop it and switch to another medication. Other doctors prefer to use low doses of many different treatments together until the patient is getting good, solid sleep regularly. I strongly prefer the latter approach. Most of a medication's benefits occur at low doses and most of the side effects at high doses. In addition, if you combine low doses of a few different sleep aids, each of them will be cleared out of your body by morning—so you won't be hung over. Meanwhile, the effective blood levels that you have during the middle of the night from each treatment are cumulative and will keep you asleep for 8 to 9 hours of solid sleep each night without waking or hangover. (You'll notice that I keep repeating this phrase.)

### *Getting Started*

My treatment checklist (see Appendix B: Pain Treatment Protocol), lists a number of natural and prescription sleep aids. Depending on your preference, you may want to start with the natural aids, see how those work, and then use the prescription ones as needed (or available). My preference is to start with at least one of the sleep medications (Ambien® and/or Klonopin®) combined with some of the natural remedies. However you choose to do it, on the first night begin with one of the remedies at a low dose.

For most of the treatments recommended, by the next morning you will know the effects (both beneficial and side effects) that it is going to have. It may, however, take 6 to 12 weeks to see the full effect of 5-HTP. In rare cases, some of these treatments have the opposite of their normal effect, activating you instead of putting you to sleep. If this happens, don't use that treatment.

Once you have tried a low dose of a single treatment, increase the dosage each night until you either get 8 to 9 hours of solid sleep without waking or hangover, you get side effects (for example, next-day sedation), or until you are at the maximum dose on the checklist. Use the lowest dose that gives you the most benefit. In other words, you may find that 50 mg of Desyrel® is just as effective as 150 mg, in which case there is no need to take the higher dose. Once you have tried one treatment, you can go ahead and add in a second one in the way I just discussed, and then a third one, and so on. You may choose to initially try each of them separately so you can see what each one does by itself, or you may choose to simply add one treatment to the next. Basically, you are trying the treatments on to see what "fits," in the same way you would try on shoes to see which one(s) **feel** the best. Once you have found the combination of treatments that feels the best, you can simply stay on that combination. If needed (to get 8 to 9 hours of solid sleep a night) you could even take **all** the medications on the checklist together at the maximum dose noted on the list.

It is not uncommon to see your sleep worsen again during periods of increased stress—whether physical or emotional—and the flaring of your pain/illness. During these times, increase the treatments as needed to maintain 8 to 9 hours of solid sleep without waking or hangover. I find that patients do not have a problem with continually having to escalate the dose, so don't worry about increasing the treatments during periods of stress or flaring of your illness. The best way to need less medication in the long run is to use **as much as it takes** to get 8 to 9 hours of solid sleep each night without waking or hangover for 6 to 18 months. When you are sleeping well and feeling better for 6 months, you can then decrease the treatments as long as you continue to get 8 to 9 hours of solid sleep each night without waking or hangover. If you need to take some of the sleep treatments long-term, that is also okay.

For all of the medications listed below, most of the side effects that you may notice will occur the first day that you take the medication. Regardless of the package insert saying to only use Ambien® for a maximum of 1 month, both research studies and the experience of many clinicians show that it can be used safely long-term. Rarely, have I seen patients develop depression after being on Ambien for over a year. In these cases, the depression has always lifted quickly within a few days of stopping the Ambien. Except for this, I have not seen any "fly now, pay later" side effects from prolonged use of the sleep medications.

## *Which Prescription Sleep Medications Should I Use?*

Although I prescribe medications in different orders for different people, depending on the cause of their pain, the most common order I use is listed below. If something is mentioned as especially good for a certain condition, you may want to try that medication first. Do not drive or operate hazardous equipment if you are sedated from the medications. As with almost everything, do not get pregnant during treatment. Although in my experience it is very uncommon, it is possible to get unusual reactions from combining these medications. If a medication causes recurring nightmares, change the dose or medication. Appendix B: Pain Treatment Protocol contains a treatment protocol that lists all of these treatments and how to use them.

1. Zolpidem (Ambien®). I like Ambien because it is short-acting (that is, less likely to leave you hung over) and less likely to cause side effects than many other medications. Because it is short-acting, it may not keep you asleep all through the night, but it will likely give you 4 to 6 hours of good, solid sleep as a foundation. The normal dosage is ½ to one 10 mg tablet, taken at bedtime. If you wake up in the middle of the night you can take an extra ½ to 1 tablet (leave it by your bedside with a glass of water) and any sedation is usually

gone by the time you are ready to wake up in the morning. One-half tablet is usually enough for the middle of the night. If you find that taking an additional dose in the middle of the night leaves you hung over, use Sonata® (see below) when you wake instead.

Studies have not shown a wearing-off effect with Ambien in most people, nor have they found addiction with long-term use.[11] What does occur, though, is rebound insomnia when you stop using this medication—that is, the need to use something else to assist your sleep for a week. Because of this, if you have taken Ambien for more than 4 months, use one of the other medications or natural sleep remedies discussed in this chapter for a week or so to assist sleep during the time when you stop the Ambien. In my experience, Ambien can be helpful for restless leg syndrome as well.

Although the use of Ambien is only FDA "recommended" for less than a month, a two-year study of 4000 patients with chronic insomnia showed that people were able to use it long term whenever they needed it without developing any significant problems.[12]

2. Clonazepam (Klonopin®). Although in the Valium® family, and therefore potentially habit forming, Klonopin can be **very** helpful for people with pain and is excellent for patients with restless leg syndrome. When used at doses of less than 2 mg a night, I have not seen significant problems with addiction. The main side effect is next-day sedation, which is fairly common. If this occurs, take a lower dose or take it several hours before bedtime. Because it is potentially habituating (i.e. may cause withdrawel if stopped abruptly), do not suddenly stop taking Klonopin if you have been on it for over 6 weeks. Instead, taper off by decreasing the dosage by 0.25 to 0.5 mg a day every 1 to 8 weeks.

3. Cyclobenzaprine (Flexeril®). This is a muscle relaxant. It can be a very helpful medication for many people, especially if the pain is severe. The usual dose is ½ to one 10 mg tablet at bedtime, but some people need to take 2 tablets at bedtime. The main side effects are sedation and dry mouth and eyes.

4. Carisprodol (Soma®). This is predominantly a muscle relaxant and I would use this earlier in treatment if you are being kept awake by severe pain. The usual dose is ½ to two 350 mg tablets at bedtime. Soma is potentially addictive, although I have almost never seen withdrawal in patients who are only using 1 to 2 tablets at bedtime (as opposed to people taking it 4 times a day for pain). The main side effect is sedation.

5. Neurontin (Gabapentin®), 300 mg (comes in 100 to 800 mg doses). Taking 1 to 3 capsules at bedtime can markedly help with both sleep and pain in many patients. Its main problem is next day sedation, which often wears off with time. It can also be taken during the day for pain relief at doses of up to 4800 mg daily.
6. Zanaflex (Tizanidine®), 4 mg tablets. Taking ½ to 2 tablets at bedtime can be helpful for both pain and sleep. It rarely causes nightmares. If this occurs repeatedly, stop the Zanaflex.
7. Gabitril®, 2 mg twice a day and increase by a maximum 4 mg daily each week to maximum of 24 mg a day. It helps both pain and deep sleep.[13] The average optimally effective dose of the Gabitril is 16 mg a day (range 10 to 24 mg a day). In one study, Gabitril decreased pain by approximately 30 percent and decreased sleep problems by approximately 40 percent. Another benefit is that the amount of time spent in deep, restorative sleep is increased.[14]
8. Zaleplon (Sonata®), 10 mg tablets. Sonata generally wears off within 3 to 4 hours, so it is best used in the middle of the night (for example, at 4:00 A.M.) if you wake up and need something to help you fall back to sleep, or if you have trouble **falling** asleep but not staying asleep.
9. Amitriptyline (Elavil®). Technically an anti-depressant, Elavil was one of the first medications to be studied for fibromyalgia and found to be effective. It is also the only medication that many doctors have heard of for treating fibromyalgia. Although Elavil can be very helpful, it has significant side effects and therefore is often one of the last treatments I try. These side effects include weight gain, dry mouth, sedation, aggravation of restless leg syndrome, neurally mediated hypotension, and abnormal heart rhythms. It is, however, especially good for nerve pain, vulvadynia (pain in the vulvar area), and, perhaps, interstitial cystitis, characterized by severe urinary frequency and burning without infection (see Chapter 18). If these are present, it is reasonable to start with Elavil or a related medication. You can take ½ to eight 10 mg tablets at bedtime. If you take more than 2 tablets, it should be tapered off and not stopped suddenly. I would not use more than 80 mg at bedtime (unless you have to) because of the side effects.
10. Trazodone (Desyrel®). In high doses, Desyrel is marketed as an anti-depressant, but at a low dose it is helpful for sleep and anxiety. Desyrel comes in 50 to 450 mg tablets, and the usual recommendation is to take ½ to 6 of the 50 mg tablets at bedtime

(most patients need no more than 2 tablets). The main side effect of Desyrel is next-day sedation, and priapism can occur in males. Priapism is a condition characterized by a painful erection that does not go away. This is unusual. Most men find that while it causes an improvement in the strength of their erections, it does so at a comfortable level, as opposed to an erection that will not go away after a normal amount of time. If you develop an erection that does not go away after an hour (despite a cold bath), stop taking the medication and go to a hospital emergency room. If erections are lasting longer than normal, you should stop the Desyrel and switch to the other medications.

11. Alprazolam (Xanax®). This is a short-acting cousin of Valium® that gives a good 3 to 5 hours of sleep with less hangover in the morning. I was pleasantly surprised to find that it improves sleep quality, because it is a cousin to Valium, which usually seems to worsen this in most people. It is very good for anxiety as well, and tends to be very well tolerated. It can be addictive however. The usual dosage is ½ to four 0.5-mg tablets at bedtime or during the night.
12. Xyrem® (GHB). This is an excellent (and possibly the best) sleep medication for pain and fibromyalgia. Because the DEA claimed (many suspect mistakenly) that it was being used as a date rape drug, it has gone from being inexpensive and over-the-counter to being tightly regulated and costing approximately $500 a month. If all else fails, this often works very well. It comes as a liquid that can dissolve your enamel and damage your teeth, so be sure to rinse your mouth well and swallow after taking the liquid to prevent this. Physicians must fill out special forms when prescribing Xyrem.

In addition to the prescription medications above, the serotonin-raising anti-depressants known as SSRIs can help improve sleep. They also have many other benefits in treating pain—even if there is **no** depression present. These medications include fluoxetine (Prozac®), paroxetine (Paxil®), and sertraline (Zoloft®).

By using a combination of the treatments discussed above, almost all people, even those with chronic pain, can get 8 to 9 hours of solid sleep a night without waking or hangover. It usually takes trial and error to find out exactly what is best for you, but it is worth being persistent. Once you are feeling well for 6 to 9 months, you usually will find that you need much less medication to get 8 to 9 hours of solid sleep without waking or hangover. At that time, you can go ahead and decrease the medication. If I have a patient who has been feeling better and then finds that their pain is coming back, one of the first things I ask is, "How is your sleep?" The usual answer is, "Not good." Many people, because of fear of addiction and concern about having to use constantly escalating doses of sleeping pills, are afraid to take enough medication to get adequate sleep. They are so grateful to get 5 hours of sleep a night that they settle for it. That's a bad idea! I recommend taking whatever you need to get 8 to 9 hours of solid sleep without waking or hangover, even if this means taking 6 of these medications at one time—or even all of the above natural remedies and/or medications.

After you're better, you may occasionally find that your sleep worsens for a while during physical and/or emotional stress. If this occurs, increase or resume your sleep medications for as long as you need and then taper them or stop them when the problem is resolved. Please be sure to do what you need to do to achieve the goal of adequate good-quality sleep. You'll be very happy you did. ■

**Important Points**

1. Getting 8 to 9 hours of solid, deep sleep a night without waking or hangover is critical to getting well.
2. Natural remedies can be very helpful for sleep, and may be safer than medications. Revitalizing Sleep Formula is excellent. Consider adding calcium, magnesium, 5-HTP, and/or melatonin as needed at bedtime.
3. Ambien®, Klonopin®, Soma®, Flexeril®, Zanaflex®, Gabitril®, and Neurontin® are excellent prescription sleep medications for patients with chronic pain. Many others are also available. (See Appendix B: Pain Treatment Protocol.) Most other medications sold as sleeping pills make you worse by keeping you in light sleep.
4. Take whatever combination of these natural and prescription sleep aids you need to get 8 to 9 hours of sleep a night. When you're feeling better for 6 months you can start to lower the dose—as long as you continue to get eight hours of sleep a night. Anytime your sleep starts to get worse, resume sleep treatments until the insomnia passes.

CHAPTER 4

# Treating Hormonal Deficiencies

Our hormonal system regulates our body's metabolism. Although most hormonal deficiencies (and sometimes excesses) can cause pain, the key players are hypothyroidism, inadequate adrenal function, and low growth hormone. In addition, for those of you whose pain began from ages 40 to 60, it is worth considering low testosterone in men and low estrogen or testosterone in women. Recent press reports about problems with the Premarin (Pre = pregnant, mar = horse, in = urine) form of estrogen were no surprise. I've been saying for over a decade that it is insane for people to take pregnant horse urine as these estrogens are markedly different from the ones your body makes. We will discuss ways to give estrogen therapy that can be much safer and may actually decrease the risk of developing cancer. For now, however, let's begin with hypothyroidism—the most important hormonal trigger for chronic pain.

## Hypothyroidism

The thyroid gland, located in the neck area, is the body's gas pedal. It regulates the body's metabolic speed. If the thyroid gland produces insufficient amounts of thyroid hormones, metabolism decreases and the person gains weight. As I mentioned earlier, it is not uncommon for chronic pain patients to put on twenty to fifty pounds during the first years of their illness. In addition to nerve, muscle, ligament/tendon, and other pains, other symptoms of hypothyroidism include fatigue, infertility, weight gain, "brain fog," constipation, and intolerance to cold.

The thyroid makes two primary hormones, including Thyroxine ($T_4$), which is the storage (inactive) form of thyroid hormone. The body uses it to make triiodothyronine ($T_3$), which is the active form of thyroid hormone. Most synthetic thyroid medications, such as Synthroid® and Levothroid®, are pure $T_4$. These synthetics are fine if the body has the ability to properly turn them into $T_3$. Unfortunately, many patients find that their bodies do not have this ability. Fortunately, natural thyroid hormone preparations, such as Armour Thyroid®, do contain active T3 as well as the T4.

## *The Problem with Thyroid Tests*

Modern medicine has gone through many generations of thyroid tests, and with each new test, we found that we missed an enormous number of cases of hypothyroidism. To make matters more difficult, if the thyroid is under-active because the hypothalamus is suppressed (as is common in chronic pain), the TSH test, which is the test most often used, may appear to be normal, or even suggest an overactive thyroid.

In two studies done by Dr. G.R. Skinner and his associates in the United Kingdom, patients who were felt to have hypothyroidism (an under-active thyroid), because of their symptoms (including pain), had their blood levels of thyroid hormone checked. The vast majority of subjects had technically normal thyroid blood tests. This data was published in the *British Medical Journal*.[1] Since that time, Dr. Skinner has done another study in which the patients with normal blood tests who had symptoms of an underactive thyroid—those who your doctor would likely say had a normal thyroid and would not need treatment—were treated with thyroid hormone. A remarkable thing happened-well, maybe it wasn't that surprising! The large majority of patients, despite being considered to have a normal thyroid, had their symptoms improve upon taking thyroid hormone (Synthroid®), at an average dosage of 100 to 120 micrograms a day. [2]

These two studies, plus another, which indicated that thyroid blood tests are only low in about 3 percent of patients whose doctors sent in blood tests (and this is at an HMO where the doctor really suspected that the patient had thyroid problems), confirm what I have been saying all along.[3] Our current thyroid testing will miss **most** patients with an under-active thyroid. Once again, doctors of decades ago were on target when they knew that one has to treat the patient and not the blood test. In fact, in November 2002 the American Academy of Clinical Endocrinologists again changed the normal range on the TSH thyroid blood test (so that a TSH over 3 warranted treatment), increasing the number of patients with hypothyroidism in the United States from 13 to 26 million. Less than a quarter of these patients have been properly diagnosed and treated.

If you have chronic pain **and** suffer from chronic fatigue, heavy periods, constipation, easy weight gain, cold intolerance, dry skin, thin hair, **or** a body temperature that tends to be on the low side of normal, you should consider asking your doctor to prescribe a low dose of thyroid hormone. In addition, family members of those with a low thyroid have about a 50 percent chance of also getting it. If your doctor won't prescribe a thyroid hormone, you may wish to consult one who is open to the idea (visit my website at www.Vitality101.com for a list of health professionals). Before seeing a new doctor, call and ask if he or she sometimes treats people with thyroid hormone despite the blood tests being normal if their symptoms show they need it. As long as you do not have underlying angina/heart disease and you follow up with a blood test to make sure that your Free T4 (do not use TSH) thyroid levels are in a safe range (going **above the upper limit** of normal may aggravate osteoporosis) a trial of low-dose thyroid hormone treatment is usually safe and may be dramatically beneficial.

Some patients have found desiccated thyroid (Armour Thyroid) to be helpful and the synthetic thyroid (Synthroid®) not to be. Some have found the opposite. What is important to know is that if you have muscle or nerve pain and an under-active thyroid that is not treated (even if your blood tests come back normal), these pains simply will not resolve. Many experts on chronic pain agree.[4-8]

I have found—either through blood testing or according to symptoms—that over 47 percent of my fibromyalgia patients have a low thyroid and that 83 percent of these patients have improved by taking a low dose of thyroid hormone.[9] In another study, 152 women were evaluated who had symptoms of an under-active thyroid despite normal blood tests. In the first phase of the study, 49 women were given a high-protein, low carbohydrate diet that eliminated sugar, wheat and dairy for one month. This group experienced an 18 percent decrease in joint pain and a 14 percent decrease in muscle pain, combined with a 21 percent decrease in fatigue. All 152 patients were then given 22 days of thyroid therapy using T3, the active form of thyroid hormone. They were given 7 ½ micrograms twice a day, slowly increased to 37 ½ micrograms twice a day and then tapered off. After 22 days, all of their symptoms decreased by an average of 39 percent. One week later, they were switched to Armour Thyroid 60 mg twice a day for 3 more months. Fatigue decreased by 60 percent, headaches by 63 percent, depression by 73 percent, insomnia by 69 percent, joint pain by 58 percent, and muscle pain by 58 percent.[10]

### *Do You Feel That Doctors Missing Hypothyroidism Is a Major Problem?*

Absolutely! To give you an idea of its importance, let's look at the situation further.

Hypothyroidism, like most other illnesses that affect predominantly women, has been dramatically under-diagnosed. [2, 3] As noted above, the American Academy of Clinical Endocrinologists (AACE), the nation's largest organization of thyroid specialists, has now confirmed this. After a 2002 meeting, the normal range for thyroid tests was dramatically narrowed. As noted in the AACE press release:

> "Until November 2002, doctors had relied on a normal TSH level ranging from 0.5 to 5.0 to diagnose and treat patients with a thyroid disorder who tested outside the boundaries of that range. Now the AACE encourages doctors to consider treatment for patients who test outside the boundaries of a narrower margin based on a target TSH level of 0.3 to 3.0. AACE believes the new range will result in proper diagnosis for millions of Americans who suffer from a mild thyroid disorder, but have gone untreated until now.
>
> "The prevalence of undiagnosed thyroid disease in the United States is shockingly high—particularly since it is a condition that is easy to diagnose and treat," said Hossein Gharib, MD, FACE, and president of AACE. "The new TSH range from the AACE guidelines gives physicians the information they need to diagnose mild thyroid disease before it can lead to more serious effects on a patient's health, such as elevated cholesterol, heart disease, osteoporosis, infertility, and depression." [11]

Now, years after the new directives have been given, doctors are still largely unaware of these new lab guidelines for diagnosis and treatment. Even the major labs doing thyroid testing have not bothered to change the now incorrect normal ranges for both diagnosis and treatment of thyroid disorders.

The normal range for thyroid hormone levels in the past have been based on statistical norms (called 2 standard deviations). This means that out of every 100 people, those with the 2 highest and lowest scores are defined as abnormal and everyone else is arbitrarily considered to be normal. That means if a problem affects over 2 percent of the population (as many as 24 percent of women over 60 are hypothyroid[12] and 12 percent of the population have abnormal antibodies attacking their thyroid[13]), then our testing system will miss most of them. In addition, our testing system does not take biological individuality into account. To translate how poorly this "2 percent equals abnormal" system works, consider this: if we applied this approach to getting you a pair of shoes, any size between a 4 and 13 would be "medically normal." If a man was accidentally given a size 5 shoe or a woman a size 12, the doctor would say the shoe sizes they were given are "normal," and there is no problem!

Simply changing the normal range for the TSH test to "less than 3" increased the number of Americans with thyroid illness from 13 million to approximately 27 million. Unfortunately, over 13 million Americans with thyroid disease remain undiagnosed, [11] and the majority of those receiving treatment are not being dosed appropriately. [12, 13] Doctors do not know that they have not been adequately trained in the proper diagnosis or treatment of hypothyroidism, and the cost in human life and devastating illness is enormous. What makes this especially tragic is how easy treatment is if doctors are given the correct information.

### What Is the Potential Cost of Missing Hypothyroidism?

1. There may be over 30,000 preventable deaths per year from heart attacks. Women with untreated hypothyroidism are more than twice as likely to have a heart attack. A study in the prestigious *Annals of Internal Medicine* noted that hypothyroidism "contributed to 60 percent of cases of myocardial infarction [heart attacks] among women affected by subclinical [even mild] hypothyroidism." It contributed more to causing heart attacks in these patients than smoking, elevated cholesterol, high blood pressure, or diabetes.[14]
2. Six percent of miscarriages are associated with hypothyroidism with 4600 miscarriages per year after 15 weeks of pregnancy and countless more before. Undiagnosed hypothyroidism is also associated with infertility. In moderate to severely hypothyroid mothers, the baby was also over six times as likely to die soon after being born.[15]
3. Children born to hypothyroid mothers have a lower IQ by an average of 7 points. They are almost four times as likely to have an IQ under 85 and over twice as likely to have learning difficulties resulting in their having to repeat a grade.[16]
4. Over six million Americans have fibromyalgia and tens of millions more have chronic muscle pain. Undiagnosed or inadequately treated thyroid disorders contribute to these unnecessarily disabling conditions.
5. Hypothyroidism is a major cause of gaining and being unable to lose weight. It also causes fatigue, dry hair, coarse skin, depression, and "brain fog" as well. Americans are currently treating hypothyroidism, which is often confused with depression, with Prozac®. This is an even bigger problem in the elderly who are being misdiagnosed with depression or Alzheimer's/ senility when what they have is hypothyroidism.

What makes this situation especially tragic is that, given the proper information, hypothyroidism can be incredibly easy and inexpensive to diagnose and treat. Instead, because of lack of awareness on the part of our medical community, Americans unnecessarily suffer from a major public health disaster.

### *Treating an Under-active Thyroid*

We are constantly learning powerful new tricks for treating hypothyroidism and there are many reasonable treatment approaches. I would recommend starting with a trial of Armour Thyroid. Our treatment protocol information checklist (see Appendix B: Pain Treatment Protocol) gives the "nuts and bolts" of how to begin and adjust all of the treatments discussed in this book.

Check a free T4 (the thyroid blood test that measures the actual level of the main hormone produced by the thyroid) about one month **after** the 90 and 180 mg levels of Armour Thyroid are reached. **Do not** check a TSH test. It will often be inaccurate and low (because of the hypothalamic dysfunction) and your doctor will incorrectly think you're on too much thyroid—even if your blood hormone levels are low normal. This will confuse both you and your doctor. Adjust the thyroid slowly to the dose that **feels** the best and **not** simply to where your blood test is above the lower limit of normal. When you find the dose that feels best, check to confirm that it is **within normal range for the free T4 blood level. The free T4 is the only thyroid blood test I would check to monitor therapy**. Your doctor may be concerned because **excess** thyroid hormone can cause osteoporosis (bone thinning). Having reviewed the medical literature, I have seen **no** studies showing any increase in osteoporosis in pre-menopausal women if the T4 thyroid blood level is kept in the normal range. Although many patients can stop taking thyroid hormone after 12 to 24 months, you can stay on Armour Thyroid or Synthroid® for as long as it is needed.

If your doctor is unwilling to prescribe Armour Thyroid (some feel it is too "old-fashioned") you can also try Synthroid (T4)®. One hundred micrograms (0.1 mg) of Synthroid "equals" 1 grain of Armour Thyroid. Often, one hormone treatment works when the other does not. Adjust the dose as noted in Appendix B: Pain Treatment Protocol.

## Adrenal Insufficiency—the Adrenal Gland, Your Stress Handler

The adrenal glands, which sit on top of the kidneys, are actually two different glands in one. Both parts are critical to your "stress response system." The center of the gland makes adrenaline (epinephrine). The outer part of the adrenal gland, called the cortex, also makes many important hormones. These include:

- Cortisol. The adrenal glands increase their production of cortisol in response to stress. Cortisol raises the blood sugar and blood pressure levels and moderates immune function, in addition to playing numerous other roles. If the cortisol level is low, the person may have fatigue, low blood pressure, hypoglycemia, poor immune function, an increased tendency to allergies and environmental sensitivity, and an inability to deal with stress. Inadequate cortisol can markedly increase pain by hindering your body's ability to deal with inflammation. In addition, recurrent drops in blood sugar (hypoglycemia) can constantly throw your muscles into spasm.

- Dehydroepiandrosterone sulfate (DHEA-S). Although its mechanism of action is not clear, DHEA is the most abundant hormone produced by the adrenal cortex. If it is low, you will often feel poorly. Patients often feel dramatically better when their DHEA-S levels are brought to the mid-normal range for a 29-year-old. DHEA-S levels normally decline with age and often drop prematurely in fibromyalgia patients. DHEA has been called the "fountain of youth" hormone. This is because gray hair sometimes returns to its original color when one takes DHEA. In fact, I didn't realize that my nephews thought I was dying my hair for years (I would never dye my hair—I like the salt and pepper look), because my normal hair color would return when I took DHEA!
- Estrogen and testosterone. These hormones are produced in small but significant amounts by the adrenals as well as by the ovaries and testicles.

## Causes of Adrenal Insufficiency

I suspect that many people have "adrenal burnout." Dr. Hans Selye, one of the first doctors to research stress reactions, found that if an animal becomes severely overstressed, its adrenal glands bleed and develop signs of adrenal destruction before the animal finally dies from the stress.

If you think back to your biology classes in high school, you may remember something called the "fight-or-flight response." This is a physical reaction that occurs during times of stress. During the Stone Age, when a caveman met an animal that wanted to eat him, the caveman's adrenal glands activated multiple systems in his body that prompted him to either fight or run. This reaction helped the caveman survive. In those days, however, people probably had a couple of weeks or months to recover before facing the next major stress. That is no longer the case. In today's society, especially with chronic pain, people often experience stress reactions every few minutes.

I suspect that many people suffer exhaustion of their adrenal glands. With the kinds of stresses common in modern society, a person's adrenal test may initially show hormonal levels that are actually higher than usual, since the adrenal gland tends to overcompensate to deal with stress. Over time, this may exhaust the adrenal reserve, that is, the adrenal's ability to increase hormone production in response to stress. Both high and low cortisol can contribute to weight gain. In endocrinologist Dr. William Jefferies' experience (and in mine as well), people with either low hormone production or a low reserve often respond dramatically to treatment with low doses of adrenal hormones.[17-18]

## *Symptoms of Adrenal Insufficiency*

If your adrenal glands are under-active, what symptoms might you experience? Low adrenal function can cause, among other symptoms:

- Pain and fatigue
- Recurrent infections
- "Crashing" during stress
- Hypoglycemia (irritability when hungry)
- Low blood pressure and dizziness upon first standing

Hypoglycemia deserves special mention. Many people become shaky and nervous, then dizzy, irritable, and fatigued when they get hungry. They then often feel better after they eat sweets, which improve their energy and mood for a short period of time. Because of this, these people often crave sugar, not realizing that it makes their blood sugar level initially shoot back up to normal, which is what makes them feel better, but then eating the sugar makes the blood sugar continue to soar beyond normal. The body responds to this by driving the sugar level back down below normal again. The effect, energy-wise, is like a roller coaster.

Dr. Jefferies has noted—and again, my experience confirms his finding—that most people with hypoglycemia have under-active adrenal glands. This makes sense because the adrenal glands' responsibilities include maintaining blood sugar at an adequate level. Sugar is the only fuel that the brain can use. When a person's blood sugar level drops, he or she feels poorly and it can flare their pain. I recommend diagnosing "hypoglycemia" based on symptoms, and, like other tests of hormonal function, I consider "glucose tolerance tests" to be incredibly unreliable.

## *Treating Adrenal Insufficiency*

People with hypoglycemia can treat low blood sugar symptoms by cutting sugar and caffeine out of their diets; having frequent, small meals; and increasing their intake of proteins and vegetables. Fruit—not fruit juices, which contain concentrated sugar—can be taken in moderation, about 1 to 2 pieces a day, depending on the amount of sugar in the fruit. Taking 250 micrograms of chromium a day (present in the vitamin powder) for 6 months often helps smooth out hypoglycemic symptoms.[19]

Treating the under-active adrenal problem usually banishes the symptoms of low blood sugar. You can begin with adrenal glandulars combined with licorice and key nutrients (all present in Adrenal Stress End®, which I helped to formulate—see Appendix C: Resources). Your doctor may consider using prescription hydrocortisone, such as Cortef® in addition. When used in doses of 20 mg or less a day (see Appendix B: Pain Treatment Protocol) Cortef is usually quite safe and can result in a dramatic decrease in many types of pain. Interestingly, some doctors are using "microdose" Cortef therapy for arthritis. Although some doctors may charge $4000 to prescribe this simple and inexpensive treatment, yours could prescribe it for free!

## Toxicity of Cortisone

Adrenal hormones are essential for life. Without them, a person dies. But, as with any hormone, too much can be dangerous. In the early studies using adrenal hormones, the researchers had no idea what dose was normal and what was toxic. When they gave injections of the hormone to patients, the patients' arthritis went away and they felt better. However, because they gave patients many times more than the normal amount, the patients became toxic and died. Because of this, the researchers became frightened and avoided using adrenal hormones whenever possible. Medical students were taught to avoid adrenal hormones unless no other treatment choices existed.

The use of adrenal hormones needs to be put into perspective, however. Imagine if the early thyroid researchers had given their patients 50 times the usual dose of thyroid hormone. Thyroid patients would have routinely died of heart attacks. The thyroid researchers, however, were fortunate enough to stumble upon the body's healthy dose early on and to skip these negative outcomes. If they had not, people today would not be treated for an under-active thyroid until they displayed symptoms of very advanced thyroid disease (myxedema) and were nearly comatose. Medical science is just beginning to learn that a person can feel horrible and function poorly even with a minimal to moderate hormone deficiency. Waiting for the person to go "off the deep end" of the test's normal scale is not healthy.

Dr. Jefferies has found that as long as the adrenal hormone level is kept within the normal range, the main toxicity that a patient might experience is a slight upset stomach due to the body not being used to having the hormone come in through the stomach.[20-21] Taking the hormone with food usually helps this. In addition, some patients gain a few pounds. This is because a low adrenal level can cause a person's weight to drop below the body's normal "set point," even if that set point is high because of their fibromyalgia. (The average weight gain in fibromyalgia is 32 pounds.) However, any weight gain often is more than offset by the weight loss resulting from being able to exercise once again.

Many physicians do not like to prescribe even low doses of adrenal hormone. If your physician is uncomfortable with Cortef, invite him or her to read Dr. Jefferies' material on the safety of low-dose cortisone as well as our recent study.[20-21,22] Most patients only need 5 to 12 ½ mg a day, equivalent to 1 to 3 mg a day of prednisone (a more dangerous and less effective synthetic form of Cortisol® that your doctor is aware of), which is a dose so low that most doctors have never prescribed it. After feeling well for 6 to 18 months, most people begin to slowly decrease their adrenal hormone dosage, eventually discontinuing the treatment entirely.

If your symptoms started suddenly after a viral infection, if you suffer from hypoglycemia, **or** if you have recurrent infections that take a long time to resolve, you probably have under-active adrenal glands.

### *Dehydroepiandrosterone (DHEA)*

The adrenal gland makes many hormones in addition to hydrocortisone. One of these is DHEA, which is often **very** low in chronic pain patients. Although DHEA's function is not yet fully understood, it appears to be important for good health, which makes a low DHEA level worth treating.[20] Some studies suggest that the higher a person's DHEA level is, the longer that person will live and the healthier he or she will be. I'm concerned that pushing the blood level **above** the upper limit of normal may slightly increase the risk of breast cancer, so keep it in the normal range. For many patients, when a low DHEA level is treated, the result is a dramatic boost in well-being and a decrease in pain.

If your DHEA-S (**not** DHEA) blood level is low (under 120 micrograms per deciliter [mcg/dL] of blood for females or 325 mcg/dL for males), I recommend beginning treatment with 5 to 25 mg of DHEA per day and slowly working up to what feels like an optimal level to you. For women, I suggest keeping the DHEA-S level at around 150 to 180 mcg/dL, which is the middle of the normal range for a twenty-nine-year-old female. For men, I keep the DHEA-S level between 350 and 500 mcg/dL, which is the normal range for a 29-year old male. The low ends of the normal ranges are normal only for people over 80. If you have side effects, such as facial hair or acne, which are uncommon, check your blood level of DHEA-S and decrease your dose. I have found that many brands of DHEA are not reliable. I recommend you use DHEA made by compounding pharmacists or by General Nutrition Center or other reputable companies.

### *Growth Hormone*

This hormone is critical for tissue repair. Many people take growth hormone by injection at a cost of over $12,000 a year, to stay young. Although it can be helpful, I almost never prescribe it because of its cost, safety concerns and the need for injections. Growth hormone can be raised in three easier and less expensive (and often more fun) ways. We have already mentioned getting 8 to 9 hours of deep sleep each night. Exercise and sex also raise growth hormone. In addition, growth hormone stimulates DHEA production, and raising the DHEA, which can be done easily, may be responsible for much of growth hormone's benefits.

## Low Estrogen and Testosterone

Many people going through midlife develop pain, fatigue, poor libido, or depression. This includes men and women alike. An under-active adrenal gland can aggravate this problem. Although the ovaries make most of a woman's estrogen and the testicles make most of a man's testosterone, in women the adrenals make significant amounts of testosterone.

### *Low Testosterone—Not Only a Male Problem*

Inadequate testosterone is a major problem in 70 percent of my male patients with fibromyalgia and/or chronic pain. It is important (again, in both men and women) to check the "free" or "unbound" blood testosterone level. This measures the **active** form of the hormone. If your result is below normal, or even in the lowest 25 percent of the normal range, I would consider a trial of testosterone therapy.

Low testosterone is associated with many problems also caused by pain, including fatigue, depression, poor stamina, muscle-wasting, osteoporosis, and poor libido. Chronic pain is routinely associated with low testosterone, further aggravating these problems. Treating men with low testosterone helped all of these conditions.[23] Although testosterone levels are normally much lower in females, testosterone deficiencies in women cause these same problems. Testosterone is critical for females, as well as for males, and I find low free testosterone levels in many female patients.

A recent study by Dr. Hillary White, an associate professor at Dartmouth Medical School, found that testosterone replacement therapy is helpful in the treatment of fibromyalgia pain. Because the study is still awaiting publication, more details are not yet available. Dr. White became interested in this problem when testosterone helped relieve her own fibromyalgia pain. She notes that it is important to use natural testosterone and not the synthetic methyl testosterone form.

## *Treating Low Testosterone*

For men, I often treat with natural testosterone cream from a compounding pharmacy (I have it made up as 100 mg of testosterone per gram of PLO gel). Most men need 25 to 50 mg rubbed onto thin-skinned areas (for example, the inner upper arms from the elbow to two inches below the armpit) 1 to 2 times a day. Androgel® 50 mg is another alternative. It is more expensive, unless you have prescription insurance.

For women, testosterone treatment is easier. Oral natural micronized testosterone (and natural estrogen and progesterone) are available through most compounding pharmacies. (For a compounding pharmacy that does mail-order prescriptions, see Appendix C: Resources.) The usual dose is 2 to 4 mg 1 to 2 times a day by mouth or in cream form. If you take the capsules and also need to take estrogen or progesterone (see below), they can be combined in the same capsule at a lower cost. I usually begin by prescribing 2 mg, 1 to 2 times a day for 6 weeks to see the effect, then raise or lower the dosage if needed. With this dosing, most women feel more energy and have thicker hair, younger skin, and improved libido.

I check free testosterone blood levels 6 to 14 weeks after starting therapy and adjust the dosing accordingly. Blood levels are not reliable, however, if you are taking synthetic methyl testosterone instead of natural testosterone. Check the test 1 ½ to 3 hours after taking the tablets or applying the cream.

## *Potential Side Effects of Testosterone Treatment*

In women, if acne, nightmares, or darkening of facial hair occurs, the dose is too high and should be decreased. These effects, which can also occur with DHEA supplementation, are generally reversible. These side effects can also be caused by an estrogen level that is too low relative to your testosterone, and may be avoided by supplementing both together. For women, it may help to begin the estrogen for 4 to 8 weeks before starting testosterone. This often decreases side effects.

In men, acne suggests the dose is too high. Monitor free testosterone blood levels, and keep them at the 70$^{th}$ percentile of the normal range. Testosterone supplementation can also elevate thyroid hormone levels in those taking thyroid supplements. If you are on thyroid supplements, I would recheck thyroid hormone levels after 6 to 12 weeks of adding testosterone, or sooner if you get a racing heart or anxious/hyper feelings.

Most studies show that low testosterone in men is associated with an increased risk of angina and that using testosterone (use the natural testosterone, not synthetic) to bring low testosterone up to the mid-normal level **decreases** angina and leg artery blockages, improves cholesterol, and may decrease diabetic tendencies.[24–29] It is not clear if taking testosterone increases the risk of prostate enlargement or cancer beyond that of any other healthy male. While I don't feel being testosterone deficient is a good way to prevent these illnesses, if you are a man over 50 who is taking testosterone, it is reasonable to do a prostate exam and prostate-specific antigen (PSA) test yearly. For many men, improvements in overall sense of wellness have been dramatic, and treating the low testosterone has been critical.

### Low Estrogen and Progesterone in Women

Although not likely to be a problem with men, deficiencies of estrogen and/or progesterone can be major problems in women with CFIDS/FMS. In a book by Dr. Elizabeth Lee Vliet, *Screaming To Be Heard: Hormonal Connections Women Suspect...and Doctors Ignore*, the role of estrogen deficiency in causing pain, fatigue, brain fog, disordered sleep, fibromyalgia, poor libido, PMS, low levels of serotonin and other neurotransmitters, interstitial cystitis, as well as other problems is reviewed in detail. She notes, appropriately, that the perimenopausal period (the period as you approach menopause) has a gradual onset, and symptoms of estrogen deficiency can occur 5 to 12 years before your blood tests and periods become abnormal.

If your pain or migraines are worse when your estrogen levels are dropping (i.e. during ovulation, which occurs about fifteen days after the first day of your period and around your period), a trial of **natural** estrogen supplementation is warranted. Other symptoms of inadequate estrogen include inadequate vaginal lubrication, night sweats, and/or hot flashes.

### Treating Low Estrogen and Progesterone

Most of the media attention and research about estrogen being dangerous relate to the use of conjugated (i.e. pregnant horse urine) estrogens like Premarin®. I prefer to use natural biestrogen (1 1/4 to 2 1/2 mg 1 to 2 times a day) from a compounding pharmacy. This contains estradiol plus estriol, a weaker form of estrogen that may actually decrease the risk of developing breast cancer. Patients with estrogen induced migraines usually get them not from the estrogen itself but from fluctuating blood levels of estrogen. They will often get relief by using estrogen patches that last for the week around their period. These give steady estrogen levels without the fluctuations.

Unless you have had a hysterectomy, if you take supplemental estrogen you **must** also take progesterone. I prefer natural progesterone—for example, 200 mg of Prometrium® a day for the first 10 days of each month, or 50 to 100 mg every day. Taking both estrogen and progesterone every day will often result in your periods going away after 6 to 9 months, and most women over 48 prefer this approach. ■

**Important Points**

1. Under active adrenals are common. Treat low or borderline adrenal function with **low-dose** Cortef® and/or DHEA (adrenal hormones). Also take adrenal glandulars with added licorice and other key nutrients (see Appendix C: Resources).
2. Hypothyroidism is very common and must be treated in chronic pain patients—despite normal blood tests. Treat symptoms of low or borderline thyroid function with Armour Thyroid®—even if your blood tests are normal.
3. Consider estrogen deficiency if your symptoms are worse around your period or if you have decreased vaginal lubrication, regardless of what your blood tests show. Whether you are male or female, consider testosterone deficiency even if the test is low-normal. Consider a treatment trial using **natural** hormones.

# Section 2

# *Eliminating the Underlying Causes/Triggers of Your Pain*

In addition to pain coming from not having the basic things your body needs for health, it can also come from outside triggers. Infections, including subtle ones that are often hidden, can be a common trigger. Tissue compression (e.g. cancer or disc disease) and structural problems also frequently cause pain. Some other causes, such as thermal/burn injuries are obvious, while toxin exposures, such as those produced by chemicals and infections (especially yeast), may be more subtle. This section reviews some of the more important triggers.

*"Man's mind, once stretched by a new idea, never regains its original dimensions."*

Oliver Wendell Holmes

# Chapter 5

# Infections

Many different kinds of infections can trigger pain. Pain can be caused by direct irritation caused by the infection, but can also be caused by the inflammation or immune activation your body creates as it attempts to fight the infection—like feeling achiness with the flu.

In some cases, such as Lyme disease, the role of infection in causing the pain is fairly well accepted. In many, if not most cases, however, the role of infections is still controversial as a source of pain.

## *What Infections Can Cause Pain?*

Although it is possible for numerous infections to be the source of pain, we will focus on the most important ones. These are:

1. Fungal infections and overgrowth. Although many doctors still believe there is no such thing as fungal overgrowth, the increase in antibiotic and sugar use in our society has made this problem more common. When it affects the skin (e.g. athlete's foot) or causes obvious vaginal infections, it can be readily seen and is therefore accepted by the medical community. Unfortunately, when it affects the bowels and sinuses there is no reliable way to test for it, and many physicians still make believe that fungal overgrowth cannot occur in these areas. It can, however, and it is very important to treat it.

2. Antibiotic sensitive infections. In traditional medicine, we like to look for things that are easy to test for. If we have no test for an infection, we make believe it does not exist. This was the case with Polio, Lyme disease, and numerous other infections until tests were developed. Physicians also like to look for infections that can be cultured. These include bacteria like staph, strep, and E. coli. For these infections, a few bacteria put on a culture dish will grow into millions overnight, and these can then be seen with the naked eye. I suspect that many kinds of inflammatory arthritis (e.g. rheumatoid arthritis) are triggered by the body's response to infections that we

cannot yet culture. Research suggests that a trial of tetracycline family antibiotics (and occasionally anti-parasitics) is warranted in the treatments of these inflammatory arthritic conditions.

## *How Can I Tell When I Should Consider These Infections?*

There are no definitive tests for yeast overgrowth that will distinguish it from normal yeast growth in the body. Nonetheless, fungal/yeast overgrowth should be considered in any of the following situations:

1. Chronic sinusitis and nasal congestion
2. Spastic colon, gas, bloating, constipation, and/or diarrhea
3. A history of frequent antibiotic use
4. Recurrent or ongoing skin, nail, or vaginal fungal infections
5. Itchy ears or anus, recurrent aphthous ulcers (painful ulcers in the mouth where the lips meet your gums that last for 5 to 10 days), and/or sugar cravings
6. The presence of widespread achiness without inflammation (i.e. fibromyalgia/chronic fatigue syndrome)

Although people most often speak of Candida as the main type of fungal infection, these infections can be caused by many different fungi/yeast. Although many tests are recommended to look for these infections, I do not consider them to be more reliable than simply looking for the six things that I noted above. If any of these are present, I believe that an empiric trial of anti-fungal therapy is warranted. Your body's response to therapy is the best indicator of whether fungal overgrowth was a problem. If your symptoms initially worsen with anti-fungals and/or improve significantly by the end of six weeks of treatment (shorter courses are unlikely to eradicate the problem), this suggests that fungal overgrowth is playing a role in your pain (and perhaps many other symptoms). A number of very effective methods can be used to eliminate a yeast problem. My preference is to treat with a mix of natural and prescription therapies (see below). If your doctor is unwilling to use prescription anti-fungals, either begin with the natural therapies or look for a doctor who **will** prescribe them.

## *Tell Me More about Fungal Infections*

Many physicians feel that yeast overgrowth causes a generalized suppression of the immune system. In other words, once the yeast gets the upper hand, it sets up a cycle that further suppresses the body's defenses.[1] Interestingly, a recent Mayo Clinic study showed that most cases of chronic sinusitis also seem to be associated with a reaction to yeast in the sinuses—something I proposed years ago. Nonetheless, as I already noted, this theory is controversial. Yeast are normal members of the body's "zoo." They live in balance with bacteria—some of which are helpful and healthy and some of which are detrimental and unhealthy. The problems begin when this harmonious balance shifts and the yeast begins to overgrow.

Many things can prompt yeast to overgrow. One of the most common causes is frequent antibiotic use. Antibiotics kill off the good bacteria in the bowel along with the bad bacteria. When this happens, the yeast no longer have competition and begin to overgrow. The body is often able to rebalance itself after one or several courses of antibiotics, but after repeated or long-term courses—and especially if the body has an underlying immune dysfunction—the yeast can get the upper hand.

Other factors are also important. Studies have shown that animals that are sleep-deprived and/or have increased sugar intake develop bowel yeast overgrowth. Many physicians feel that eating sugar stimulates yeast overgrowth in people as well. Sugar is food for yeast. Yeasts ferment sugar in order to grow and multiply. Yeast overgrowth due to the overuse of sugar also seems to cause immune suppression, which facilitates bacterial infections, requiring even more antibiotic use. Poor sleep also results in marked suppression of your immune function.

## *How Do I Treat Suspected Fungal Overgrowth?*

### Natural Yeast Treatments

The first thing you need to do is to stop feeding the yeast. Yeast grow by eating sugar and other sweets. You can enjoy one or two pieces of fruit a day, but you should not consume concentrated sugar sources such as juices, corn syrup, jellies, pastry, candy, or honey. Stay far away from soft drinks, which often have 10 to 12 teaspoons of sugar in every 12 ounces. This amount of sugar has been shown to markedly suppress immune function for several hours.

Using stevia as a sweetener is a wonderful substitute for sugar. Stevia is safe and natural, and you can use all you want. There are even cookbooks available for using stevia. Most brands are bitter, and I don't recommend them. Two brands taste great, however. These are the ones made by Body Ecology® (from 1-800-4stevia or my web site) or the Stevita Company®.

Other healthy natural sweeteners include maltitol (used in many sugar free chocolates), inositol, and xylitol. The yeast do not appear to be able to ferment these. In addition, inositol can decrease nerve pain and anxiety. Xylitol also appears to decrease osteoporosis. Be prepared to have withdrawal symptoms for about one week when you cut sugar out of your diet. Several excellent books have been written on the yeast controversy and offer additional dietary methods to try. One of the best is *The Yeast Connection and the Woman* by Dr. Crook, a physician who did a spectacular job of advancing our understanding of the problems caused by fungal overgrowth.

Acidophilus—milk bacteria, a healthy type of bacteria for the bowel—helps restore balance in the bowel. Acidophilus is found in yogurt with live and active yogurt cultures. Indeed, eating 1 cup of yogurt (with live bacterial cultures) a day can markedly diminish the frequency of recurrent vaginal yeast infections.[2] Acidophilus is also available in many forms. Unfortunately, recent tests of many brands showed that the quality control is very poor. The only forms of acidophilus that I currently recommend are those that have a pearl coating to protect the bacteria and keep them alive such as Acidophilus Pearls® or Probiotic Pearls (see Appendix C: Resources). Take 2 pearls twice a day for 5 months. This will help to restore the healthy bacteria in your colon that were destroyed by antibiotic use. Some people like to continue on 1 pearl a day long-term to help maintain healthy bowel function. If you are on antibiotics (**not** anti-fungals), take the acidophilus at least 3 to 6 hours away from the antibiotic dose.

Another effective natural anti-fungal is Citricidal®. Derived from grapefruit and grapefruit seeds, it can be quite powerful at inhibiting fungal growth and the growth of other infections. Take one or two 100 mg tablets twice a day. Do not use the liquid form, as it tastes vile. Many natural anti-fungals are available, but using a strong enough dose often causes stomach irritation and reflux. By combining several anti-fungals at lower doses, one can increase their effectiveness with fewer side effects. Phytostan® by NF Formulas (available from healthcare practitioners and at www.vitality101.com) is an excellent mix of natural anti-fungals. These include grapefruit seed extract, Pau d'arco, caprylic acid, undecylenic acid, rosemary, and thyme. The recommended dose is one tablet, 3 times a day or 2 tablets, twice a day.

## *Medical Treatments for Yeast Overgrowth*

Nystatin®, an anti-fungal medication, has been helpful in the treatment of yeast overgrowth. Unfortunately, some fungi seem to be developing resistance to nystatin. In addition, nystatin is poorly absorbed, which means that it has little impact on the yeast outside of the bowel. Other anti-fungal medications, such as Diflucan® and Sporanox®, seem to be effective systemically (throughout the body) but they have two main drawbacks. First, they are expensive, costing more than $450 to

$900 for a two-month course. Happily, Diflucan just wen can now be found for $40/month. Second, any effective a initially make the symptoms of yeast infection worse. If you tion, start your treatment with Acidophilus Pearls, a sugar-fi Phytostan® for a few weeks before beginning the Nystatin a ucan.

Although it is uncommon, Diflucan and Sporanox can also cause liver inflammation. If you are taking Diflucan or Sporanox for more than 6 to 12 weeks, I would consider intermittent blood tests to check liver function—specifically checking blood levels of ALT and AST, two inexpensive and good indicators of injury to the liver. If you have preexisting active liver disease, you should be cautious about using Diflucan or Sporanox—or do not use them at all. I recommend taking 200 to 300 mg of lipoic acid a day whenever you take Sporanox or Diflucan. This is a natural supplement that helps to protect and heal the liver (and can also be helpful for nerve pain). I also recommend lipoic acid for anyone with nerve pain (200 to 300 mg 2 to 3 times a day) or **active** liver disease (e.g. hepatitis), at doses up to 1,000 to 3,000 mg a day, as it may prevent and/or help treat cirrhosis (lipoic acid is not in the vitamin powder).

## *Avoiding Yeast Overgrowth*

The best thing you can do to combat yeast overgrowth is to try to avoid it in the first place. When you get an infection, immediately begin treating it naturally. (See "Treating Infections without Antibiotics" below.) Hopefully, you will be able to prevent it from turning into a bacterial infection that might require an antibiotic. Ask your doctor what other measures you can take before resorting to antibiotics. The article below can help you to decrease the need for antibiotics dramatically.

If you find that you must take an antibiotic, all is not lost. You can still lessen the severity of yeast overgrowth by avoiding sweets and by taking Nystatin plus Acidophilus Pearls (again, not within 3 to 6 hours of an antibiotic).

## *What If the Yeast Comes Back?*

It is normal for yeast symptoms to resolve after treatment. After 6 weeks on the Sporanox® or Diflucan® many people feel a lot better. However, symptoms may recur soon after stopping the anti-fungal. If this happens, I would continue the Sporanox® or Diflucan for another 6 weeks or for as long as is needed to keep the symptoms at bay. More frequently, people feel better after treatment and stay feeling fairly well for a period of 6 to 24 months. At that time, it is common to see a

*Continued on page 52*

## reating Infections without Antibiotics

Many people do not realize how many things they can do before resorting to using an antibiotic to clear an infection. If you feel you are coming down with a respiratory infection such as a cold or the flu, I recommend that you try the following:

- Take a natural thymic hormone mimic. This is available as a product called ProBoost®, which is a very effective immune stimulant (see Appendix C: Resources). At first sign of any infection, dissolve the contents of one packet under your tongue three times a day and let it absorb there (any that is swallowed is destroyed). I have found that using it for 2 or 3 days at the onset of an infection can shorten the length of the infection dramatically and often stops it on the first day.
- Take 1,000 to 8,000 mg of vitamin C a day—enough to get diarrhea, then cut back to a comfortable level.
- If you have a sore throat, suck on a zinc lozenge 5 to 8 times a day. Make sure that the lozenges have at least 10 to 20 mg of zinc per lozenge. Less than this will not be effective. Zinc lozenges have been known to speed the time it takes to recover from a cold by about 40 percent. General Nutrition Center sells a very good one.
- Take 1,000 mg of olive leaf extract (available in most health food stores) 3 times a day for 3 to 7 days. Although probably not as effective as ProBoost, olive leaf extract seems to be helpful against viral respiratory infections and, perhaps, yeast infections. It seems most helpful in fighting the common cold. In my experience, it has been very helpful for about half the people who try it—the cold is gone in 24 to 36 hours. If it causes nausea, cut the dose in half.
- Drink plenty of water and hot caffeine-free tea (or hot water with lemon) and rest.
- Take Oscillococcinum®, a homeopathic remedy available at most health food stores and some supermarkets, if you have flu-like symptoms such as chills, fever, achiness, and/or malaise. It speeds healing and eases discomfort. It is best taken early in the infection—as soon as you have any symptoms.
- If you have a sinus infection, try nasal rinses. Dissolve 1/2 teaspoon of salt in a cup of lukewarm water. Inhale some of the solution about one inch up into your nose, one nostril at a time.

Do this either by using a baby nose bulb or an eyedropper while lying down, or by sniffing the solution out of the palm of your hand while standing by a sink. Then gently blow your nose, being careful not to hurt your ears. Repeat the same process with the other nostril. Continue to repeat with each nostril until the nose is clear. Rinse your nasal passages at least twice a day until the infection improves. Each rinsing will wash away about 90 percent of the infection and make it much easier for your body to heal. Colloidal silver nose sprays can also help. Also ask your doctor to prescribe the "sinusitis nose spray" from Cape Pharmacy (See Appendix C: Resources). In addition, see the section below on treating sinusitis.

- Try using a humidifier or vaporizer in your bedroom. You can also make a steam room by running a hot shower in your bathroom and then breathing in the steam. Or try using a steam inhaler, such as the one available from Bernhard Industries. This is also wonderful for alleviating chronic and acute sinusitis.

If, in spite of these measures, nasal and lung mucus is yellow after 7 to 14 days, or if you are feeling worse after 3 to 4 days, you may have to consider taking a course of antibiotics. If you do, you should take Nystatin® while on the antibiotic. Erythromycin antibiotics such as azithromycin (Zithromax®) and clarithromycin (Biaxin®) are usually preferable to penicillin antibiotics. Interestingly, my patients have sometimes found that pain and many other symptoms (not just the cold) improve while they are taking an erythromycin or tetracycline antibiotic. If that happens, I recommend a 6 to 24 month course of Zithromax 250 mg per day, or 100 mg of doxycycline twice a day. If you feel better on the antibiotic (take thymic hormone/ProBoost, echinacea, and the anti-fungal Nystatin® in conjunction with it), keep repeating 12 week courses until the symptoms stay gone. I would also check for Lyme disease, although the tests are not reliable. For most of my patients who repeatedly get respiratory infections that take forever to go away, I consider an empiric trial of prescription hydrocortisone (Cortef®) at a dosage of 7 1/2 mg in the morning and 5 mg at noon for 2 to 3 months (see adrenal insufficiency above).

To treat or prevent bladder infections caused by E.coli (the most common cause) use the natural supplement D-Mannose. (See Appendices B and C.)

recurrence of symptoms, especially if they are eating too much sugar or are taking antibiotics.

The best marker that I have found for recurrent yeast overgrowth is a return of sinusitis or bowel symptoms, with gas, bloating, diarrhea and/or constipation. If these symptoms persist for more than 2 weeks, especially if there is even a mild worsening of pain, fatigue, or mental cloudiness, it is reasonable to re-treat yourself with 6 weeks of acidophilus, Nystatin®, and Sporanox® or Diflucan®. In addition, I would also resume treatment if there is a recurrence of vaginal yeast or other fungal infections. You may repeat this regimen as needed. By using some of the natural remedies listed earlier in this chapter, however, you may be able to avoid repeated use of anti-fungals and the possible risk of becoming resistant to them.

## *When Should I Consider Treating with Antibiotics?*

Having just talked about the problems of fungal overgrowth that occur with long-term or frequent antibiotic use, it may seem odd that we will now talk about the benefits of ongoing antibiotic use in some pain patients. This simply helps to remind us that things are neither all good nor all bad. What is important is to use the right tool in the right situation.

As mentioned above, pain may be a signal from your body that there is an underlying infection that is problematic. In other cases, the pain is not caused by the infection but by your body's reaction as it attempts to fight the infection. I suspect that this is the case in rheumatoid arthritis and possibly in some other auto-immune illnesses as well. Unfortunately, the more commonly used antibiotics (penicillin, Keflex®, sulfa) may be ineffective against the slow-growing infections. These infections are more likely to respond to tetracycline, Cipro®, and erythromycin family antibiotics. I am most likely to consider a trial of 6 to 12 months (or more) of these antibiotics in the following situations:

1. If you have recurrent low-grade fevers (which I define as anything over 98.6 degrees) and/or chronic lung congestion without your doctor finding an underlying cause

2. If your pain or other chronic symptoms improved (even briefly) while you were taking antibiotics for something else

3. If you have rheumatoid arthritis or other inflammatory arthritis (i.e. where your joints are red, hot, and swollen) of unknown cause

4. If you have persistent sinusitis, skin/scalp pustules, or other chronic infections that persist after 6 weeks of anti-fungal therapy

People with these symptoms seem to be more likely to have bacterial, mycoplasma, or Chlamydia infections that respond to special antibiotics.

The following antibiotics are most likely to have an effect on these organisms:

- Doxycycline or minocycline (Minocin®), usually at dosages of 100 mg 2 times a day, especially in patients with rheumatoid arthritis
- Ciprofloxacin (Cipro®), 500 mg twice a day. When treating males, Cipro has the additional benefit of treating hidden prostate infections, as does doxycycline. You should not take oral magnesium or any supplement containing magnesium (such as the vitamin powder) within 6 hours of taking Cipro or you won't absorb the antibiotic
- Azithromycin (Zithromax®), 250 mg a day **or** clarithromycin (Biaxin®), 500 mg 2 times a day. They may work against infections missed by doxycycline and Cipro.

Although all these antibiotics can be effective, it is not uncommon for infections that are sensitive to one to be resistant to the others. Therefore, it is best to try either doxycycline or Cipro first. If they are not effective, then try Zithromax or Biaxin. Antibiotic treatments should be taken for at least 6 months. If there is no improvement in 2 to 4 months, switch to, or add, the other antibiotic or simply stop the treatment. If you have a low-grade fever (i.e. over 98.6) that drops with the antibiotic, it suggests that you do have one of these nonviral infections and the antibiotic is helping. This would encourage me to continue the antibiotic trial—even if it takes up to 18 months to see an improvement in your symptoms.

As with the yeast treatments, it is not uncommon to get what is called a Herxheimer (die-off) reaction that includes chills, fever, night sweats, and general worsening of your symptoms when the antibiotic first kills off the infection.

## Bowel Parasite Infections

The symptoms of parasitic infections can include pain. As immune dysfunction may be present in chronic pain patients, I believe that **all** parasites should be treated.[3–7]

I am most likely to test for parasites in patients who have gas, bloating, diarrhea, and or constipation—especially if the symptoms do not resolve with anti-fungal therapy, or if the person traveled overseas (or develop the bowel symptoms) in the weeks to months before the chronic pain began.

## *Diagnosing Bowel Parasites*

Most laboratories miss parasites when they do stool testing. The only labs (by mail) that I use for stool testing are the Parasitology Center and the Great Smokies Diagnostic Laboratory (for more information, see Appendix C: Resources). The appropriate treatment for many bowel parasites depends on which organism is causing the problem. My website at www.vitality101.com gives the treatment protocol, which includes treatments for the more common parasites. Prevent parasitic infection by filtering your water with an effective filtration unit (most are not effective). I recommend the Multi-Pure® filter (see Appendix C: Resources).

## *Other Infections*

We will discuss specific infections such as sinusitis, bladder infections, and prostatitis in the chapters on localized pain below (e.g. headache, pelvic pain syndromes, etc.). In addition, many things determine how likely your body is to react with a severe inflammatory response, and how much damage this response is likely to do. Nutritional factors such as essential fatty acids, antioxidants, and hormonal factors such as inadequate cortisol levels can dramatically modify your body's inflammatory response.

## *Detoxification*

Although an extensive discussion of detoxification is beyond the scope of this book, there are several simple things you can do that can be very helpful:

1. Sweating can remove toxins, especially if you shower soon after. Because of this, saunas can be very helpful for health. With many of the newer saunas, called "far-infrared," a ½-hour sauna 3 to 7 times a week can help detoxification.

2. Some of you may be more comfortable with hot baths. This recipe was given to me by a wonderful osteopathic practitioner (Anette Mnabhi, D.O. in Montgomery, IL):

   **Detox Bath Recipe** (helps with general muscle aches and pains)

   Epsom Salt - 2 cups
   Baking Soda - 1 cup
   Hydrogen Peroxide- ⅓ cup

Fill tub with hot water and add the above ingredients. Soak for 20 to 30 minutes. You will sweat in the tub and lose toxins (which causes you to lose some water as well). It is important to drink plenty of water while you soak. Some people like to add fresh lemon juice to their drinking water. If you have a tendency to get light headed easily, be cautious when getting out of the tub, or have someone nearby the first time you take a detox bath. Take a lukewarm to cool shower after getting out of the tub to rinse off the salts or you may itch. Rest for 30 minutes after the bath.

Dr. Mnabhi's patients love it. She has seen one or two instances of nausea, vomiting and diarrhea after the bath. In these cases, the patient felt much better the next day.

3. There are two excellent products that can be used intermittently to eliminate toxins. These are the Whole Body Cleanse® and Metal Magnet® (see Appendix C: Resources). Simply follow the labeled instructions.

## *A Simple Way to Determine What You Need from the First Five Chapters*

I know that analyzing your medical history and lab results to determine all of the different nutritional, hormonal, sleep, or infectious problems that can be driving your pain can be complex. Because of this, I have created a sophisticated computerized educational program on my website (www.Vitality101.com) that can analyze your medical history (and laboratory test results, if available) to determine the most important underlying metabolic problems in your case. It will create a treatment protocol tailored to your case that you can institute on your own and will assist and support your doctor in giving you the best possible care. The "long form" can also create a complete medical record of your case for your physician. ■

**Important Points**

1. Chronic pain may be associated with disordered immune function, which opens the door to repeated infections, repeated treatment with antibiotics, and yeast overgrowth. Suspect yeast overgrowth if you have chronic sinusitis/nasal congestion or spastic colon. Even hidden infections can often cause pain.
2. Treat yeast overgrowth by avoiding antibiotics and sweets. Many patients have found nystatin and other anti-fungal medications, such as Diflucan® and Sporanox®, to be helpful. Acidophilus (milk bacteria) Pearls and natural anti-fungals such as Phytostan® are also often useful.
3. Check for parasites if bowel symptoms persist after anti-fungal treatment. However, most laboratories do not adequately detect parasites through stool testing. To get an accurate test result, use a laboratory that specializes in stool testing. (See Appendix C: Resources).
4. Prevent parasitic infection by filtering your water with an effective filtration unit. I recommend the Multi-Pure filter (See Appendix C: Resources).
5. If you have body temperatures over 98.6°F and/or chronic lung congestion, if your symptoms improved (even temporarily) in the past while taking an antibiotic, or if you have rheumatoid arthritis try long-term treatment with Cipro® or doxycycline. Take Nystatin® while on the antibiotic to prevent yeast overgrowth.
6. Pain caused by inflammation can be modified using nutrients and hormones that suppress inflammation, anti-inflammatory medications, or treating the underlying cause of the inflammation (see Chapter 11).

**CHAPTER 6**

# *Body Work, Structural Issues, and Trauma*

*Bren Jacobson, a gifted Rolfer, writes this chapter about body work and ergonomics. He practices in Annapolis Maryland, and I send people to him if I can't get rid of their pain.*

## Body Work, Ergonomics, and Stress Reduction

**by Bren Jacobson**

### Body Work

The term "body work" generally refers to various types of massage and therapies performed on one's body. I will use it in a much broader sense, which will include anything that affects and improves the body. This embraces exercises and various therapies.

Most pain is part of a cycle that originates with stress. This stress can be physical, emotional, psychological, or spiritual or any combination of these. Any kind of stress causes muscle tension and stiffness. This ultimately leads to permanent muscle tightness and eventually to immobility. This state of chronic contraction of the muscles and connective tissue leads to reduced blood flow and oxygenation, along with an inability to get rid of toxic waste products. All of these factors put strain on the body and cause it to constantly work harder with less efficiency. This causes pain that interferes with sound, deep sleep. A lack of sleep lowers one's stress threshold and this can become a downward spiral with pain levels increasing exponentially.

To reverse this cycle of stress, muscle tightness, pain, loss of sleep and further stress, it is good to interrupt the cycle in as many places as possible. I have found that prayer, meditation, counseling, lifestyle coaching, exercise, love making, and doing those activities that one enjoys are all effective ways of reducing stress. Poor sleep can be counteracted by herbs, medicine, hot baths, soothing music, a glass of wine or warm milk. Muscle tightness as well as stress and pain can all be dealt with and alleviated with body work, stretching, exercise, and all the other suggestions presented in this book.

Here are a few general suggestions that apply to all forms of body work:

1. If you try any form of body work and find that you feel worse after a fair trial, or it causes you continuing discomfort, or you simply don't like it, stop and find something you enjoy more and you feel helps your situation. By a fair trial I mean that if after one yoga lesson you feel sore and stiff the next day, you don't give up. Try it regularly, more slowly, for shorter periods of time and more gently for a month and then if you don't feel that it is helping, stop it and try something else.
2. Always start gradually. Don't start with three or four hours of exercise a day. Twenty minutes of yoga every day is better than five hours on the weekend. A daily walk around the block is better than running a marathon once a year. Do only what feels good and do it only as long as it is enjoyable.
3. To find a good therapist or teacher, ask friends for references, check the person's credentials, and talk to the person to see if you are compatible.
4. If you have any sort of medical condition, check with your doctor to see if the type of body work you are considering is appropriate and has no potential to do harm.
5. Always listen to the messages that your body and intuition give you. Try to pay more attention to what your body is telling you. You live in your body and have a very intimate knowledge of what is good or bad for it. People often get into trouble when they ignore what their bodies are trying to tell them. When one doesn't listen to one's body, it often gives louder, more insistent and harder to ignore messages in the form of pain or disabilities that prevent one from doing damage (like a fuse blowing to prevent a fire in an electrical system). The Chinese have a saying which is applicable, "A stumble very often prevents a fall."
6. Never push yourself, never show off, and never, never compete with anyone while exercising. If you are in a yoga class and the person on the mat next to you is doing a forward bend with her hands flat on the floor and her head touching her knees, and you can barely

touch your toes, it doesn't matter at all. The purpose of the exercise is not to touch the floor or your toes but to stretch the muscles of your back and forcing yourself can cause severe injury.

7. Forget the adage "no pain, no gain." It has no truth and often causes painful injuries. "Slow, gradual, and comfortable" is a much better and safer approach.
8. Always warm up with slow gentle movements and stretches before leaping into any form of exercise. This is one of the best ways to avoid injury. It is equally important to cool down the same way after exercise. Some form of complete relaxation is a good way to end your workout.
9. Any natural activity that uses your entire body, does not involve extreme exertion, does not involve high impact, and which is fun is probably good for you. Some examples of this are walking (one of the best, easiest, cheapest, and most readily available activities for almost everyone), swimming, dancing, making love, gardening, and bicycling. It is a good practice to alternate these activities so as to achieve a good balance in your body. Some of the activities that I have found to cause pain and injury are lifting heavy weights, running, and ballet. Running often causes lower back pain, disc compression and damage (the impact on the spine when running is three times the body weight), stress fractures, torn ligaments, and knee damage (knees incur five times the amount of force when running than they do when walking). I have worked with numerous ballet dancers and weight lifters and have seen many who are totally disabled and many who are in constant, unbearable, and intractable pain.

Because of limited space, I will simply give a basic overview of a few types of body work. More in depth information on these healing modalities is readily available on the internet and I will recommend some books as I go. What I can assure you is that all of these techniques can be effective in relieving pain. If you have trouble deciding which form of body work is most likely to help you, I am available as a consultant to help you choose (phone 410-224-4877).

The most complete and time-tested system of exercise is yoga. It combines balance, stretching, resistance, breathing, and focus. Today, yoga has gone from being an esoteric spiritual practice to being commonplace. There are many different types of yoga being taught today and most of them have benefit. I feel that a good type of yoga for anyone starting out is a gentle form of Hatha yoga. Sivananda yoga, a popular and comprehensive form of Hatha yoga, is described in Swami Vishnu Devananda's *Complete Illustrated Book of Yoga* and in *The Sivananda Companion to Yoga*. The Sivananda organization has centers throughout the world that give classes, train teachers, and offer yoga "vacations" and retreats. More information can be found online at www.Sivananda.org. The advanced student can go on to try Bikram yoga, Iyengar yoga (explained in the book, *Light on Yoga*), Astanga yoga, Kundalini yoga and Anusara yoga. Ideally, the student will not just use yoga as a series of exercises, but will also become acquainted with the yoga diet, philosophy, lifestyle, breathing exercises, and meditation. All of these comprise a system that is extremely effective in relieving, as well as preventing, pain. It is possible to begin practicing yoga from a book, but it is much better to start by taking a class from a certified teacher. It is important to begin gently, never compete, never force a posture to the point of pain, and to do all of the exercises mindfully. Done properly, yoga will be enjoyable.

In yoga as well as all forms of exercise, correct breathing is of the utmost importance. Breath is a link between the mind and body. When the body is in pain, or the mind is frightened, breathing is short, rapid, and irregular. If a person is relaxed and in a state of enjoyment, breathing is long, slow, deep, and regular. It is possible to change one's state of being by simply focusing on and changing one's breathing. Practitioners of Zazen, one of the most effective forms of meditation, as well as Vipassena meditation use this concentration on their breath as a major part of their practice. A powerful way of dealing with pain is to visualize the breath as a colored healing stream of energy and to concentrate on directing the breath to the part of the body where the pain is. Imagine the healing energy of the breath dissolving the pain and carrying it out of the body with each exhalation.

Another breathing practice that can be useful and which is an essential part of a complete yoga practice is called Pranayama. This consists of a series of powerful breathing exercises that arouse and control the flow of energy in the body. In any exercise it is important when bending forward to exhale and to inhale when bending backward. It is also good to coordinate the breath with the motion so that when you begin to bend forward, you begin to exhale, ending the exhalation when you reach the limit of your forward bend.

Another wonderful system of body work is Tai Chi Chuan. It is, all at the same time, an exercise, a dance, a moving meditation, a system of energy generation and regulation, breath control, and a martial art. It was developed over thousands of years by Chinese monks and is practiced throughout China by millions of people. It consists of a series of many "hands" or postures and movements linked together in a very slow, harmonious and graceful dance. Today there are numerous books and video tapes that offer to teach various forms of Tai Chi, but it is very difficult to learn it that way. My advice is to join a class that proceeds slowly and rigorously. For health and pain relief purposes, it is better to avoid schools that teach Tai Chi as a martial art.

Similar to Tai Chi is another Chinese practice called Chi Gong. This is a type of healing that can be performed by a practitioner and is also a system of exercise, similar to Tai Chi with more emphasis on healing and controlling the flow of energy in the body. An excellent introduction to its philosophy, history, and practice can be found in books by Ken Cohen.

Pilates is a system of body work that is enjoying increasing popularity in the U.S. It complements the other systems of body work that I have mentioned and is taught in many gyms and spas. It is somewhat vigorous and should be done by someone who is already in a fairly healthy state. As with other forms of body work, it is of the utmost importance to work with a properly rained and experienced teacher.

There are various other forms of body work that focus on proper and efficient ways to move and use one's body. These include Feldenkrais work, the Alexander technique, Rolf movement work, Trager Mentastics, and Aston patterning.

Some types of body work performed by a practitioner focus primarily on the physical body and others concentrate on the body's energy system. In all cases, however, there is an overlap. For example, acupuncture is primarily a way of enhancing the proper flow of energy in the body, but it also affects physical change. Likewise, Structural Integration/ Rolfing, which works only on the physical body, always affects the energy system. Furthermore, anything that changes the body physically not only changes a person's structure and physiology, but also changes the person emotionally and psychologically. We are all familiar with the expression "psychosomatic." The reverse phenomenon of physical improvement causing a corresponding psychological improvement, i.e. "somatopsychic" is not as universally recognized. An analogy I use to illustrate this phenomenon is that the body and the mind are like the back and the palm of the hand. Both are separate, distinct, different, and distinguishable, but it is impossible to move or in any way change one without a corresponding change in the other. In other words, they are inextricably linked.

Before discussing various types of body work and massage, I would like to give a few cautionary notes. Anyone with open sores, an infectious disease, severe psychological imbalance, a fracture or other serious injury, an acute illness, or a pain or other symptom that is increasing in frequency or severity should see a physician before trying any of the following therapies. If you have acute appendicitis or hepatitis, for example, an acupuncturist, chiropractor, or reflexologist would not be the appropriate therapist to go to.

Over a period of 35 years I have studied and practiced many forms of body work worldwide and I now work with my own fusion of all of them. If, however, I were to be asked which single form of body work I find most profoundly effective in relieving pain as well as enhancing well being and vitality, I would recommend Structural Integration This is a holistic system of balancing and integrating the body that was developed by Dr. Ida P. Rolf and which was has been called Rolfing by many of its practitioners to honor her. It is also known in its other incarnations or variations as Heller work and Aston work.

I had the great honor of studying advanced Rolfing with Dr. Rolf and have practiced it for over 30 years. I find it to be the most holistic, long lasting, and transformative form of body work available. An excellent source of information about structural integration is available online at www.Rolfguild.org. Excellent books on the subject are available Two of the best are *Rolfing: Reestablishing the Natural Alignment and Structural Integration of the Human Body for Vitality and Well-Being* and *Rolfing and Physical Reality*, both by Dr. Rolf.

Structural Integration involves ten sessions of work with most of the work being done with connective tissue to straighten and balance the body so that it gets support from gravity, rather than being torn down by it. The results that most people get are reduced pain, more energy, better posture, less anxiety, as well as easier, more efficient, and more graceful movement. A fairly common remark by people who have had this work done is that they feel more comfortable in their own skin. Because so much pain and dysfunction is caused by imbalance and structural problems, such as one leg being shorter than the other, uneven hip heights, the head being forward, the pelvis tilted or the shoulders rotated, this is an extremely effective approach for alleviating these problems and the pain caused by them.

A broad category of body work involves hands on manipulation generally referred to as massage. It is one of the oldest forms of healing and has been used from time immemorial. Today there are scores of different schools of massage and one of the best introductions to the various types is the book *Hands on Healing*.

One wide group of massage techniques uses stroking, friction, kneading, and vibration. This relaxes muscles and increases blood and lymph flow, while increasing oxygenation of the tissues of the body. This type of work generally relieves muscular tension and leaves the person feeling relaxed and energized at the same time. This category includes Swedish massage, sports massage, Esalen massage, Tuina (a type of Chinese massage), and lymphatic drainage massage.

Other forms of body work focus on regulating and directing the flow of energy in the body. These include acupuncture, reflexology, Shiatsu, acupressure point massage, polarity work, do-in, and applied kinesiology. Thai massage is explained well in the book *Thai Massage – Sacred Body Work* by Ananda Apfelbaum.

Various types of body work mobilize joints and release muscles, while straightening and balancing the spine. These include chiropractic work, osteopathy, Trager, and cranial-sacral work. The latter two are both very gentle and powerful.

Any and all of these systems and techniques will help to relieve pain but obviously no person has the time, money, or energy to do them all. Nor are all types of work suited to all people. It is best to talk to other people and health practitioners as well as read more about these healing modalities and then try one. If it helps, keep doing it and if not, try another.

Never get discouraged. Each type of body work will help in some way and each will teach you something about yourself.

I would like to note that many of the things I have mentioned are synergistic. This means that they work together and enhance each other so that the total effect is greater than each done separately. In other words the total effect is greater than the sum of the parts. A combination that I have found to be particularly effective is yoga, structural integration, meditation, and Tai Chi.

## Ergonomics

Ergonomics refers to the science of engineering, adapting, and designing machines, tools, and furniture to suit people and increase efficiency. I will use the term here in its broader sense to include the ways in which individuals adapt themselves to their environment and work.

Even very subtle imbalances in our bodies or in the way we use them can cause severe pain. Dr. Rolf taught that the connective tissue in the body forms a continuous web so that any injury, strain, or inflammation was instantly and lastingly communicated to the entire body. She often used the analogy of trying to straighten out a wrinkled bed sheet; as soon as one tugs on one corner of the sheet to get rid of a crease, it causes another crease somewhere else.

A more practical example of this principle is illustrated in what happens to a woman's body when she wears high-heeled shoes. The most energy efficient and comfortable way to stand is vertically. When high-heeled shoes are worn, the woman's weight is shifted forward to a fairly small area on the ball of the foot. To make matters worse, the toes are jammed into the front of the shoe, causing bunions that are both painful and unattractive. In addition, there is excess tension in the ankle which causes immobility in the joint. Because of the elevation of the heel, the calf muscle and Achilles tendon shorten causing increased stress on the knee. With the weight and therefore the pelvis being shifted forward, the shoulders come back and the head goes forward to compensate. The pelvis also tilts forward creating a lordosis (sway back) and causing the abdomen to protrude—making the person look many pounds heavier than she actually is. The long-term effects of simply elevating the heels a few inches are almost invariably lower back, upper back, and neck pain as these are the parts of the body that have to constantly do extra work to compensate for the imbalance created by the shoes. A whole constellation of secondary pains and other symptoms can arise from this apparently simple cause, including headaches, knee pain, imbalance and pain in the jaw, poor digestion, and fatigue. The feet are the only interface that we have with the earth. They are, in other words, our sole foundation and the support for the entire body. If we do not have proper weight distribution, flexibility, contact, and support from our feet, our entire body will suffer. We will become "ungrounded."

As an interesting example of synchronicity, just after finishing this paragraph I stopped writing to read the *New York Times*' science section and came across the article "In the Relentless Pursuit of Fashion, the Feet Pay the Price." The article quoted the president of the Podiatric Medical Association as saying, "the current trend in fashion is very bad for woman's feet." He and other medical experts said that poorly designed and fitting shoes that included not only high heels, but flip-flops, some running shoes, and platform shoes cause the problems that I have already mentioned as well as causing nerve damage. These shoes make the wearer more prone to accidents and ankle sprains. They upset the stabilizing mechanics of the foot, contributing to arthritis, inhibiting range of motion, causing lose of toe strength, causing shin splints and foot deformities such as bunions and hammer toes as well as plantar fascial tears and fasciitis (pain along the soles of the feet).

Another example of an ergonomic problem is that of a man who came to see me in Holland. For over 12 years he had suffered extreme and constant pain in his neck, shoulders, and between his shoulder blades, as well as unbearable migraine headaches. He had gone to over 40 healers, including neurologists and surgeons and shamans and hypnotists. No one had helped him. As I took his history, I asked what kind of work he did. He replied that he played cello for the Amsterdam Concertebau Orchestra and he practiced four to six hours a day. I then asked him to pretend that he was playing his cello so that I could see how he was using his body. When he did this, I observed that he bent forward at the waist, hunched his shoulders and brought his head forward. All of this was obviously the cause of his problems and I asked him why he didn't sit erect. He replied that the cello was low and he was tall and hence he had always played hunched over. I suggested that he was intelligent enough to figure out a way to raise the cello. As it turned out there is a peg under the cello that adjusts its height. He went home and adjusted the height of his cello. He called me a week later and said that by simply sitting erect while playing, his pain had gone from being tortuous to only a mild annoyance, his headaches had disappeared and that his teacher had remarked that his playing was much improved (because he was no longer "wrapped" around the instrument and because he had more freedom in his arms and shoulders).

I could go on with endless examples of people that I have worked with who have suffered years of torment because of a poorly placed computer monitor, a piece of furniture that didn't suit them, an activity that they performed in the wrong way, or they tried to do a job with an inappropriate or poorly designed tool; but I would rather suggest the following guidelines to help you avoid these problems:

1. Keep a daily journal. Rate whatever pain or discomfort you have on a scale of one to ten, with one being no pain and ten being excruciating pain. This can be done at any time of the day but the end of the day is a good time and it is preferable to do it at the same time each day if possible. On any day that your pain level is low (one to three) or high (seven to 10) try to figure out, examine, and record any variables that might make that day different from others. Some things you might consider are:

   A. Is it a work day or a holiday? Do you have a new job, different work, or increased responsibilities?

   B. Are you on vacation or just returning from one?

   C. Have you been doing a different activity than usual or are you doing a normal activity in a different way or with a different tool?

   D. What have your interpersonal relationships been like that day?

   E. Have you been using a different piece of furniture than usual? It is particularly important if you have pain, to notice if you are better or worse when sleeping away from home on a different bed.

   F. What types of stress have you been subjected to that day? Are any of them new or different? If you have encountered your usual stresses, have you reacted to, or dealt with them any differently?

G. Is the weather (barometric pressure, temperature, wind, or humidity) particularly different?

H. Has your diet changed in either type of food, quantity, or quality?

I. Has anything in your work or home environment changed? This could be anything from more noise to new furniture, lighting, carpeting, or paint.

J. Are you using a different car, bike, golf clubs, tennis racket, telephone, shoes, etc?

When you are able to identify any variable that affects your level of pain, vitality, wellness, and sense of well-being, avoid it, change it, or do more of it as is appropriate.

You may be think that the above points are obvious and not worth wasting time with, but I can assure you that this is not the case. I have counseled thousands of people and could tell hundreds of stories like the one above about the Dutch cellist who relieved years of pain by playing detective and finding the factors that caused his pain. It is particularly important to keep a written journal on a daily basis, because on the days that the pain is severe it can be so distracting that you wouldn't think of trying to track down the causative factors of your pain. On days when you feel good, it is common to forget that you ever had pain and you don't want to expend the energy to think about it.

2. Vary your work and play and the way you do it. One of my teachers said that "the best vacation is a change of work." There is much truth in the saying. Instead of spending a whole day cleaning the house and another day gardening and yet another day doing paperwork, it is far preferable to spend a shorter time doing each and then switching. This enables you to not only use different muscle groups, but different mind functions. It also creates a relaxing change of pace as well as preventing ennui. Equally important is to intersperse work periods with time spent in play, relaxation, exercise, entertainment, and meditation or reverie. One of the most invigorating and healing practices is a 20-minute afternoon siesta or nap. Not everyone has the luxury to indulge in this, but even having lunch in a park or quiet place instead of a busy restaurant can be beneficial.

3. At the risk of sounding repetitive I will say that one of the most important things you can do is to listen to your body. I am not referring to the various noises emanating from it (although doing so can reveal such conditions as lactose intolerance), what I mean is that

people need to be more aware of what is happening in their bodies. Our bodies communicate with us through aches, pains, pleasures, resistances to certain activities, or reactions to different conditions. The body has its own wisdom and very often, even though it doesn't have warning lights like your car, it will through various means attempt to communicate with you its owner. To expand this car analogy, if you race your engine constantly or subjecting it to long periods of disuse, use the wrong fuel, ignore regular checks, tune ups and services, and preventative maintenance—you will eventually encounter a breakdown. If this seems a silly analogy, consider that many of the people that I work with routinely checked their car's tire pressure but have never had their blood pressure checked. Others wouldn't think of using low-test gasoline but regularly eat junk food. Still others never go more than six months without having their automobile serviced but haven't had a physical checkup in years.

I have learned over the years that when the body gives a subtle hint or message that is ignored by its owner, it will continue to give the same message in a different way or at increased volume. If it is still ignored it will continuously try to make its message clear. If the person still does not pay attention, it will try to make it impossible for the person to persist in the activity that may be endangering him. One example is the person who is overexerting himself on a constant basis. The body's first message might be lethargy, discomfort or mild digestive upset. When that person ignores these conditions and continues to work too long, too hard, or too constantly, the pain, tiredness, and indigestion will most certainly grow worse. If these indications are ignored, the body in its wisdom realizes that the path that the person is persisting on may lead to severe repercussions such as a nervous breakdown, loss of job or relationship, or even a life threatening occurrence such as a heart attack. At that point the body puts into play some form of circuit breaker that forces the person to stop what they are doing. This can take the form of headaches, back pain, chronic fatigue, fibromyalgia, or irritable bowel syndrome, etc. It is much better to heed the early warning signals we get from our bodies and moderate our behavior, than it is to deal with these more serious conditions.

You are your body, and if you pay close attention to that part of yourself you will often be able to become aware of problems long before a diagnostic test, x-ray, or doctor's exam will. This doesn't mean that you should not talk to your doctor about your concerns. As many spiritual traditions have held, the body is the temple of the soul. It should never be disregarded and anyone who does, does so at their own risk.

4. Use you body and enjoy it. The same goes for your mind and spirit. Don't become a couch potato. One of the best ways to stay healthy and young is to constantly try new activities, meet new people, explore new places, try new foods, keep in touch with old friends and family, read new books, and be of service to those who are less fortunate or capable than you. **Use it or lose it**. I would not be so presumptuous as to believe that I know what the true meaning of life is, or what the ideal way to live is, but I am absolutely sure that it is not about doing as little as possible while accumulating as much as possible. I am sure that service, knowledge, home, family, friends, community, and relationships in general are much more important than most other things that people strive for. They are also more healing and bring more happiness. Many spend their lives striving for wealth, thinking that money will bring happiness. True wealth, however, is not getting what you want but wanting what you have.

   After 35 years as a healer I can say with great conviction that the four best medicines for pain are laughter, sleep, tears, and loving, although not necessarily in that order. They also are necessary to create true health, wholeness, and happiness.

5. If doing any activity causes pain or strain, and you must do it or can't find someone to do it for you, find a better way to do it. Today there are many devices that make various activities—from opening a bottle to digging in the garden—easier. These devices can be found in various catalogues or on the internet. For example, I found (in the Museum of Modern Art gift shop, of all places) a short handle that could be attached to the longer handle of a shovel. When digging this device enables me to pull up on the shovel handle instead of lifting. This gives me a great mechanical advantage and reduces my effort by half. Sometimes a little bit of ingenuity goes a long way. Very often by using a lever, wedge, or pulley, you can reduce the effort necessary to do a job to a fraction of what it might have been. When lifting, keep your back straight and your feet apart to give yourself a broad stable foundation. When lifting things, turn your entire body, using your legs rather than twisting your spine. If you can push or pull or slide instead of lifting, do that. If you can put something under the object to be moved to reduce friction, do so. It will then require a small fraction of the work necessary to move the thing.

6. Remember the adage that "one man's meat is another's poison." There is not any one shoe, mattress, diet, therapy, exercise program, climate, job, or lifestyle that is perfect or even right for every-

one. I remember a man that I worked with in Spain. He suffered severe burning and pain on getting up in the morning. I suspected a bad mattress and suggested to him that this might be the source of his problem. He was positive the mattress could not possibly be the problem because it had cost $6,000 dollars, been designed by Germany's most famous orthopedic surgeon and had been prescribed by Spain's top back specialist. He even brought me to his home to examine it and try it out. I laid down on it and it was a very comfortable, supportive, firm mattress and I had to agree with him that it was probably not the cause of his pain. He got rolfed, which was beneficial for his general well being and his back, but he still had the burning sensation when he woke up. He later tried chiropractic, acupuncture, Mezier work, and physical therapy with the same results. I ran into him a year and a half later and he told me that the burning sensation had disappeared. I immediately thought that the rolfing, which usually takes a full year after the work is finished to manifest its full benefit, had finally done the trick. He told me that what had really made the most difference was going to a hotel that had cheap, soft, sagging mattresses, which evidently suited him better then the super expensive one that he had imported from Germany.

Always buy for comfort, adjustability, and functionality rather than cost, an expert's opinion, a brand name, appearance, or fashion. Much of the furniture that is available today is over-stuffed and too soft to give proper support or it is of an extreme shape that would look good in an art museum but is not suited to the human body. Very often the best chair is a simple old fashioned straight-backed chair. Instead of buying the fanciest sports car, buy one that you can drive without getting back pain. A simple rule of thumb is to "try before you buy" (or be sure that you can take it back if it turns out to be unsuitable). If you are buying a car, try renting that model first and drive five hundred miles, and see how your back feels at the end of the trip. If you are buying an office chair that you might spend 20 percent of the rest of your life in, go to the store and sit in every chair until you find the one that is most comfortable. Sit in that one for an hour and read a magazine and see how you feel at the end of that period. Shoes, which I have already spoken of at length, can cause more problems than any other item that people use. They should always be chosen for comfort before any other consideration.

Another good general rule is to buy the item that is the most adjustable and customizable. If you buy a computer desk, for instance, buy one where the height of the monitor and the keyboard can be adjusted independently. With the office chair, look for one that can be adjusted for the height of the seat, the height of the arms, the height and amount of lumbar support, and the amount of tilt as well as the force needed to change the tilt. Likewise, the more separate adjustments an automobile seat has, the easier it is to make it comfortable for your body. The more customizable anything is, the easier it is to get it to work efficiently with your body.

7. Try to bilaterally balance physical activities. For example, if you are carrying something like a shopping bag, switch hands frequently (the tendency is always to use your dominant or strong side, which increases imbalance), divide the load into two bags, use a back pack, or, ideally, use a wheeled cart. One of the most common problems that I see is neck and back pain caused by office workers holding their telephone headset with their shoulder while at the same time using a keyboard. This is very easily dealt with by getting a head set from a store like Radio Shack, Best Buy, or Circuit City. Almost all cordless and cellular phones have jacks for a headset, and Radio Shack has phones with headsets that can be plugged into the wall. Another solution is using a speaker phone, and G.E. makes one with good sound quality that I bought for $12.

## Stress Reduction

### *The Benefits of Meditation*

I mentioned meditation several times and want to be more specific about what I mean by this. Many associate meditation with someone who shaves his or her head, and bangs a tambourine in an airport or someone who sits in a cave contemplating his naval. The truth is that every religious and spiritual tradition worldwide advocates and uses some form of meditation. There are also many individuals with no religious or spiritual aspirations who meditate for reasons that are as varied as lowering their blood pressure to improving their golf game.

What I mean by meditation is "one-pointed, focused, mindfulness and awareness." This can be visual concentration on a candle flame or religious icon or an auditory input, such as wholeheartedly listening to a Gregorian chant or the waves on a beach. Some people find that verbal or silent repetition of a mantra is most effective. Other people find the repetition of a word helpful, which is talked about in Benson's book *The Relaxation Response*. Others recite the rosary or a phrase like "Om," or they repeat their name over and over as did Alfred Lord Tennyson. Mindful meditation can involve a kinesthetic experience such as walking or doing an everyday task such as gardening or washing dishes with full attention and awareness. The secret is to "do one thing." In other words when you are washing dishes, focus only on doing the dishes. Be aware of the sound of the water, the feel of the dishes, the way your body works to accomplish the task, the smell of the soap, and the appearance of the soap bubbles. If your back becomes tired, be aware of that in an observant rather than a judgmental way. When you are doing the dishes think "I am doing the dishes." Try not to let the usual useless mind chatter take over, such as, "boy, I wish I didn't have to do the dishes; I wonder what's on television; I wish I had said such and such to so and so earlier today; wouldn't it be great if I had a dishwasher; maybe I should use paper plates." If these thoughts intrude, just let them go without judging yourself and get back to "washing the dishes."

Observing, concentrating, and "becoming one" with one's breathing are all part of another form of meditation. One of the best practical manuals for this form of meditation, called Zazen, is Phillip Kapleau's *Three Pillars of Zen*. Another very good introduction to meditation is *Mindfulness Meditation: Cultivating the Wisdom of Your Body and Mind* by Jon Kabat Zinn.

## *The Benefits of Sex*

Last, but not least, I have several times alluded to the benefits of sex. I would like to expand on what I mean by this. To begin with, I am talking about more than a simple orgasmic release. I am speaking about all forms of physical give and take in a loving relationship. This can range from wild sex to a simple foot massage. There have been an increasing number of studies from such conservative bastions as Johns Hopkins and Dartmouth as to the physical and emotional health benefits of this kind of relationship and its ability to maintain well-being and reduce pain. Part of this has to do with the release of neurotransmitters such as endorphins and oxytocin, but the cardiovascular benefits, not to mention the pleasure derived cause a cascade of health promoting effects from better sleep to improved immune function. There is even proof that frequent sex increases growth hormone levels, resulting in less pain, weight loss, and a more youthful appearance, and even an increase in life expectancy!

*Reverend Bren Jacobson has spent the last 35 years studying and practicing healing around the world. He offers advanced Rolfing, pastoral counseling, life style coaching, and ergonomic consulting (by phone at 410-224-4877). He also consults on water purification options. He has been the Director of the Buffalo Meditation and Philosophy Center, the Berkley Center for Health Maintenance Practices, and the Annapolis Rolfing and Health Center. He has worked, taught courses, counseled and led groups at*

*Esalen Institute, The Human Dimensions Institute, the Amherst Counseling Center, The Stichting Center in Amsterdam, the Buffalo Suicide Prevention Center, the Ardennes's Health Center in Belgium, the Amethyst Center in Dublin, as well as clinics in Brazil, Venezuela, England, Spain, France, Germany, and Sweden. He owes a debt of gratitude to a large number of teachers who are too numerous to mention.*

## A Brief Note On Trauma

Trauma can also cause pain by many mechanisms. Initially it can cause inflammation or direct tissue injury. If bleeding occurred into the area, the iron in the blood can actually continually trigger inflammation (iron is "pro oxidative"). This ongoing inflammation can be shut down by using antioxidants. Nutritional and sleep remedies also support the healing of injuries. Often, an injured muscle can get stuck in a shortened position, causing years or decades of pain.

Using some simple techniques (e.g. stretch and spray), the shortened muscles can often be released in a matter of seconds or minutes—often with instantaneous relief of what had been chronic pain. Sometimes this is all that is needed for permanent pain relief. Other times, the muscle again contracts to the shortened position, causing pain. This problem often responds beautifully to nutritional, sleep, and hormonal support, and to eliminating underlying infections as we have discussed in this book. It is also important to treat the structural abnormalities. ■

# Section 3

## *Types of Pain*

In this next section I discuss the common types of pain, their causes, how to recognize and evaluate them and how to treat them. Section 4 will teach you how to evaluate and treat pain based on its location.

CHAPTER 7

# The Biochemistry of Pain

New research suggests that pain affects men and women differently. This likely occurs in part because of hormonal differences related to estrogen and testosterone. For example, male animals injected with estrogen appear to have a lower pain threshold while giving testosterone to female animals increases pain tolerance. How pain is transmitted in our bodies also contributes to the differences in how pain is felt by men and women. Both sexes have a natural ability to suppress pain but the mechanisms are different. For example, a pain receptor called kappa-opioid is more active in women. Because of this, some medications such as Stadol® are more effective in females.

Societal factors may also play a role. Women are quicker to seek medical help and less likely to allow pain to control their lives. They are also more likely to ask for help from their friends.

A person's age also plays a role in pain. One out of five older Americans takes a painkiller on a regular basis. Because they are prone to medications' side effects, such as bleeding ulcers from NSAIDs, finding alternative and safer remedies is especially helpful for older patients.[1]

The biochemistry and anatomy of pain is fairly complex, and it is not necessary that you understand these to use the information in this book. For those of you who are "science phobic," feel free to skip this section.

When following pain pathways, it is good to start with the skin. Receptors on the skin trigger a series of electrical impulses that go to the spinal cord. Signals may be ignored, amplified, or changed in other ways before being sent to the brain. The back of the spine (called the dorsal horn) is important for receiving sensation and pain signals. In order to send the pain signal, the nerve cells have gate-like passages called "channels" that allow them to transmit the information. Blocking these channels allows us to also decrease pain.

Once the pain signal is sent from the spine to the brain it often goes to the thalamus and then to the cortex where it is interpreted as thought. This transmission process requires many chemicals called neurotransmitters, which transmit nerve impulses from one nerve cell to another via receptors specific for that neurotransmitter/chemical.

Some neurotransmitters/receptors seem to increase pain transmission. These include glutamate, NMDA, and substance P (for pain). Others, such as opiate/opioid receptors, turn on pain inhibiting circuits, decreasing pain. Neurotransmitters that appear to act as natural painkillers in the body include serotonin, norepinephrine, opioid-like chemicals, and endorphins. Endorphins are the natural painkillers that are released during jogging, resulting in a "runners high." Disturbingly, nicotine may also affect endorphins, and a chemical (from an Ecuadorian frog) that resembles nicotine is highly toxic but a powerful analgesic (working on acetylcholine receptors). This raises the possibility that some people who are addicted to cigarettes may be self-anesthetizing themselves for pain. Although I've seen no studies done on this, and have not tried it in my practice out of concern over its addictiveness and health risks, it is possible that nicotine patches might also decrease pain.

Once we travel outside of the brain and nervous system, other hormones, which affect pain can be modified. For example, prostaglandins simulate nerves at the site of injury resulting in inflammation. Medications such as NSAIDs (e.g. Motrin®) and COX (Cyclooxygenase®) 2 inhibitors such as Celebrex® work by blocking the enzyme required to produce prostaglandin. Unfortunately, doing so also blocks the beneficial effects of prostaglandins (such as preventing stomach ulcers). Other chemicals used by the immune system called cytokines can also trigger inflammation. This allows another avenue to help decrease pain. ■

**Important Points**

1. New research suggests that pain affects men and women differently. This likely occurs in part because of hormonal differences related to estrogen and testosterone.
2. A person's age also plays a role in pain. One out of five older Americans takes a painkiller on a regular basis.
3. Some neurotransmitters/receptors seem to increase pain transmission. These include glutamate, NMDA, and substance P (for pain). Others, such as opiate/opioid receptors, turn on pain inhibiting circuits, decreasing pain. Neurotransmitters that appear to act as natural painkillers in the body include serotonin, norepinephrine, opioid-like chemicals, and endorphins.

# Chapter 8 Neuropathic (Nerve) Pain and Reflex Sympathetic Dystrophy (RSD)

The term "neuropathic pain," or nerve pain, refers to a wide range of problems that cause diseases of, or injury to, the nervous system. It is a category of pain syndromes and not a single problem. Neuropathic pain can come from malfunction of nerves or the brain associated with illness (e.g. diabetes, low thyroid, etc.), infections (e.g. shingles), pinched nerves, nutritional deficiencies (e.g. vitamin B6 and B12), injury (e.g. stroke, tumors, spinal cord injury, and multiple sclerosis), and medication/treatment side effects (e.g. radiation and chemotherapy, AIDS drugs, Flagyl®). It is estimated that 50 to 80 percent of diabetics will develop some nerve injury with 30 to 40 percent of these having painful diabetic neuropathy unless preventive measures are taken such as nutritional support. Neuropathic pain affects approximately 0.6 to 1.5 percent of the U.S. population and 25 to 40 percent of cancer patients.[1] This represents over two million Americans.

Neuropathies are characterized by pain that is burning, shooting (often to distant areas), or stabbing. It also has an "electric" quality about it. "Tingling or numbness" (paresthesias) and increased sensitivity with normal touch being painful (allodynia) are also commonly seen. Ongoing pain is often continually present regardless of what the patient does or does not do. In some cases, pain comes in sudden attacks without any apparent trigger. Diagnosis is made predominantly by history and physical examination, as testing often offers little benefit clinically unless the testing is looking for a treatable cause.

As with other pain problems, neuropathies are both expensive and poorly-treated. In one study of 55,686 patients with neuropathic pain, health care charges were three-fold higher than they were in the overall population ($17,355 vs. $5,715 per year, respectively). Use of relatively ineffective therapies such as NSAIDs (e.g. Motrin®) and opioids was widespread, while relatively few received anti-epileptic drugs, tricyclic anti-depressants, or any of the many other medications that are often much more effective in relieving neuropathic pain.[2]

In the presence of nerve pain, it is especially important to look for treatable causes. Lab testing should include:

1. A blood count (CBC) and an inflammation/sedimentation rate (ESR)
2. Thyroid testing with a Free T4 and TSH
3. Vitamin B12 level
4. Screening for diabetes with a morning fasting blood sugar and a glycosylated hemoglobin (HgBA1C)

The medical history should be assessed for excess alcohol use, vitamin deficiencies, hereditary factors, or treatment with medications that can cause nerve injury. A neurological examination may also give an indication of the cause.

Nerve pain is often associated with a process called pain-sensitization. The nerves and brain are like wires that carry information. When they become over-stimulated with chronic pain, it may make the whole system over-excitable. In these situations normal touch and other usually comfortable contact can be painful. This is called allodynia. Medications that stimulate the "calming (GABA) receptors" in the brain, such as a number of anti-seizure medications, can help settle the system and decrease pain.

### Postherpetic Neuralgia (PHN)

Postherpetic Neuralgia follows a rash called herpes zoster. Often called shingles, it is caused by the same virus that causes chickenpox. The first time you get chickenpox, the virus remains in your nerve endings even after the chickenpox is gone. This usually causes no problems. If the virus re-activates in one of the nerve endings, however, it causes a rash all along the distribution of the nerve. The rash of herpes zoster is characterized by being painful and being in a line totally on one side of the body. If it extends past the midline of your body, the rash is probably coming from something else. If the pain persists after the rash is gone, continuing for weeks to years (over one year in half of elderly patients), it is called Postherpetic Neuralgia (PHN). The pain tends to be burning, electric, or deep and aching. PHN affects between 500,000 and 1 million Americans—most of which are elderly. It can severely disrupt one's life, but fortunately can now be effectively treated in most cases.[3]

### Painful Diabetic Neuropathy (PDN)

This is the most common cause of neuropathy in U. S. Alterations in sensation are common, and the feet, which are most often affected, may feel both numb and painful at the same time. There are many factors contributing to nerve injury in diabetes, including decreased circulation, accumulation of toxic byproducts, damage from elevated sugars, and nutritional deficiencies. There are also changes in NMDA and opiate receptors.[3]

Research has shown that many people who are labeled as having diabetic neuropathy actually experience neuropathic pain caused by vitamin B6 or B12 deficiency. In addition, the nutrient inositol has been shown to improve nerve function. The nutrient lipoic acid has also been shown to be very helpful for diabetic nerve pain.

### Nutritional Deficiencies

Neuropathic pain can also be caused by deficiencies of vitamins B12, B1, B6, E, and zinc. A number of studies have shown that different kinds of nerve pain can improve by supplementation with high dose B vitamins. Excess vitamin B6 (over 500 mg a day for years), however, can also cause neuropathy.

In patients with long-standing shingles pain, one study showed that taking 1600 units of vitamin E (use the natural form) daily before a meal for 6 months was markedly helpful in eliminating the pain.[4] Another study showed that taking lower doses for less than 6 months was not effective.[5]

### Hormonal Deficiencies

Hormonal deficiencies, especially an under-active thyroid, can also cause neuropathic as well as muscular pain. A therapeutic trial of thyroid hormone is reasonable for anybody who has the symptoms of low thyroid including fatigue, cold intolerance, achiness, having low body temperatures, or unexplained inappropriate weight gain.

### Nerve Entrapments

A pinched nerve can cause nerve pain in many places in the body. Two of the more common ones are low back pain from sciatica and pains in the hand and sometimes wrist from carpal tunnel syndrome. Sciatica usually goes away without surgery by using intravenous colchicine (see Chapter 14), and carpal tunnel syndrome usually resolves after 6 to 12 weeks with vitamin B6 (250 mg a day), thyroid hormone, and wrist splints (see Chapter 19).

### Trigeminal Neuralgia

Also known as tic douloureux, this causes excruciating attacks of pain in the lips, gums, cheek, or jaw. It usually occurs in the middle-aged and elderly and seldom lasts more than a few seconds or minutes. The painful attacks recur frequently throughout the day and night for several weeks at a time. They can be triggered by stimulating certain areas on the face.

Tegretol® eliminates the pain in 75 percent of patients. Begin with 100 mg a day (taken with food), increasing slowly up to 200 mg 4 times a day as needed. Other treatments listed below can also be helpful. If these treatments fail, surgical options are available.

Several studies have shown that giving niacin (nicotinic acid 100 to 200 mg intravenously daily for several days) [6] and vitamin B1 intravenously with other dietary changes[7] can also be markedly effective in treating trigeminal neuralgia.

**Reflex Sympathetic Dystrophy (CRPS)**

This usually manifests as horribly severe pain in one hand or foot but can certainly spread elsewhere. See the end of this chapter for effective treatment.

**How Can I Make the Neuropathic Pain Go Away?**

Neuropathic pain occurs biochemically, making it a very fluid system that can often be quickly modified, resulting in pain relief. Many different chemicals (neurotransmitters) in your body may be involved in your pain, and therefore it is worth trying different types of medications to see which ones work best in your case. For many, treating the nutritional and thyroid deficiencies and eliminating the muscle spasms, which are compressing your nerves, may be enough to eliminate your pain. Others may need to take medications to suppress the pain while we look for ways to eliminate the underlying cause. The best way to tell which chemicals are involved in your nerve pain is to simply try different medications (individually and, if needed, in combination) to see what eases your pain. Basically, it is like trying on different shoes to see what fits best. The good news is that we have a large assortment of "shoes" that you can try on and that are likely to help you.

It is, of course, critical to begin by eliminating the underlying causes of neuropathy and giving the nerves what they need to heal. This includes the nutritional support we've discussed. In addition, the involvement of free radicals in nerve excitation was found in 1995, supporting the use of antioxidants in nerve pain.[8] Since that time, the antioxidant lipoic acid (300 mg 3 times a day) has been shown to be helpful in diabetic neuropathy and should be tried in other neuropathies as well. You will be amazed at how much benefit you may get over time simply from optimizing nutritional support.

In addition, if you are tired, cold intolerant, experience achiness, have low body temperatures, or have weight gain I think it is reasonable to consider a therapeutic trial of natural thyroid hormone regardless of your blood levels. It may take 3 to 6 months for the thyroid and/or nutritional therapies to begin working, but regardless of the cause of your neuropathy, this treatment may result in nerve healing. It is reasonable to begin medications along with the nutritional support so that you can get pain relief as quickly as possible. If only a small area is involved, it makes sense to begin with a Lidocaine® patch. Otherwise, I prefer to begin with Neurontin® and/or tricyclic anti-depressants. All of the recommended oral nutrients discussed in this chapter, except lipoic acid and the 1600 unit mega dose of vitamin E, are contained in the Energy Revitalization System vitamin powder and B-complex. For carpal tunnel syndrome, add 200 mg of B6 to the powder.

Let's look at each of the different categories of treatments that can be helpful for nerve pain. Begin with the nutritional and thyroid support as noted above. You can then add the medications below in the order that they're listed. For all medications discussed in the book, directions for use can be found in Appendix B: Pain Treatment Protocol.

1. Lidocaine® patch, 5 percent. This Novocain®-like patch is applied directly over the area of maximum pain. It can be cut to fit the area, and up to four patches can be used at a time (although the package insert says only three). It is left on for 12 hours and then removed for 12 hours each day, although recent reports have suggested that the patch can be left on up to 18 hours and stiil be safe and effective. [3] Results will usually be seen within 2 weeks. Because the effect is local, side effects are minimal. The most common side effect is a mild skin rash from the patch. It should not be used if you have an allergy to Novocain/lidocaine.

   The patches are most likely to be helpful if the pain is localized to a moderately-sized area. Even in a large area, however, patches can be used on the most uncomfortable spots. The main downside of the patches is that they are expensive. If you have prescription insurance, however, they will usually be covered.

2. Neurontin® and other seizure medications. Newer anti-seizure medications, and some of the older ones, can also be very helpful for neuropathic pain. Neurontin has been shown to be helpful for both shingles and diabetes pain.[9–11] Common side effects include sedation, dizziness, and sometimes mild swelling in the ankles when first starting therapy. These side effects can often be avoided by starting with a low dose and raising the dose slowly. A common total dose for Neurotonin is 600 mg, 3 to 4 times a day.

   For trigeminal neuralgia, Tegretol® has been the drug of choice for over 30 years. Tegretol is not especially effective however for diabetic or post-herpetic nerve pain and has many more side effects than the newer medications. Dilantin® can also be helpful if other medications fail or cost is a problem (see below).

3. Tricyclic anti-depressants. These include medications such as Elavil®, Tofranil®, nortriptyline, or doxepin. Tofranil may be more effective than Elavil. Sedation, constipation, dry mouth, and weight gain are the most common side effects, although dizziness can also occur. Other side effects include urinary retention, sweating, and abnormal heart rhythms. As most of the benefit occurs with the first 10 to 50 mg, and most of the toxicity occurs with higher doses, if adequate relief is not attained at a low-dose, before uncomfortable side effects occur, I then add the next treatment or switch to another tricyclic instead of pushing the dose to higher levels. If it gave no benefit, I would, of course, stop the tricyclics when I began the next treatment. These can be very helpful for nerve pain and have the added benefit of being inexpensive (if you buy the generic form of the drug).

4. Topical Gels. A wonderful new addition to the treatment of pain in general, and especially nerve pain, is the use of prescription topical gels. New gels have been developed that markedly increase the absorption of medications through the skin. By using a low dose of many different medications in the cream, one can get a powerful effect locally with minimal side effects. It is best to have a knowledgeable compounding pharmacist (see Appendix C: Resources) guide you and your physician in the prescribing of these creams and gels.

   For example, studies have shown that for longstanding, persistent (average 31 months) nerve pain that occurs after shingles (post-herpetic neuralgia - PHN), using a 5 percent Ketamine gel applied 2 to 3 times daily over the painful skin areas decreased pain significantly in 65 percent of cases—usually within days and without side effects, except for occasional mild skin irritation. Other studies have also found topical Neurontin, opioids, and capsaicin to be effective.[12] Lidocaine patches resulted in a "highly significant" decrease in pain, which was seen within one week.[13] I find the Lidocaine patches to be more effective than the Lidocaine topical gels.

   To explore an example of how to treat with these creams combined with nutritional support, let's use the example of diabetic neuropathy. One must, of course, begin with proper control of the elevated blood sugars. Nutritional support with high levels of vitamin B12, B6, and inositol are also important in diabetic nerve pain as are many other nutrients, such as vitamins C and E, magnesium, antioxidants, and bioflavonoids. In addition, lipoic acid 300 mg 3 times a day has been shown to be helpful for diabetic neuropathy. A compounded gel containing Ketamine 10 percent, Neurontin® 6 percent, clonidine .2 percent, and nifedipine should be added to painful areas (apply 1 g 3 times a day as needed). The nutritional support can actually make the pain go away over time, while the cream/gel can add symptomatic relief. Other medications discussed in this chapter can then be added as needed to assist in the neuropathic pain.

In addition, another excellent cream for neuropathic pain is a combination of lidocaine 10 percent, amitriptyline 7 percent, Ketamine 5 percent, and Tegretol 7 percent used 2 to 4 times a day as needed. If results are not seen within 14 days, speak with the compounding pharmacist (or your physician if they are familiar with pain creams) about modifying what is in the cream. Start with having the pharmacist make up relatively small amounts of the cream until you find a mix that works well for you.

To give an idea of the effectiveness of topical gels, one study used amitriptyline (Elavil®) topically and found that it markedly anesthetized that area.[14] Other studies have shown that Doxepin® cream is also very helpful for neuropathic pain, including diabetic neuropathy. In one double-blind study of 200 adults, positive effects were seen with minimal side effects.[15-17] The gels can be used in combination with oral medications. Although it is generally not recommended that the gels be used "under occlusion" (i.e. putting Saran Wrap® or a patch over the gel to force it into the skin) because this may raise blood levels of the medications causing side effects, I think the benefit of increased effectiveness may outweigh the risks. I feel it is reasonable to put the Lidocaine patch over an area where you have applied the pain gels (once the gel has dried). If you get unacceptable side effects, remove the patch and use the patch and creams/gels separately.

5. Other anti-depressants. Although anti-depressants can be helpful for pain, even if **no** depression is present, they seem more likely to help nerve pain when they also raise adrenaline (norepinephrine) and not just serotonin. For example, the medication Effexor® reduced diabetic nerve pain by 75 to 100 percent in one open study of 11 patients.[18] In another study of 40 patients with multiple areas of nerve pain, Effexor 225 mg a day decreased pain scores by 20 percent on average. Patients with diabetic neuropathy and those who had higher blood levels of the medication had the greatest effect.[19] I recommend use of Effexor early in your treatment if you have depression associated with your pain. Higher doses (225 mg a day) seem more effective for nerve pain than the lower doses used for depression.

6. Ultram (Tramadol®). This is an interesting medication that works on many areas of pain and in many different types of pain. It has been shown to be effective for nerve pain in a placebo-controlled study after four weeks.[20] It blocks both norepinephrine and serotonin re-uptake and also stimulates the narcotic receptors. Main side effects include dizziness, nausea, constipation, sedation, and lightheadedness on standing. These are more likely to occur when the dose is raised rapidly. Lower doses should be used with anti-depressants and other medications that can raise your serotonin levels. Begin with a dose of 50 mg twice daily and increase to a maximum of 100 mg 4 times a day. Most people find that 100 mg twice daily is wonderful and higher doses cause uncomfortable side effects.

7. Topamax (Topiramate®). Although studies have shown mixed results using Topamax, many people get marked improvement. In one study of diabetic neuropathy, 36 percent of patients had at least a 50 percent decrease in painful diabetic neuropathy after 12 weeks (much more effective than placebo).[21] This medication is usually given twice a day at a total daily dose of 50 to 100 mg/day for migraines and 200 to 300 mg a day for nerve pain, although lower doses can be effective. This is a medication that I have seen work wonderfully in patients who failed numerous other treatments. It is best to start with a low dose (e.g. 25 to 50 mg twice a day) and increase by 25 mg per week as able and needed. Side effects include numbness and tingling (paresthesias), cognitive dysfunction, and weight loss (which most people like).

8. Lamictal (Lamotrigine®). This drug also can be effective for many kinds of neuropathic pain including that which comes from AIDS and central brain pain coming from stroke.[22–23] Lamictal is a seizure medicine that acts as a sodium channel blocker with some calcium channel blockade. In one study with patients who had severe refractory neuropathic pain (especially disc pain) who had failed at least two other treatments, there was an average 70 percent drop in pain in 14 of 21 patients.[24]

   In early studies where lower doses of 200 mg a day or less were used, the effects were marginal. Doses of 200 to 400 mg a day divided through the day are more effective for some kinds of pain. Start with a low dose and increase by 25 mg a week to decrease the probability of side effects. The most worrisome side effect is a rare rash (called Stevens-Johnson Syndrome), which can be fatal. If you develop a rash, stop the medication immediately and let your doctor know. The vast majority of the time it will not be this dangerous type, but better safe than sorry.

9. Zanaflex®. If the other medications do not work adequately, try Zanaflex as it treats the pain from a totally different direction. In one study (not placebo-controlled) 23 patients with neuropathic pain were given Zanaflex. After eight weeks at an average dose of 23 mg a day there was an average 25 percent decrease in pain. 68 percent felt that their pain was improved or much improved. Side effects were very common with over 50 percent experiencing fatigue, one third having gastrointestinal upset, and one percent having liver inflammation.[25] Although it is worth trying, I would try the other medications we discussed first, using Zanaflex for muscle/myofascial pain where it seems to be more effective at lower doses.

10. Gabitril (Tiagabine®). This anti-seizure medication has been shown to increase GABA by inhibiting re-uptake in the same way that Prozac® raises serotonin. Studies also find that it improves deep sleep.[26] Gabitril was given at a dose of 2 mg twice a day and increased by a maximum 4 mg daily each week to maximum of 24 mg a day. The main side effects are sedation, dizziness, and gastric upset, although overall it seems to be fairly well tolerated. The most common effective dose of Gabitril is 8 to 16 mg a day. Gabitril decreased pain by approximately 30 percent and decreased sleep problems by approximately 40 percent. It has also been helpful for neuropathic pain, sleep, and anxiety in several other studies.

    In a study of cancer patients with neuropathic pain, Gabitril decreased pain by approximately 30 percent.[27] Although I use it later than other medications because it is newer, it is rapidly moving up my list, and I often try it right after Neurontin.

11. Keppra®. This is another new anti-seizure medication that we are just starting to explore; it has been effective when other treatments have not helped.

12. Trileptal ® (oxcarbazepine). This is a cousin to the medication Tegretol®, and both medications are helpful for trigeminal neuralgia. In a small study of four patients with neuropathic pain of unknown cause, pain was decreased by approximately 50 percent after 3 weeks at a dose of 150 to 300 mg twice a day. The side effects (sedation, blurred vision) decreased after the initial 3 weeks of treatment.[28]

13. Dilantin®. This is another older seizure medication that also can be helpful in many cases of refractory pain and is relatively inexpensive. It is safer and better tolerated than Tegretol®. The usual

dose is 200 to 400 mg day, and I recommend checking blood levels with it. It can cause hair growth on the earlobes and overgrowth of gum tissue, which needs to be trimmed away by your dentist. This side effect can actually be helpful for those with receding gums.

14. Capsaicin®. This natural compound from hot red peppers can be helpful for nerve pain when applied as a cream. It basically irritates the area so much that it depletes the chemicals that transmit pain. When first using it, it can actually increase pain. In addition, it needs to be taken on a regular basis to prevent the pain chemicals from building back up. Despite it being a natural compound, I prefer to use other treatments.

15. Narcotics. These have been found to be helpful in neuropathic pain. The most common side effects include constipation, sedation, and nausea. Because of side effects and concerns with habituation, as well as the legal issues involved, it is usually best to begin with the other medications we've discussed. Narcotics are only modestly helpful but are considered an accepted treatment for neuropathic pain.

16. Amantadine®, 100 mg. Taking 1 to 3 tablets each morning may help nerve pain, and it is also an anti-viral. In studies using it for pain, the medication was administered intravenously, although this may have been because an oral form was not available in those countries.[29] The most common side effects include visual blurring, dizziness, and nausea. Both effectiveness and blood levels can increase over a 2 week period, so if you get side effects lower the dose.

17. Zonegran®, 100 mg. This is an anti-seizure medication. Begin with 100 mg a day for 2 weeks and then increase to 2 tablets a day. The maximum dose is 400 mg daily, although most of the benefit occurs at the first 200 mg. Because there have been rare occurrences of a life-threatening rash (most rashes caused by the medication are not, however), stop the medication immediately if you get a rash.

18. Benadryl® (diphenhydramine). Sometimes we get help from unexpected places. Studies have shown in both humans and animals that antihistamines can help pain—in spite of our not knowing why this works. It has even been found to be helpful in patients who failed treatment with heavy narcotics. It is recommended that you start with 25 mg every 6 to 8 hours and adjust the dose to the optimum effect.[29A]

**Table One—Some Modes of Action of Medications Used for Neuropathic Pain (Many Medications Have Multiple Actions)**

Glutamate antagonist—Neurontin®

Sodium channel blockers—Dilantin®, Neurontin®, Tegretol®, Depakote®

NMDA-calcium channel blockers—Ketamine®, dextromethorphan, Symmetrel®

Alpha 2 agonists—clonidine, Zanaflex® (Tizanidine®)

GABA agonists—baclofen, Gabitril® (tiagabine)

Norepinephrine increasers—doxepin

Alpha one antagonists—minipres

Substance P. blockers—opioids

Many of these medications can be taken in many ways, including tablets, injections, gels, nasal and suppository forms. Some medications enhance the effectiveness of others. For example, taking dextromethorphan can decrease the tolerance that occurs with the use of opioid medications (Goodman and Gilman's, *The Pharmacological Basis of Therapeutics, Ninth Edition*, 1996, pp 525 to 556) and Zanaflex can increase the effectiveness of opioids. Opioids by themselves are only modestly effective for neuropathic pain.

## *Sympathetically Maintained Pain*

Reflex Sympathetic Dystrophy (RSD) is a nasty and chronic pain disorder affecting as many as 1.5 million Americans. It often begins with severe pain in one hand or foot. It is also referred to as Complex Regional Pain Syndrome (CRPS), although I still prefer to use the name Reflex Sympathetic Dystrophy. The name was changed because it is not entirely clear that over-activity of the sympathetic nervous system is involved. It was first called Causalgia in 1864 during the Civil War. Soldiers noted burning pain, progressive skin changes, and decreased function in an affected limb.[30] CRPS is called type 1 (RSD) when there is no clear damage to the nerve. Type 2 CRPS (Causalgia) occurs when there is actual damage to the nerve instead of only to the affected limb. When I first meet a patient, and I see that he or she immediately moves her hand or foot out of the way to be sure that it is not touched, I quickly inquire about symptoms suggesting RSD.

The Reflex Sympathetic Dystrophy Association of America defines the disorder as a multi-system, multi-symptom syndrome that usually affects one or more extremities and can affect the entire body. There are many pain patterns, but the pain is often very severe and much greater than one would expect from the precipitating injury. Any number of traumas, including accidents, fractures, surgery, or even mild injuries such as IV insertions, can trigger RSD in one's hands or feet. Interestingly, injury of the hip can cause foot pain, and injury in the shoulder can cause hand pain. A heart attack can also trigger RSD in the hand. Pain is usually burning or stinging and the skin has exquisite sensitivity to even the lightest touch. It is sometimes associated with swelling, color and temperature changes in that hand or foot, and unusual sweating. Muscle spasms, tremor, and/or weakness may also be present. Although it is classically considered to affect just one extremity, according to one survey as many as 70 percent of people with RSD had noted spreading of pain beyond the hand or foot to other parts of the body.

The most common pattern of spread is for pain to move over the same extremity. It may continue to spread or move to the opposite extremity or other distant sites. Early diagnosis with prompt treatment may result in the problem being more easily reversed.

Many pain specialists use a combination of treatments, including physical therapy, medication, electrical nerve stimulation, nerve blocks, and/or emotional support with counseling. It is best to avoid surgery or further injury to the area, if at all possible, as it will usually result in worsening of the symptoms. Casting and immobilization can also worsen symptoms and should be avoided as well. Unfortunately, there's no definitive test for the illness as nerve pain does not show up on x-rays or standard diagnostic tests. Because of this, most people with RSD have not been properly diagnosed, resulting in further psychological trauma. The level of pain can be anywhere from mild to devastating. Patients sometimes choose to have the extremity amputated because of the pain, only to find that the pain still persists! In addition, it is suspected that people who have had RSD once are at greater risk of developing it again with future injury.

The good news is that in addition to new treatments, there is also a simple preventive measure. In one study of 123 adults with wrist fractures, half of the patients were given 500 mg of vitamin C daily and the other half were given placebo for 50 days. RSD occurred in 22 percent of the patients in the placebo group, but only 7 percent of the vitamin C group.[31]

For more information on RSD, visit the web site of the RSD Syndrome Association of America at www.rsd.org.

CRPS has three stages: Stage 1, the acute stage, usually lasts about 3 months and is characterized by severe burning, aching pain, redness, swelling, increased nail and hair growth, and warmth. Stage 2, which lasts approximately 3 to 6 months, is called the dystrophic stage. It is characterized by diffuse pain, hair loss, spotty osteoporosis (bone thinning), increased joint thickness, muscle wasting, brittle and grooved nails, skin changes, pale and cold skin, and reduction in range of motion. In stage 3, called the atrophic stage, pain may spread to the entire limb or body. There is extreme weakness of joints, atrophy of muscles, and bone loss.

The first stages of the disease may be treated with a combination of sympathetic nerve blocks and physical exercise. This combination has been reported to relieve pain and increase mobility in 80 percent of patients treated during Stage 1. In the first year of the illness, surgical intervention (to the nerves leading to the pain, not to the area having pain) may be helpful. In one study, 7 of 7 patients recovered after having had a sympathectomy during the first 12 months after injury, while only 44 percent recovered with this procedure after two years past the injury.[31 - 32]

Ketamine® (an NMDA receptor antagonist anesthetic) can also be helpful for neuropathic pain. Unfortunately, many patients experience the side effect of intoxication, including hallucinations, which may be uncomfortable. This problem can be avoided in most cases by giving the Ketamine as a topical gel. In one study of five patients with refractory reflex sympathetic dystrophy, pain was temporarily relieved by 65 to 100 percent within three minutes of applying Ketamine gel (1 to 9 mg Ketamine per kg of body weight) to the painful area without significant side effects. All patients chose to continue treatment. The dose needed to maintain the benefit ranged from 50 to 600 mg, 3 to 6 times daily.[33]

Since this study was conducted, reports have been published of permanent elimination of severe RSD using an IV infusion of Ketamine continuously for 6 days. The IV Ketamine was started in one patient at 10 mg per hour and increased by 10 mg per hour every 2 hours as tolerated, with the maximum infusion rate of 30 mg per hour. A higher dose was not used, as the patient wished to remain "in control" without being overly intoxicated from the medication. By day 3 her pain was decreasing and by day 5 it was gone. Cessation of the pain continued after the treatment was stopped. This medication holds great promise for the treatment of this devastating problem.[34]

Dr. Argo , a pain specialist at the Pain Management Center at Columbia Rose Medical Center, Denver, has found that Paxil® can be helpful for reflex sympathetic dystrophy where other SSRIs are not.[35] In another clinic, a combination of Neurontin® and Clonidine® creams decreased RSD pain by one third. ■

**Important Points**

1. Neuropathies are characterized by pain that is burning, shooting (often to distant areas), or stabbing. It also has an "electric" quality about it. "Tingling or numbness" (paresthesias) and increased sensitivity with normal touch being painful (allodynia) are also commonly seen.
2. Neuropathic pain can come from malfunction of nerves or the brain associated with illness (e.g. diabetes, low thyroid, etc.), infections (e.g. shingles), pinched nerves (e.g. from muscles or disc disease), nutritional deficiencies (e.g. vitamin B6 and B12), injury (e.g. stroke, tumors, spinal cord injury, and multiple sclerosis), and medication/treatment side effects.
3. Nutritional support is critical! I recommend using the vitamin powder/B-complex plus lipoic acid 300 mg 3 times a day.
4. Do blood testing to check for diabetes, low thyroid, or vitamin B12 deficiency.
5. Many medications can be very helpful for nerve pain. For small areas, begin with the Lidocaine patch and topical gels. For large areas, or if these are not effective, use the oral medications we've discussed.
6. If you have severe pain in 1 hand or foot, consider RSD. Ketamine by cream or IV, Neurontin, and other treatments can be helpful to reduce or eliminate RSD pain.

# Chapter 9 Myofascial (Muscle/Ligament/Tendon) and Fibromyalgia Pain

Fibromyalgia (FMS) and myofascial pain syndrome (MPS) occur when your muscles get stuck in the shortened position. In fibromyalgia, this also results in reversible changes in how your brain processes pain. You would think that if muscles do not have the energy they need, they would get limp and loose. The opposite is true. When muscles do not get the nutrients, sleep, or hormonal support they need, or if underlying infections exist, the muscles can't release.

This makes sense when you think about what occurs when someone dies. Instead of the muscles going limp, they become rigid as a board (rigor mortis). In addition, fibromyalgia patients have suppression of a major control center in the brain called the hypothalamus. This is basically like blowing a fuse in your brain. The good news is that our research has shown that 91 percent of patients can turn the hypothalamic "circuit breaker" back on by treating four key areas we discussed in previous chapters. Doing this can make both fibromyalgia and myofascial pain go away.

These key areas are:

1. Disordered sleep. Most patients with these illnesses find that they are unable to get 7 to 8 hours of deep sleep a night without taking medications. In part, this occurs because hypothalamic function is critical to deep sleep. **For patients to get well, it is critical that they take enough of the correct sleep medications to get 8 to 9 hours sleep at night!** These medications include Ambien®, Desyrel®, Klonopin®, Xanax®, Soma®, and, if you don't have restless leg syndrome, Flexeril® and/or Elavil®. In addition, natural remedies can help sleep. An excellent natural compound is the Revitalizing Sleep Formula® (see Appendix C: Resources). It contains theanine, Jamaican dogwood, wild lettuce, valerian, passionflower, and hops. (See Chapter 3 and Appendix C: Resources for other sleep therapies.) In the first 6 months of treatment, it is not uncommon to require 6 to 8 different products **simultaneously** to get 8 hours of sleep at night. After 6 to 18 months of feeling well, most people can come off most sleep (and other) medications. I'm

starting to believe that, to offer a margin of safety during periods of stress, it may be wise to stay on ½ to 1 tablet of a sleep medication or herbal for the rest of your life. Your doctor may initially be uncomfortable with this. Nonetheless, my experience with over 2,000 patients and two research studies has found this approach to be safe and critical to people getting well. When one recognizes that fibromyalgia and its disabling cousin chronic fatigue syndrome (CFS/FMS) are hypothalamic sleep disorders—not poor sleep hygiene—this approach makes sense. Otherwise, it is as if your doctor would immediately try to stop blood pressure or diabetes medicines every time the patient was doing better!

2. Hormonal deficiencies. The hypothalamus is the main control center for most of the glands in your body. Most of the normal ranges for our blood tests were not developed in the context of hypothalamic suppression. Because of this, and for a number of other reasons, it is usually necessary, albeit controversial, to treat with thyroid, adrenal (very low dose Cortef®, DHEA), and ovarian and testicular hormones—despite normal blood tests. These hormones have been found to be reasonably safe when used in low doses. (See Chapter 4 Treating Hormonal Deficiencies and Appendix C: Resources for more information on hormonal therapies.)

3. Unusual infections. Many studies have shown immune system dysfunction in Fibromyalgia/CFS. Although there are many causes of this, I suspect that poor sleep is a major contributor. The immune dysfunction can result in many unusual infections. These include viral infections (e.g.HHV-6, CMV, and EBV), parasites and other bowel infections, infections sensitive to long-term treatment with the antibiotics Cipro® and Doxycycline® (e.g. mycoplasma, chlamydia, Lyme, etc.) and fungal infections. Although the latter is controversial, both my study and another recent placebo-controlled study found treating with an anti-fungal to be very helpful with the symptoms seen in these syndromes. Avoiding sweets (stevia is OK) and taking Acidophilus Pearls (a healthy milk bacteria), 2 pearls twice a day for 5 months, can be helpful. I often also add prescription anti-fungals as well. (See Chapter 5 and Appendix C: Resources for more information on infections.)

4. Nutritional supplementation. As discussed in Chapter 2, nutritional deficiencies are widespread in fibromyalgia. I recommend taking the vitamin powder long-term. I also recommend adding NAC, 500 to 650 mg; Coenzyme Q10 (use the Vitaline® form), 200 mg; and Acetyl l-carnitine, 1000 mg a day for 3 to 4 months if you have fibromyalgia. These are all readily available.

The above four areas are discussed at length earlier in this book. For an in-depth look at how to eliminate fibromyalgia and myofascial pain, I invite you to read my best-selling book *From Fatigued to Fantastic!* My double-blind, placebo-controlled study showed a 91 percent improvement rate when these four areas were treated.[1] The full text of the study can also be seen on my web site at www.vitality101.com.

While treating the underlying causes of muscle pain that we discussed above, it is also helpful to have other treatments to keep you comfortable. NSAIDs like Motrin are minimally effective, only helping about 10 percent of fibromyalgia patients. Interestingly, Celebrex® is more likely to be helpful—despite having similar mechanisms of action. Safety concerns have been raised about this family of medications as well, however. Other medications that are very helpful include Ultram®, Skelaxin®, Neurontin®, and Baclofen®. Zanaflex® has also been helpful in many patients, and most only need a 4 mg tablet at bedtime.[2] Zanaflex also helps to decrease levels of substance P in the spinal fluid. This pain messenger is 300 percent of the normal level in fibromyalgia patients.

Permax (Pramipexole®), a medication used for Parkinson's disease, has also been found to be helpful in fibromyalgia. In one study of 166 severe fibromyalgia patients, 22 percent discontinued treatment within the first two weeks because of mild to moderate side effects. Of those who tolerated the medication, increasing as tolerated over two months to an average dose of 1.5 mg at bedtime, 29 percent became pain-free, 43 percent had minimal pain, and 76 percent were improved. A larger study is currently underway. The medication is begun with ¼ mg at bedtime and increased by ¼ mg each week to a maximum dose of 2 mg at bedtime. If stomach pain occurs, Nexium® or similar medications are used during the first month. If restless leg syndrome worsens, Klonopin® is also added at bedtime. Both of these side effects generally go away as the dose is increased.[3] Pregabalin® is another medication that is helpful for fibromyalgia pain. It was scheduled to be released in late 2004, but may not be allowed because of safety concerns.

Another non-drug pain treatment that is currently being studied is Flexyx®. This medication is a brainwave biofeedback and treatment system. (See www.flexyx.com for more information.) ■

**Important Points**

1. Fibromyalgia and myofascial pain syndrome are associated with shortened, tight muscles.
2. To release the muscles and eliminate pain four key areas need to be treated. These are sleep, hormonal support, nutritional support, and treating underlying infections.
3. For nutritional support take the vitamin powder long-term (see Appendix C: Resources). It is also reasonable to add NAC 500-650 mg, coenzyme Q10 (use the Vitaline form) 200 mg, and acetyl l-carnitine 1000 mg a day for 3 to 4 months.
4. For sleep, take the Revitalizing Sleep Formula® herbal combined with medications as needed. Excellent medications for sleep include Ambien®, Klonopin®, Trazodone®, Soma®, Zanaflex®, Doxepin®, and Elavil®.
5. Most patients with fibromyalgia benefit from a trial of thyroid hormone. If you have low blood pressure, experience irritability that goes away with eating, crash with stress, or have an elevated sedimentation rate blood test, I also recommend adrenal support with Adrenal Stress End® and very low dose Cortef®.
6. Treat the underlying infections—especially yeast. If you have bowel symptoms or nasal congestion/sinusitis, yeast overgrowth is especially likely—although controversial. Treat yeast by avoiding sugar ( except for chocolate) and taking Acidophilus Pearls®, Phytostan®, and Citricidal®. It is also reasonable to take prescription antifungals like Nystatin® and Diflucan®.
7. If you would like more information, my previous book *From Fatigued to Fantastic!* can make you an expert on treating these problems.

CHAPTER 10

# Arthritis Pain

Joint pain, known as arthritis, comes in many forms. The most common type is osteoarthritis, known as "wear and tear arthritis." The joints mainly affected by osteoarthritis are the finger, knee, and hip joints.

A more severe form of arthritis is rheumatoid arthritis, which is inflammatory and results in hot swollen joints. It is an autoimmune disorder that causes the body's immune system to attack the joints. I suspect that infections are common triggers for this attack.

The American College of Rheumatology has defined the following criteria for rheumatoid arthritis:

- Morning stiffness of over 1 hour
- Arthritis and soft-tissue swelling in over 3 of 14 joints or joint groups
- Arthritis of hand joints
- Symmetric arthritis
- Subcutaneous nodules
- Rheumatoid factor at a level above the 95th percentile
- Radiological changes suggestive of joint erosion

At least four of these criteria need to be met, although patients are sometimes treated despite not meeting these criteria. The childhood form of this disease is called juvenile rheumatoid arthritis.

In addition to using long-term antibiotic therapy with minocycline in rheumatoid arthritis, it is worth considering dietary changes as well. Diet can play a major role in inflammatory arthritis. A recent study tested the role of diet in 60 patients with rheumatoid arthritis. 30 patients were given a standard American diet and the other 30 an anti-inflammatory diet low in meat and high in fish oil—with supplements given to supply approximately 2 g of omega 3 fish oils daily—for 8 months. The patients on an anti-inflammatory diet had a 28 percent decrease in the number of tender joints.[1] In addition, decreasing inflammation by giving borage seed oil (supplying 1.4 g of GLA—Gamma Linolenic Acid) decreased the swollen joint score by 41 percent in the active group vs. a 40 percent worsening in the placebo group. No patients had to withdraw because of side effects.[2] Many other nutrients, including pantothenic acid, vitamin A, vitamin C, vitamin E, boron, copper, zinc, and selenium have been found to be deficient and/or helpful in the treatment of rheumatoid arthritis. In addition, see Chapter 11 for more information on treating rheumatoid arthritis with diet and supplements. High doses of fish oil (e.g. 1 to 2 Tbsp a day for at least 3 months) have been shown to be especially helpful in over six studies. As always, use fish oil that is mercury and lead free (see Appendix C: Resources).

### *Other Types of Arthritis:*

**Psoriatic Arthritis**. Psoriatic arthritis is non-destructive symmetrical inflammation of joints, which occurs along with the skin disease psoriasis. A clue to its presence is "pitting" in the fingernails, which looks like someone stuck a needle tip into several places in the nails.

**Gouty Arthritis and Pseudo Gout**. Gout is arthritis caused by the accumulation of uric acid crystals in the joints. The big toe joint is most commonly affected. Gouty arthritis is very painful. The diagnosis is made when crystals are found in fluid aspirated from the affected joint, although a clinical diagnosis is often made by an elevated uric acid blood test and sudden pain and swelling in the joints (especially the big toe). It is treated in the acute phase (first week) with NSAIDs. If attacks happen more than twice a year, Allopurinol® is often prescribed, after the acute attack settles down, to decrease accumulation of uric acid. Colchicine® can also be used for acute attacks. Although attacks of gout can be slightly decreased by avoiding organ meats, seafood, beans, and peas, the benefit is modest and I don't know if it is really worth bothering with. I think it is worthwhile, however, to avoid fructose, beer and excess alcohol (beer is more of a problem with gout than other types of alcohol).[3]

**Pseudo Gout (calcium pyrophosphate deposition disease)**. This is a very similar disease, but the crystals look different under the microscope, and they are not uric acid.

**Systemic Lupus Erythematosus and Other Auto-immune Diseases**. These can also cause arthritis. See Chapter 11 for information on how to treat this disease.

**Hemochromatosis**. Arthritis of the hand joints occurs in the disorder of excess iron called hemochromatosis. Its treatment is iron elimination by donating blood regularly and avoidance of iron supplements. It often occurs in association with diabetes and/or liver inflammation. Suspect this if you have elevated iron (check an "iron percent saturation and ferritin"). If elevated, see a gastroenterologist or liver specialist. If caught early, it is easy to treat. If caught late, it can kill you. It is often familial/

genetic, so if one family member has it, everyone in the family should be checked for it. It is not rare, and missing this diagnosis is tragic. In fact, it is enough of a problem that we elected to leave iron out of the vitamin powder (for this and other reasons).

As baby boomers begin reaching the age of retirement, the number of Americans developing arthritis-type disorders is expected to soar. This increase will add to already significant arthritis rates. According to the Centers for Disease Control, one out of four American adults has been diagnosed with arthritis and another 17 percent may be suffering from it without having been diagnosed. In 2002, the percentage of those diagnosed with one or more forms of arthritis (including rheumatoid arthritis and gout), lupus, or fibromyalgia ranged from a low of 17.8 percent in Hawaii to a high of 35.8 percent in Alabama. Thirty-six million workdays are lost each year because of osteoarthritis. A CDC (Center for Disease Control) arthritis expert stated that the number of cases of arthritis in America is huge compared to most other diseases. Fortunately, there are many natural and prescription therapies that can be effective.

## Natural Therapies

I prefer using natural rather than prescription therapies for osteoarthritis. The most common prescription medications in use (NSAIDs like Motrin®) kill over 16,000 Americans yearly and do not slow, and may actually hasten, the progression of the arthritis. I recommend you begin with a natural treatment program that will decrease inflammation and help repair the joints.

This natural treatment program has four main components:

1. Repair
2. Prevent Damage
3. Restore Function
4. Rule Out and Treat Infections and Food Allergies

### *Repair*

The joint cartilage can be repaired using a combination of glucosamine sulfate, Condroitin®, and MSM. It is also critical that you get comprehensive nutritional support, as discussed earlier, to promote wound healing. Glucosamine, a cartilage compound that has been shown to actually heal your joints, is as effective as NSAIDs (e.g. Motrin® and other anti-inflammatory drugs). In addition, a recent animal study showed that glucosamine and the anti-inflammatory drugs work synergistically. This means that when the two are taken together, it is much more effective than simply taking either one alone. Using glucosamine can therefore allow you to stop the anti-inflammatory drugs, or at least lower the needed dose. This can improve the safety, effectiveness, and cost of treatment dramatically.[4]

Because of this, for tissue repair I recommend Glucosamine **Sulfate**, 500 mg, 3 times per day. Also consider MSM, 1.5 to 3 grams a day for 2 to 5 months, and Chondroitin, although these last two are less important. MSM supplies the Sulfur amino acids needed for healing in general. Although most of the research on MSM and arthritis has not been placebo-controlled, two studies were. One showed an 80 percent decrease in arthritis pain after 6 weeks using 1500 mg in the morning and 750 mg at lunchtime. Another showed that Glucosamine and MSM are synergistic for reducing pain and swelling in arthritic joints. One hundred and eighteen patients with mild to moderate osteoarthritis were treated 3 times daily with either 500 mg of glucosamine, 500 mg of MSM, a combination of both, or placebo. After 12 weeks, the researchers found that the combination treatment had a faster effect on decreasing pain and inflammation compared to Glucosamine or MSM alone.[5, 5A]

Glucosamine sulfate is a cartilage building compound that has been found to be helpful in arthritis in many studies. Although its exact mechanism of action is not yet fully understood, it is a major component of the cartilage that is damaged in arthritic joints. Glucosamine taken by mouth is incorporated in the molecules that make up this cartilage, likely contributing to the healing of arthritis. As you may have noted above, I recommend the sulfate form (as opposed to Glucosamine hydrochloride) because the sulfate can also help with wound/joint healing.

Unlike aspirin/NSAIDS that do not slow down destruction of joints in arthritis, Glucosamine has been shown to actually help stabilize, and often heal the joints, as shown on x-ray. Doses of less than 1000 mg a day do not affect symptoms, and the standard dose is 500 mg 3 times a day. It can also be taken as 1500 mg once a day. It can be taken with or without food, and had no more side effects than placebo.[6] Chondroitin sulfate is sometimes added to Glucosamine or taken by itself. Its benefits are modest because less than 10 percent of it is absorbed, as opposed to 90 percent for Glucosamine sulfate.[7] Because of this, I rarely use Chondroitin®. On the other hand, 1200 mg a day can be helpful in slowing down arthritis and is worth trying if you do not get adequate relief with the other treatments. It can be taken all at once or 400 mg 3 times a day with equal effectiveness.

Overall nutritional support is also critical. For example, low concentrations and low intake of vitamin D seems to be associated with an increased risk of progression of osteoarthritis of the knee.[8] In addition, SAM-e can be helpful. This nutrient is produced from methionine (an amino acid) in combination with multiple nutrients, including B vitamins, folate, and inositol. It was initially tested and found to be effective in treating depression. Researchers also noted that it improved patients' arthritis as effectively as anti-inflammatory medications (NSAIDs). A number of studies were done including one that gave 600 mg a day for 2 weeks followed by 400 mg daily for 2 years. Pain and stiffness decreased within 1 week and the improvement continued throughout the 2-year trial.[9] A study that reviewed 7 other studies was inconclusive. A major problem with SAM-e products is that they are not stable and break down easily, with many products not really delivering what they claim. In addition, it is quite expensive. A better alternative is to take the nutrients your body needs to make SAM-e. Combining the nutrients found in the vitamin powder and B complex resulted in increased blood levels of SAM-e similar to those found in people taking 400 to 800 mg of SAM-e daily.

These are only a few of many examples of the importance of overall nutritional support in treating arthritis. Dozens of other important nutrients can help arthritis (e.g. niacin, pantothenic acid, B complex, vitamin C, vitamin E, boron, selenium, and zinc). As you can tell, it important to get optimal nutritional support. The vitamin powder makes this easy to do.

## Prevent Damage

I recommend a mix of several natural remedies, many of which can be found in combination. The formulation that I like the most combines boswellia, willow bark, and cherry. These are combined in an excellent new product called End Pain (see Appendix C: Resources). Using these three together can powerfully decrease many kinds of pain while preventing damaging inflammation. Take 2 tablets 3 times a day until your pain subsides (approximately 2 to 6 weeks) and then you can often lower the dose to 1 tablet 2 to 3 times a day, or as needed. Curcumin can also be a healthful anti-inflammatory but requires the addition of piperine from black pepper for the curcumin to be adequately absorbed. I do not generally recommend that you use these if you take any prescriptions, however, because piperine may potentially also increase the absorption of other medications, causing them to reach toxic levels. Fish oil (see Appendix C: Resources), ½ to 1 Tbsp daily, also has strong anti-inflammatory properties.

## Restore Function

Restore function with stretching, exercise, and heat. Exercise at least 20 minutes a day. Swimming, walking, and yoga are good choices. Use a heating pad or moist heat for up to 20 minutes at a time to give relief.

Diet, exercise, and lifestyle can be important in the treatment and prevention of osteoarthritis. For example, losing 11 pounds will reduce a woman's risk of developing arthritis of the knee by 50 percent over a 10 year period.[10 - 11] Adding exercise may further decrease arthritis pain.[12]

### *Rule Out and Treat Infections and Food Allergies*

These can aggravate arthritis. New techniques that combine acupressure and applied kinesiology can be a very powerful way to eliminate allergies and sensitivities. I recommend using a brilliant technique called NAET. It was developed by Dr. Devi Nambudripad (see www.NAET.com for more information). If you also have osteoarthritis or rheumatoid arthritis, I recommend using a spin off-of this technique called JMT (see www.jmt-jafmeltechnique.com for more information). For rheumatoid arthritis, I also use long-term antibiotics (Minocycline) because I feel this is an infectious disease in many cases, and research has shown antibiotics to be effective. One type of food sensitivity to be aware of in arthritis that has not responded well to other treatments is reactivity to foods in the nightshade family. These include tomatoes, potatoes, eggplant, peppers, paprika, cayenne, and tobacco. If you do not experience relief after one month of being off these foods, reintroduce them to see if they affect your symptoms. Also avoid the artificial sweetener Aspartame (NutraSweet®).

In addition to these four treatment areas, although it may seem silly, copper bracelets have actually been shown in a blinded crossover study to be helpful in relieving arthritis, and I have also seen patients get better using them .[13]

## Other Natural Therapies

As noted above, I recommend that you begin with the End Pain formula and glucosamine/MSM/ chondroitin. You may also want to try this popular home remedy:

> **Purple Pectin for Pain**. Purchase Certo® in the canning section of your local grocery. It is the thickening agent used to make jams and jellies. Certo contains pectin, a natural ingredient found in plants. Take 1 to 3 Tbsp of Certo in 8 ounces of grape juice 1 to 2 times a day (1 to 2 Tbsp a day is enough for most people, but you can try more). If it's going to help, you'll likely know in 7 to 14 days. As the pain disappears, the dose can be reduced to 1 tsp in grape juice once or twice a day as needed. Many people have found this simple, safe, and cheap treatment to be effective.

Although I prefer nutritional and herbal therapies, many **homeopathic remedies** can also be helpful for arthritis—especially if given by a well-trained homeopath. For those of you not familiar with homeopathy, the concept is that an extraordinarily diluted amount of a substance does the opposite of the high-dose when prepared properly. There have actually been a number of studies showing that this approach can be very helpful.

Homeopathy is not based on the diagnosis (e.g. osteoarthritis) but rather on the specific nature of the symptoms. Homeopathic remedies have the benefits of being very safe and also rather inexpensive. Because it is so diluted, one drop of a substance can make thousands of gallons or many thousands of tablets of the homeopathic remedy. For the homeopathic remedies below, look for a 6, 12, or 30 C potency, and take it 4 to 6 times a day. Only take it as long as it is helping. Below are some of the better known homeopathics for different kinds of arthritis pain (for more information, see Dana Ullman's book *Homeopathic Family Medicine*, available online at www.Homeopathic.com.):

1. Rhus Tox (poison ivy). This is a commonly used homeopathic for acute arthritis pain. It is especially helpful when the pain is worse on first waking and decreases after you've moved around awhile. Morning stiffness is one example of this. It is especially helpful for those of you who tend to be sensitive to wet and cold weather and feel worse at night. If this does not work, try rhododendron.

2. Bryonia. This remedy is best used when your pain is activated by moving around, especially if the pain is severe and helped by heat and laying still.

3. Apis. This remedy is best used if you have great swelling in your joints with hot burning, stinging pain, and pain that is aggravated by hot compresses and eased up by cold.

4. Belladonna. This remedy is best used if you have red, hot, swollen joints that are aggravated by touch or motion and have rapid onset and relief with hot compresses (e.g. gout and perhaps rheumatoid arthritis).

5. Ruta. Consider using this if your pain developed at the site of an old injury, is aggravated by motion and cold, and is worse in the morning.

6. Kalmia (Mountain Laurel). This remedy is most helpful for sudden onset of severe arthritis that moves from joint to joint, is aggravated by cold and helped by heat, and is associated with numbness, weakness, and heart conditions.

7. Caulophyllum (Blue Cohosh). This remedy is best used if your arthritis predominantly affects the small joints in your hands or feet, and closing one's hands creates a lot of pain.
8. Arnica. Although more often used for acute traumatic injury (my favorite is a cream called Traumeel®), it can also be helpful for arthritis pain.

My favorite companies for homeopathics are Heel and Boiron (see Appendix C: Resources).

## Prescription Therapies

Prescription therapies include NSAIDs such as Motrin®, and COX 2 inhibitors such as Celebrex®, Tylenol®, and Ultram®. Because most of you and your physicians are well aware of these, and they are discussed in Chapter 22, we will not go into more depth about them. A recent study also showed that the Lidoderm® patches were helpful in decreasing pain by approximately 30 percent in 2 weeks, with many patients experiencing over a 50 percent drop in pain. Except for headache and an occasional skin rash where the patch was applied, treatment was well tolerated.[14]

Although I have been using natural cortisol (Cortef®—by prescription) in doses of up to 20 mg daily for decades, some recently touted techniques have been adapting the protocol to use low-dose pulse therapies. The main concern with cortisol is that too high a dose can be toxic and it also suppresses the adrenal glands. Doses of up to 20 mg daily (approximately equal to 4 to 5 mg of prednisone but safer) have been shown to be safe even when used for extended periods.

If the arthritis persists despite natural therapies, it is worth trying the following:

Give the Cortef in 7 to 9 day cycles:

- On day 1 and 2, give 20 mg twice a day
- On day 3 and 4, give 10 mg twice a day
- On day 5, give 5 mg twice a day
- Take no Cortef for the next 2 to 4 days

Keep repeating the cycles, looking for benefit to occur within 3 months. At that time, you can try lowering the dose. If inflammatory arthritis is present (and in severe cases even if it is not), consider Minocycline, 100 mg twice a day (an antibiotic), long-term as discussed above. ■

**Important Points**

1. Do not presume that joint pain is arthritis. It can also come from the muscles, tendons, and ligaments around the joint. This is so even if the x-rays are abnormal.

2. The most common type of arthritis (osteoarthritis) is known as "wear and tear arthritis." The joints mainly affected by osteoarthritis are the finger, knee and hip joints. There may be joint deformities, but there should not be inflammation.

3. If inflammation is present, consider rheumatoid or infectious arthritis. In either of these situations, in addition to standard treatments, I recommend adding the antibiotic minocycline 100 mg twice daily, and an anti-inflammatory diet low in meat and high in fish oil. It is a good idea to take fish oil, 1 to 2 Tbsp daily (see Appendix C: Resources) and borage seed oil supplements. Many other nutrients are also critical and are present in the vitamin powder.

4. If you have psoriasis, or "pitting" in the fingernails, which looks like someone stuck a needle tip into several places in the nails (even without the skin changes/rash), your arthritis may be from the psoriasis.

5. If you have an elevated uric acid blood test and sudden pain and swelling in the joints (especially the big toe) consider gout. The NSAID medications plus colchicine can work well for the acute phase. Allopurinol® can be used to prevent further attacks. Your doctor is very likely familiar with the treatment for gout.

6. I recommend you begin with a natural treatment program which will decrease inflammation and help to repair the joints. This has four main components:

   A. Repair. The joint cartilage can be repaired using a combination of glucosamine sulfate (most important—500 mg 3 times a day for at least 6 weeks), Chondroitin (less important), and MSM (1.5-3 grams a day). It is also critical that you get the other nutrients discussed above ( present in the vitamin powder), which promote wound healing and naturally increase your SAMe levels. They have also been shown to help arthritis. After 6 weeks, these also decrease pain.

*Continued on next page*

**Important Points** *(continued)*

B. Use other anti-inflammatories to prevent damage and decrease or eliminate pain. I recommend a combination of several natural remedies, many of which can be found in combination. The mix I like the most combines boswellia, willow bark, and cherry (all included in the End Pain formula—see Appendix C: Resources). This acts like a natural COX-2 inhibitor (like Celebrex), but much safer. It takes 6 weeks to see the full effect.

C. Restore function with stretching, exercise, weight loss, and heat. Exercise at least 20 minutes a day. Swimming, walking, and yoga are good choices. Use a heating pad or moist heat for up to 20 minutes at a time to give relief.

D. Rule out and treat infections and food allergies, which can aggravate arthritis. Most food allergy blood tests (except the ones from Elisa Act Technologies—see Appendix C: Resources) are not reliable. NAET (see www.NAET.com) is a wonderful way to test for and eliminate food sensitivities. A related technique called JMT (see www.jmt-jafmeltechnique.com) is also an excellent way to treat rheumatoid and osteoarthritis naturally using energy medicine. Homeopathics can also be helpful.

**7.** For symptomatic relief, prescription therapies, including NSAIDs such as Motrin®, COX 2 inhibitors such as Celebrex®, Tylenol®, Lidoderm® patches and Ultram®, can all be helpful. NSAIDs and Celebrex may have significant toxicity, however, and natural remedies are safer.

CHAPTER 11

# Inflammatory Pain

Inflammation is your body's response to what it perceives to be an outside invader or irritant (e.g. gout).When caused by infections, the inflammation can sometimes be rather obvious as occurs with pneumonia. Other times, it can be very subtle.

Keep in mind the following key points regarding inflammation and pain:

1. Treat the underlying infections or irritants when able.
2. Often the inflammation causes more harm than good. It is often worthwhile to simply decrease the inflammation using natural remedies, nutrients, ultra low-dose cortisol, and anti-inflammatories such as aspirin and Motrin® family medications.
3. Sometimes the inflammation is obvious because it causes redness, heat, and swelling. At other times, it can be quite subtle and needs to be looked for.

There are many different autoimmune and inflammatory illnesses. Lupus (Systemic Lupus Erythematosus or SLE) is a common autoimmune disease that often results in significant fatigue and pain. What most rheumatologists don't realize is that **the secondary fibromyalgia caused by lupus and many other rheumatologic diseases (including rheumatoid arthritis) may be a source of many, if not most, of the symptoms and much of the disability in these patients**. Flaring fibromyalgia may also be misinterpreted as a flaring of lupus, or other inflammatory disease, activity.[1] In addition, both of these illnesses can be associated with marked vitamin D deficiencies.[2] Vitamin D deficiency has also been associated with muscle pain. The Energy Revitalization System vitamin powder contains a large amount of vitamin D (600 Units).

When one treats the associated fibromyalgia, patients often find that their lupus is actually a minimal problem. In addition, several studies have shown that taking DHEA, 200 mg a day, significantly improves the outcome of lupus and allows the patient to get by with a lower dose of prednisone. The main side effects of a too high DHEA level are darkening of facial hair and acne. If either of these occurs, lower the dose. It is unnecessary to follow blood levels of DHEA at this dose, because this is a very high dose and you can assume the blood level will be high. Lower doses, however, are not as effective as 200 mg a day.[3] As many, if not most, inflammatory and/or autoimmune illnesses can cause a secondary fibromyalgia, and fibromyalgia is now treatable, it is important to keep this possibility in mind. **If you have widespread pain, fatigue, and insomnia, look for and treat the associated fibromyalgia!**

## Inflammation (in General)

Inflammation is a common cause of pain and many other medical problems that we experience in Western society. For example, anything that ends in the letters "itis" means that the problem is inflammatory. This includes things like arthritis, tendonitis, bursitis, spondylitis, appendicitis, etc. Inflammation is obviously a major cause of pain.

Our body's armies of inflammation are often on high-alert when they don't have to be. Much of this occurs because of the high amounts of animal fats relative to fish and vegetable oils in our diets. Land animal fats tend to contain arachadonic acid (in the "omega 6 fatty acids" family), which stimulate inflammation. Fish oils and some vegetable oils, such as flaxseed, contain what are called "omega 3 fatty acids." These decrease inflammation. Over the last few hundred years, we have markedly decreased anti-inflammatory omega 3 fatty acids and increased proinflammatory omega 6 fats in our diet. This often results in our bodies being on "inflammatory overdrive" unnecessarily. This excess inflammation has been associated not just with an increased tendency to pain, but at times with increases in heart attacks and other diseases as well. You can sometimes see this tendency to over-inflammation in yourself when you get a paper cut. Sometimes the paper cut heals so quickly that you barely notice it's there. At other times, the same type of cut will be red and inflamed and will continue to hurt beyond the initial few seconds of the cut.

### *How Do I Decrease My Tendency to Excess Inflammation?*

Medically, we do this by using steroids such as prednisone or the Non-Steroidal Anti-Inflammatory Drugs (NSAIDs—e.g. medications in the Motrin® family). Unfortunately, both of these can be fairly toxic. In the long run, using diet and nutrition is a much safer and more effective way to get your inflammatory system into balance.

A recent study, for example, showed that taking a multivitamin can reduce inflammation with vitamin C and B6 seeming to play the largest role.[4] Many other natural therapies (see below) are also helpful in decreasing inflammation.

For acute injury, remember the old standbys. These have the initials R.I.C.E., which stand for Rest, Ice, Compression, and Elevation. These are the standard treatments recommended by coaches, trainers, and other professionals to treat muscle or joint injuries such as sprains or strains. When combined with enzymes such as Megazyme or Ultrazyme and homeopathic creams such as Traumeel® (one of several wonderful products for traumatic injuries that contains arnica), acute injuries heal much more quickly (see Appendix C). Adding another supplement called MSM can help when tissue healing is necessary (e.g. sprains or broken bones). The vitamin powder can give overall support for healing as well.

Inflammation is part of our natural healing process. Whenever there is injury, our body puts out "cytokines" in those areas to bring in white blood cells to knock out any infections and bring in other cells to begin the healing process. Because of this, healthy inflammation is a very beneficial tool that our body uses to heal. The cells come in, eliminate any infections, fix the problem, and then dissipate. When healthy, it is almost always localized and short-term.

Inflammation can become unhealthy, however. In these situations it is often generalized throughout the body. In addition to causing pain and disability, it can also cause premature aging. As noted above, anytime you see the letters "-itis" at the end of the word, it tells you that unhealthy inflammation is present. Excess inflammation is very common. For example, over 40 million Americans have arthritis. The inflammation can then damage the joints, causing deformity. Allergic rhinitis, which causes swelling of the nasal passages, is also common, affecting approximately 40 million Americans. Gastritis and colitis, which cause abdominal pain, are two other examples. Dermatitis, including psoriasis and eczema, are inflammatory illnesses of the skin. Even Alzheimer's disease and heart disease have been associated with increased inflammation. Asthma, with its associated bronchitis, is also an inflammatory condition—and one that has doubled in frequency during our lifetime. In treating these allergies and asthma, we sometimes mistakenly focus on the trigger. But the trigger is not the main problem because most people don't have problems when they come in contact with that trigger. It is more important to look at the cause of the overall reactivity in each individual.

## What Mediates Inflammation?

As noted above, the body creates inflammatory chemicals called "cytokines" in response to injury. These attract the different cells that mediate inflammation. In people with excess inflammation, the cytokine levels are elevated. Although there are a very large number of different cytokines (it is not necessary to go into all the different ones), two simple tests will tell you whether you have excess inflammation. These are the sedimentation rate (costs approximately $15) and the C Reactive Protein (CRP, which costs approximately $70). In fact, people with an elevated CRP may be three times as likely to have a heart attack—making it more sensitive than cholesterol as a predictor of future heart attacks. A normal CRP is one or less. Between one and two is considered mildly elevated. Over two is considered very elevated. Elevated CRP can also be seen in strokes, cancer, colitis, autoimmune diseases (e.g. Lupus), Alzheimer's, and many other medical problems.

All this tells us that there is a balance point where inflammation serves us, but if it is out of balance it can wreak havoc. Again, it is important not to confuse the trigger for the inflammation (e.g. inhalation and food allergens, dust, wear and tear, etc.) with why your body is prone to the inflammation. Being overly prone to inflammation, or "pro-inflammatory," means that the chemicals in your body that regulate inflammation are out of balance. Conventional medicine uses anti-inflammatory drugs to poison parts of the inflammatory system. These can be effective, but they can also result in high levels of toxicity and do not seem to prevent long-term damage like the natural approaches.

We are now beginning to understand why we are so much more prone to inflammation these days than we were in the past. As noted above, clues for understanding this can be found by looking at how the modern diet has changed over the last several thousand years.

Research shows that prehistoric hunter gatherers were much less likely to have degenerative diseases; their main problems were infection and trauma. They had a high-protein, high complex carbohydrate, and high-fiber diet. Most importantly, their diet was high in omega-3 fatty acids and low in inflammation stimulating omega 6 fatty acids (e.g. fats from meat, saturated and trans fats,shortening, margarines, and grains). Their diet was also high in antioxidants, nutrients that put out the "inflammatory fires." Foods were also unprocessed and low in refined sugar.

As society became more farming-based, our diet included more grains, and cattle were more likely to be grain fed. All this resulted in higher levels of the omega 6 pro-inflammatory fats. These omega 6 fats stimulated cytokines and inflammation. At this time, inflammation began to increase. This problem had been seen once before in recorded history in ancient Egypt. This civilization also had the osteoporosis and inflammatory diseases seen today.

Our current diet has continued to degenerate to where we are getting **12 to 20 times** as many inflammatory fats in the diet as we used to! In addition, we have a massive amount of sugar, potatoes, and white flour in our diet. This stimulates insulin resistance and release, further increasing the production of pro-inflammatory hormones (arachadonic acid) from these omega 6 fats. At the same time, our intake of antioxidants to put out these fires has markedly decreased.

### *What Does Modern Medicine Do about This?*

Doctors give anti-inflammatories like Motrin® and Celebrex®, which block conversion of the omega 6 fats to the pro-inflammatory cytokines by blocking the enzyme cyclooxygenase. Unfortunately, these also block your body's ability to make anti-inflammatory messengers. This is one reason why over 15,000 Americans a year die from these medications. We also use high dose steroids as anti-inflammatories, which used long-term, can be highly toxic. Other treatments include new tumor necrosis factor blocking medicines for rheumatoid arthritis that cost $10,000 a year. We focus on prescription medications because that's where the money is—so the pharmaceutical industry makes sure that we learn about them!

### *What Natural Alternatives Do We Have That Are Safer and Effective?*

Substituting olive oil for other oils can be very helpful. In addition, increasing fish, nuts and seeds, berries, free range chicken and grass fed meats, spices and herbs, and green leafy vegetables (not potatoes and grains) can be a very helpful start. For more information on this, there is an excellent book you can read, *The Inflammation Syndrome: The Complete Nutritional Program to Prevent and Reverse Heart Disease, Arthritis, Diabetes, Allergies, and Asthma* by Jack Challem. In addition to this book, an excellent set of two cassette tapes will help you understand excess inflammation in more detail. *Inflammation and Aging* by Ronald E. Hunninghake M.D. (Tapes 1 and 2) are available by calling 1-800-447-7276.You can either pay $10,000 a year to use the new tumor necrosis factor blocking medicines for rheumatoid arthritis, or you can take fish oil and other nutrients and clean up your diet (do it in ways that taste good)! Which one do you think the drug companies will be encouraging your doctor to recommend?

Does that mean you should only eat things that you hate? Of course not. You may find that substituting a wide variety of nuts such as peanuts, cashews, walnuts, etc. for chips and sugary snacks actually tastes better. Eating more salmon and tuna is not a big deal if you like these. If you don't like them, don't eat them. You can always add fish oil (see Appendix C: Resources) instead. Take 1/2 to 2 Tbsp daily. When you feel better you may be able to drop to 1 tsp a day.

When you're shopping for meat, go to Whole Foods Market, Wild Oats, Sprouts, or a similar store where you can get free range chicken and grass fed beef. Although it is a bit more expensive, it tastes much better, will not make you put on as much weight, and will save you a fortune on doctor bills. Olive oil is also tasty and can be used for frying, cooking, and instead of butter on your bread. Substitute stevia or saccharin for sugar. Use sugar-free chocolates (Russell Stover® makes a delicious line and there are now an enormous amount of yummy sugar-free options for those on the Atkins' diet). They taste just as good as foods with sugar but will not make you sick. In addition, as a general rule of thumb, the more colorful a vegetable the healthier it is. For example, sweet potatoes or carrots are a lot healthier than white potatoes. The vitamin powder will also supply extensive antioxidant support, simplifying the process dramatically.

The effects of treatment with diet are not subtle. In a study done at the University of Washington, it was found that women who ate 1 or 2 servings of fish a week were 22 percent less likely to have rheumatoid arthritis. Those who had more than 2 servings a week were 43 percent less likely. Those who had deep fried fish (usually fried in omega 6 fats), however, were **more** likely to have rheumatoid arthritis. In another study done in Scotland, 64 men and women with rheumatoid arthritis were given fish oil. They began to feel better in three months. By one year, they had decreased NSAID medicine use by 40 percent. There is also evidence suggesting that fish oil helps heal the joints and may decrease osteoporosis as well.

Unlike prescription medications, which can result in quick results (but some such as like steroids and NSAIDs cause long-term toxicity), natural and dietary therapies take longer to see the full effect. They are more likely, however, to build up and heal your system. I find that benefits usually start to be seen by 6 to 12 weeks and continue to build over years as the person gets healthier and healthier. Because of this, I tend to use medications as an initial "band-aid," while the natural therapies heal the underlying problem over time.

### *What Natural Anti-inflammatories Can I Use?*

In addition to using fish oil, it can be very helpful to use the End Pain formula, which contains willow bark, boswellia, and cherry (see Appendix C: Resources). These natural elements can wonderfully decrease both pain and inflammation.

### *Can You Summarize What I Need to Do?*

If you have excess inflammation, your body can often repair the damage over time. This means decreasing sugar and simple carbohydrates (keep chocolate but make it sugar free), increasing protein and healthy oils (e.g. fish, olive, nuts), and getting optimal nutritional support (e.g. the vitamin powder). Use the End Pain formula to decrease inflammation. Your dietary changes can actually be simple (similar to the Atkins' diet but using healthy fats), and will leave you younger-looking, thinner, healthier, and feeling great! ■

**Important Points**

1. Inflammation is a common cause of pain and many other medical problems that we experience in Western society. For example, anything that ends in the letters "itis" means that the problem is inflammatory. This includes things like arthritis, tendonitis, bursitis, spondylitis, appendicitis, etc.
2. Many inflammatory problems can cause a secondary fibromyalgia, which may be causing most of the symptoms. **If you have widespread pain, fatigue, and insomnia, look for and treat the associated fibromyalgia.**
3. Much of our increased tendency to inflammation occurs because of the high amounts of animal fats relative to fish and vegetable oils in our diets. Increasing fish, nuts and seeds, berries, free range chicken and grass fed meats, spices and herbs, and green leafy vegetables (not potatoes and grains) can be a very helpful start if you want to decrease inflammation.
4. For acute injury, remember the old standbys. These have the initials R.I.C.E., which stand for Rest, Ice, Compression, and Elevation.
5. In addition to dietary changes, natural remedies can be helpful in settling down inflammation. These include antioxidants, which are abundantly present in the vitamin powder. In addition, fish oil can be helpful. Begin with 1 to 2 Tbsp daily. You can then lower the dose to 1 tsp a day after 2 to 6 months as the inflammation settles. Many herbals such as willow bark, boswellia, and tart cherry, which are available in the End Pain formula, are also excellent.
6. Anti-inflammatories such as Motrin® and Celebrex® can be helpful but are more likely to cause side effects and long-term problems. Natural therapies are safer and more likely to help heal the body over time, while also decreasing pain.

**CHAPTER 12**

# Other Pains—Osteoporosis and Cancer Pain

## Osteoporosis and Bone Pain

Osteoporosis, or decreased bone density/strength, can worsen with age, inactivity, and hormonal deficiencies (estrogen, testosterone, and DHEA). Currently, the rate of osteoporosis among older women is estimated to be about 29 percent. Yet only 13 percent of older women have been diagnosed with the disease. Osteoporosis can be easily diagnosed by performing a test called a DEXA scan. Fortunately, many treatments can be effective at restoring bone strength and eliminating osteoporosis pain.

Although using calcium to increase bone density has received most of the media attention, it is actually a rather small player when it comes to improving bone strength. In addition to weight-bearing exercise and natural estrogen, many other nutrients and treatments can dramatically improve bone density and decrease bone pain. Sadly, except for calcium, most doctors only hear about expensive prescriptions such as Fosamax® and calcitonin (200 units twice a day—**use only in severe cases**). Although these can be helpful, I would certainly start first by adding the nutrients that your body needs to make strong bones.

If you already have osteoporosis, I would take Fosamax® or a related medication in addition to the treatments below. The usual dose is 70 mg once a week on an empty stomach taken with a full glass of water. It is best to take it immediately on waking and then stay upright for 30 minutes so gravity helps it get past the stomach quickly (it can irritate the stomach). For those of you on the 35 mg a week prevention dose, you should be aware that the 35 and 70 mg tablets cost exactly the same amount; you can save half the cost with a 70 mg tablet by breaking it in two. The same price for both low and high dose tablets is commonly seen with many medications.

There are many other nutrients that are critical for bone production. These include magnesium, boron, folic acid, copper, manganese, zinc, and vitamins B6, B12, D, and C. All of these are present in the Energy Revitalization System vitamin powder. In addition I recommend adding:

1. Calcium, 1000 to 1500 mg daily. Be sure you get a form that dissolves in your stomach. Unfortunately, most calcium tablets are chalk (calcium carbonate) and do not dissolve. Because of this, they go in your mouth and out the other end, doing no good along the way. If you get one that is a chewable, powder, or liquid, this is not a problem. If you get a tablet, put it in some vinegar for an hour and see if it dissolves. If it does not, it will not dissolve in your stomach either, and I recommend that brand not be used. If you are taking thyroid hormone supplements, do not take the calcium within 2 to 4 hours of the thyroid hormone or you will not absorb the thyroid hormone. In addition, make sure that your Free T4 thyroid blood test (**not** the TSH test) is not above the upper limit of normal because too high a thyroid dose can also cause osteoporosis. You may choose to take your calcium at meals and bedtime (e.g. 500 mg at lunch, dinner, and bedtime) because it is better absorbed with food, and calcium taken at night can help you to sleep.

2. Strontium. This mineral is highly effective at improving bone density. I am not speaking about strontium-90, the very dangerous radioactive compound released during nuclear testing. The strontium available in health food stores is non-radioactive and very safe—even in high doses. Studies using strontium in the treatment of 353 osteoporosis patients showed a dramatic 15 percent increase in lumbar spine bone mineral density (BMD) over 2 years in patients using 680 mg of strontium (2000 mg of strontium ranelate) a day.[1] They then repeated the placebo-controlled study with 1649 osteoporotic women. New fractures decreased by 49 percent in the first year of treatment, and bone mineral density in the lumbar spine increased by an average of 14.4 percent after 3 years. There was an 8.3 percent increase in hip BMD as well.[2] Other forms of strontium have shown similar benefits, and 680 mg of elemental strontium daily appears to be a good dose (see Appendix C: Resources). Strontium gluconate is better absorbed than strontium carbonate. If possible, take the strontium on an empty stomach and at a different time of day than the calcium, as calcium can block strontium's absorption. Early data also suggests that the strontium may also be helpful in the treatment of osteoarthritis. Although it took 3 to 36 months of therapy, taking strontium was associated with a marked reduction in bone pain in osteoporosis patients.[3]

3. Hormonal support (See Chapter 4: Hormonal Support). Make sure that your DHEA and testosterone levels are optimized, since these hormones also can improve bone density considerably. These are discussed in the section on hormonal therapies. It seems that even very low dose transdermal (by patch) estrogen replacement therapy improves bone density in menopausal women. The findings come from a study of 400 postmenopausal women aged 60 to 80 with thinning bones who received either the patch containing natural estradiol or a placebo. The results showed that women in the treatment group had improved bone density in the spine and hip and experienced reduced bone turnover. The lead investigator stated that the ultra-low dose estrogen patch offers a more natural approach to menopausal hormone therapy, because it is replacing circulating estrogen rather than increasing it. This study's results were presented at the 52nd Annual Clinical Meeting of the American College of Obstetricians and Gynecologists (ACOG) 2004 held in Philadelphia.
4. Fish oil (see Appendix C: Resources). Fish oil also may decrease osteoporosis. You can either increase your intake of salmon and tuna or use fish oil 1 to 2 tsp a day.[4]

## Cancer Pain

It is unacceptable for cancer patients to be in pain, and the treatments discussed in this book can be very helpful in eliminating cancer pain as well. Most pain is coming from tissue invasion or muscle spasm. Treat these pains as discussed elsewhere in the book. In addition, nutritional deficiencies are rampant in cancer patients and can contribute markedly to the pain and disability. I strongly recommend that most cancer patients take the vitamin powder (see Appendix C: Resources; one can lower the dose if diarrhea is present). As an aside, there are many treatments that can help cancer that your oncologist may not be aware of (usually because they are too <u>in</u>expensive). I recommend that any patient with a significant cancer order a search of medical studies done on their specific type and stage of cancer from Health Resources. They do a spectacular job (call Jan Guthrie at 800-949-0090 for more information). This report routinely turns up valuable treatment options that most doctors are not aware of. I have seen "incurable cancers" go away when the patient combines the best of the standard and complementary therapies that are found in the printout's studies. As an example, my research associate has now been cancer-free for over five years despite having had an ovarian cancer metastatic to her neck!

Here are a few additional thoughts for treating cancer discomfort:

A. For uncontrollable nausea, use ABHR cream applied to an area of soft skin, such as the wrist. This prescription cream contains lorazepam, Benadryl®, Haldol®, and metoclopramide, and can be made by compounding pharmacists (who can also guide you in its proper use). Nausea often settles within 15 to 30 minutes after applying the medication. The cream can be reapplied every 6 hours as needed. Promethazine® 25 mg per 1/2 cc of cream is also helpful for nausea.

B. In addition to causing severe pain, cancer that has spread to bone to can also make the bones weak and susceptible to fracture. Because of this, treatments that improve bone density (see information on osteoporosis above) may decrease bone pain as well. If you have breast cancer, do not use DHEA without your doctor's approval. In one study of patients with bone metastases from breast or prostate cancer, strontium gluconate (the healthy form—not the radioactive one), 274 mg daily, increased bone re-growth in areas of tumor, and often resulted in patients feeling better and gaining weight.[5] I would use the 680 mg a day dose discussed above (see Appendix C: Resources).

C. Cancer often triggers muscle/myofascial pain, and treating this (see Chapter 9 on fibromyalgia/myofascial pain) can result in more comfort and the patient needing less pain medicine and therefore having less side effects. In addition, a study by Dr. Neoh Choo Aun, a wonderful acupuncturist and friend in Taiwan, showed that using acupuncture to treat the trigger points in cancer patients was very beneficial.[6]

D. In one study of 12 patients with very severe neuropathic, or nerve pain, due to the cancer pushing on major nerve centers, IV magnesium was given. Half the patients received 500 mg and the other half 1000 mg given over 10 minutes. Aside from producing a mild feeling of warmth at the time of the injection, the IV was well-tolerated. 10 of the 12 patients experienced significant relief that lasted approximately four hours.[7] I would give 2 grams of magnesium over 30-60 minutes. Most patients with neuropathic pain will not need this—although it can easily be given if they have an IV in place—if they simply use the medications we discuss in Chapter 8 on neuropathies.

E. It takes much less medication to prevent pain than to make it go away once it occurs. Because of this, if you have chronic pain, take the medication before you expect the pain to occur, or at the first sign of it coming back, instead of waiting for it to be severe. You'll need less pain medicine and have fewer side effects. If narcotic side effects are problematic, ask your doctor to use the other pain medications we discuss in the book as well so you can find a combination that is more comfortable. In addition, Chapter 22 on prescription therapies discusses how to treat many narcotic side effects. Using Fentanyl® patches can be very helpful because they give steady release of pain medication, are powerful, and can be taken even if nausea or confusion is present. ■

**Important Points**

**Osteoporosis and Bone Pain**

1. Taking calcium plays a modest role in improving bone strength. Take 1000 to 1500 mg/day with meals or at bedtime, and not within 2 to 4 hours of taking thyroid hormone.
2. Also take the Energy Revitalization System vitamin powder, because magnesium, boron, folic acid, copper, manganese, zinc, and vitamins B6, B12, D, and C are all important in treating osteoporosis.
3. Take strontium 680 mg/day as well. This nutrient can amazingly increase bone density by over 7 percent a year safely and inexpensively. It can also help osteoarthritis.
4. DHEA, testosterone and estrogen replacement (using the safer **natural forms**) can also help with bone pain.
5. Fosamax® (Rx) 70 mg once a week can also be worthwhile in relieving bone pain.

**Cancer Pain**

1. It is unacceptable for cancer patients to be in pain. Treatments discussed in this book can be very helpful in eliminating cancer pain as well. Most pain is coming from tissue/nerve invasion or muscle spasm. Treat these pains as discussed elsewhere in the book (see Chapter 22 on prescription therapies).

*Continued on next page*

**Important Points** *(continued)*

2. It takes much less medication to prevent pain than to make it go away once it occurs. Because of this, if you have chronic pain, take the medication before you expect the pain to occur, or at first sign of it coming back, instead of waiting for it to be severe. You'll need less pain medicine and have fewer side effects.
3. I recommend that any patient with a significant cancer order a search of medical studies done on their specific type and stage of cancer from Health Resources (Call Jan Guthrie at 800-949-0090 for more information). I have seen "incurable cancers" go away when the patient combines the best of standard and complementary therapies.
4. For uncontrollable nausea, use ABHR cream applied to an area of soft skin, such as the wrist. This prescription cream can be made by compounding pharmacists, who can also guide you in its proper use, and contains lorazepam, Benadryl®, Haldol®, and metoclopramide.
5. Treatments that improve bone density may decrease bone pain as well.

# Section 4

# *Evaluating and Treating Common Pains Based on Their Locations*

*The person who says it cannot be done should not interrupt the person doing it."*

-Chinese Proverb

### *Another Cause of Headache*

A pirate walks into a bar and the bartender says, "Hey, I haven't seen you in awhile. You look terrible. What happened?"

*"What do you mean?" replies the pirate, "I feel fine."*

"What about the wooden leg? You didn't have that before."

*"Well, we were in a battle and I got hit with a cannonball, but I'm perfectly fine now."*

"That's good," says the bartender, "but what about that hook? What the heck happened to your hand?"

*"We were in another battle. I boarded a ship and got into a big sword fight. My hand was cut off so I got fitted with a hook. I'm fine, really."*

"Well, what about that eye patch?"

*"Oh, one day we were at sea and a flock of birds flew over. I looked up and one of them birds pooped in my eye."*

"You're kidding," says the bartender, "You couldn't lose an eye just from some bird poop."

*"It was my first day with the hook."*

CHAPTER 13

# Headaches and Facial Pain

## Headaches

Headaches are a major source of chronic pain. Although most people get an occasional headache, as many as 45 million Americans get them on a regular basis. Headache related lost work and medical expenses costs $50 billion per year in the U.S. alone. Over $4 billion a year is spent on over-the-counter headache relievers.[1-2] Headaches are problematic in about 10 to 18 percent of the general population, and 10 percent of patients identified headache as the reason for their doctor visits.[3]

### *Tension Headaches*

Tension headaches account for about three quarters of all headaches. They cause moderate pain on both sides of, and across, the forehead, tend to both start and fade away gradually, and are the result of muscle tightness coming from the sternocleidomastoid muscles in the neck. These muscles begin behind the bottom of the ear and come around the neck to the top of the collar bone (clavicle). They are the muscles that turn your head from side to side. With tension headaches you can often find a tender knot right in the middle of the muscle. This knot, called a "trigger point," refers pain and tenderness to the sides of your forehead (the temple area), and then sends the pain across your forehead. Although putting a hot compress or the pain creams on the temples and across the forehead may help temporarily, they are more effective when placed over the tender knots in the muscles on both sides of the neck.

Occasionally, tension headaches are felt at the base of the skull, on the top of the head, and/or behind the eyes. For these headaches, the pain is often coming from the muscles where they attach to the base of the skull at the top of the back of your neck. If you push on those muscles (called the sub-occipital muscles) where they attach at the base of the skull during a headache, they will be very tender and can make the headache better or worse. When the pain is reproduced by pushing on the area, you know that these muscles are part of the source of that headache. If this is the case, use heat and the pain creams over those tender areas.

### How Can I Make the Headaches Go Away and Stay Away?

Because tension headaches are muscular, the same treatments (discussed in Chapter 9 on myofascial and fibromayalgia pain) that cause your muscles to relax will often eliminate the recurrence of these headaches. These are nutritional support, hormonal support, getting at least eight hours of sleep at night, and treating underlying infections. Paying attention to structural factors can also help (see Chapter 6: Body Work, Structural Issues and Trauma).

While you are treating the underlying causes of your muscle pain, many medications can also be used to prevent chronic tension headaches. Anti-depressants can help headache and other pains as well as depression. In one study comparing Elavil® 25 mg at bedtime with Remeron 30 mg at bedtime, both groups had less headaches but the Remeron® group had fewer side effects.[4] Both of these medications are likely to be more effective for tension headaches than Paxil 40 mg daily, which had only a mild effect.[5]

### What Can I Do for the Acute Pain?

Herbal remedies such as the End Pain formula (see Appendix C: Resources), which contains willow bark, boswellia, and cherry, can be very helpful for acute attacks as can the natural and prescription pain gels (see Chapters 20 and 22). A physical therapy technique called stretch and spray, which approximately 10 percent of physical therapists are familiar with, is also an excellent and pain free way to release your muscles and eliminate a tension headache. When the underlying metabolic (e.g. infections, sleep, nutritional and hormonal deficiencies) and structural factors have been treated, stretch and spray may result in permanent relief of the pain. In addition, there are, of course, the old standbys of chiropractic and body work as well as Tylenol® and Motrin®/Advil®. Other medications that can be quite helpful include Midrin® and Ultram®. I would begin with the natural therapies first, however, as I think these are both more effective and much safer.

### Migraines

These headaches can be very severe and often leave people crippled for days. They may afflict as many as 28 million Americans. Migraines are often preceded by an "aura," which may consist of visual disturbances such as flashing lights. The headaches are often associated with nausea, sweats, dizziness, and slurred speech. Light and sound sensitivity can also be severe.

There is still marked debate over the cause of migraines. For decades, researchers thought that these occurred because of excessive contraction and expansion of the blood vessels in the brain. Others thought that this blood vessel problem occurred because of inadequate serotonin, the neurotransmitter that controls sleep and mood, which also plays a role in how blood vessels expand. Low serotonin also amplifies pain by increasing the pain neurotransmitter called substance P. Muscle spasm and nutritional imbalances and deficiencies can also contribute to migraines as can food sensitivities. Most likely, it is a common endpoint for many different underlying problems.

Effective migraine treatment is important. Not only are migraines horribly painful for many people, but they are expensive as well. The average amount of work missed by those with migraines is 19.6 days a year, costing employers $3000 per year per employee. It is also undertreated, with 31 percent of migraine patients never having sought treatment.[6]

## *What Medications Can I Take to Get Rid of an Acute Migraine Headache?*

In the U.S., medications in the Imitrex® family still remain the first choice. This new family of medications, called triptans, has dramatically increased our ability to treat migraine headaches effectively. Imitrex comes in 25, 50, and 100 mg tablets, and up to 100 mg may be taken at a time. If pain persists at 2 hours, another dose of up to 100 mg can be taken. In addition, it is also available by nasal spray, using a dose of up to 20 mg initially, followed by one more spray of up to 20 mg 2 hours later if needed. Another alternative is a 6 mg subcutaneous injection, which can also be repeated 1 hour later if needed. It is reasonable to try these different forms to see what works best for your migraines. You may also want to try a newer cousin called Amerge®. Use 2.5 mg initially. This dose may be repeated 4 hours later if needed. Your physician may also use other related medications such as Zomig®, Axert®, or Relpax®.

Imitrex has been found to be effective in eliminating an acute migraine attack in 34 to 70 percent of patients within 2 hours. Unfortunately, at least 30 to 40 percent of patients remained unsuccessfully treated.[7] Axert® (almotriptan 6.5 to 12.5 mg, which can be repeated in 2 hours) is similar in effectiveness to Imitrex but less expensive ($10.50 vs. $16.50).

Other treatments may be effective for acute migraines when Imitrex is not. Aspirin family medications do not work well in migraines because the absorption of aspirin is delayed during the migraine attack. To combat this problem, medications that enhance absorption can be added to the aspirin and/or it can be given by suppository. For example, a combination of indomethacin (a "super-aspirin"), prochlorperazine (for nausea and to enhance absorption), and caffeine in suppository form were compared with Sumatriptan® rectal suppositories for acute migraines. Forty-nine percent of patients were pain free at 2 hours on the first treatment as compared to 34 percent with the Sumatriptan.[8] Another study using a similar approach had the same result. Aspirin (lysine acetyl salicylates 1620 mg—equivalent to 900 mg of aspirin) was combined with Metoclopramide®, 10 mg. The latter medication returns the absorption of aspirin to normal during migraine attacks and also combats nausea and vomiting. In the two placebo-controlled studies, this combination was more effective than 100 mg of Imitrex by mouth and was better tolerated.[9-11] These combinations can be made by compounding pharmacists (see Appendix C: Resources). It is quite likely that regular aspirin, especially if chewed, would be as effective as the form used in the study. Metoclopramide is readily available.

Other medications can also be helpful for acute migraines. Many patients get relief with Midrin®, which is a mix of three medications. Take 2 capsules immediately followed by 1 capsule every hour until the headache is relieved (to a maximum of 5 capsules within a 12 hour period). It can also be helpful for tension headaches in a dose of 2 capsules up to 4 times a day, as needed. Many patients find this to be quite helpful and it is not addictive. Fiorinal® can also be effective but is addictive, and I prefer not to use this medication.

A fascinating study can guide you as to when to use Imitrex family medications vs. when to go with other therapies. At last years' American Academy of Neurology meeting, Dr. Burstein of Harvard Medical School noted that 75 percent of migraine patients get painful sensitivity to normal touch (e.g. from eyeglasses) around their eyes. This pain is created in a different part of the brain than the throbbing pain that gets worse with movement or coughing. The study found that if you use Imitrex before you get the tenderness/pain around the eyes, it will knock out the migraine 93 percent of the time. If the pain/tenderness around the eyes had already set in, Imitrex only eliminated the migraine 13 percent of the time (although it still helped the throbbing). In other words, if you are one of the lucky ones who does not get pain around the eyes, the Imitrex can knock out your migraine at any time. If you are one of those who gets pain/tenderness around the eyes, it is a race against the clock to take the Imitrex before that pain starts. This means that you need to take the Imitrex early in the attack (within the first 5 to 20 minutes), before the skin hypersensitivity gets established. For example, use it at the earliest warning signs like painful scalp or discomfort from wearing your glasses, shaving or wearing earrings. If the pain has already fully set in before you take the Imitrex, consider using one of the other acute treatments we've discussed.[12]

Because of the nausea and light/sound sensitivity, anti-nausea medications can also be helpful. Phenergan® or Compazine® suppositories are two such medications.

## What Natural Remedies Can I Use to Knock Out an Acute Migraine?

Two natural treatments can knock out an acute migraine. The first, which you can take at home on your own, is butterbur. This herb can both prevent and eliminate migraines. Take 50 mg 3 times a day for 1 month and then 50 mg twice a day to prevent migraines. You can take 100 mg every 3 hours to eliminate an acute migraine. Use only high quality brands (see Appendix C: Resources). Many others that were tested had impurities and did **not** contain the amount of butterbur the label claimed (i.e. they don't work).

In a hospital emergency room or a doctor's office, intravenous magnesium can effectively eliminate an acute migraine. In one study of 30 patients with moderate or severe migraine attacks, half received 1 g of magnesium sulfate IV over 15 minutes and the other half placebo. Those in the placebo group who were not better at a one half-hour were then treated with the magnesium. Immediately after treatment, at 30 minutes, and at 2 hours, 86 percent in the magnesium group were pain-free with the other 14 percent showing a reduction in pain. Associated symptoms such as nausea, light sensitivity, and irritability also resolved, and none of the patients in the magnesium group had a recurrence of pain within 24 hours. In the placebo group, no patient became pain free, and only one had a reduction in pain. When patients in the placebo group were later given the magnesium, responses were similar to subjects in the other magnesium treated group. Mild side effects, which are a normal effect of magnesium working to open blood vessels, such as a burning sensation in the face and neck, flushing, and a drop in blood pressure of 5 to 10 mm systolic occurred in 86 percent of the patients. None of these side effects was serious, and no patient had to discontinue the treatment.[13] These results were similar to those in previous reports.[14–15]

## What if I Still Can't Make the Migraine Attack Go Away?

Unfortunately, sometimes the treatments discussed above are not effective. Because of this, and largely because most people are not aware of all the treatment options, over 800,000 Americans per year visit hospital emergency rooms for treatment of their migraines. This is an expensive proposition; it often runs over $500 per emergency room visit. In addition, the average time spent in the emergency room is four hours. Because the person usually needs to have somebody drive them, this can be multiplied by 2. Therefore, it is helpful for people to have "rescue medication" that they can use instead of having to go to the emergency room. A number of options are available to serve this purpose. One such remedy is the use of "Fentanyl lollipops," known as "oral transmucosal fentanyl citrate" (OTFC, ACTIQ). Fentanyl lollipops (ACTIQ) should be intermittently sucked on, not chewed or swallowed. In between being sucked on, the lollipop should be left between the cheek and lower gum. Time the sucking so that it takes approximately 15 minutes for the medication to be absorbed into your cheek. This makes it more effective. ACTIQ comes in six strengths (200 to 1600 mcg). It begins to work within 5 to 10 minutes, with pain relief lasting approximately 3 hours. Its effectiveness is similar to 2 to 16 mg of intravenous morphine. The most commonly used doses are 400 and 800 micrograms. Because these medications are only approved by the FDA for use in patients who are on chronic narcotics, it is reasonable to have you (if you are not already on chronic narcotic pain medications) take the first dose in a doctor's office to make sure that it does not cause a dangerous level of sedation. Like other narcotics, this medication can be highly habituating. Because of this, it should only be used as a rescue medication when other medications have failed. Once you have tried the 200 and 400 mcg doses and know that they are not too sedating, begin with a 400 micrograms dose over 15 minutes. If adequate pain relief is not achieved 10 minutes later (i.e. 25 minutes after beginning the first lollipop), use another 200 or 400 mcg unit every 25 minutes until adequate pain control is achieved or you reach 1200 micrograms. The average dose needed is 800 micrograms.

In one study using this approach, all 28 of the patients in the study were able to avoid having to go to the emergency room, with 27 of the 28 patients routinely getting significant relief from pain (decreasing to a "mild" level). The medication was well tolerated with the main side effect being nausea in 18 percent of patients. A few patients had itching that was easily relieved by Benadryl®. Side effects were much less than normally experienced with the usual "rescue medication" (Demerol®).[16]

### *I'm Happy I Can Eliminate an Acute Migraine Headache, but How Can I Prevent Them?*

In addition to being able to treat acute migraines more effectively, many medications can prevent them. Together, these medications reduce the number of headache days per month by an average of 50 percent.[17]

These medications include beta-blockers (Inderal®), calcium channel blockers, Neurontin®, Depakote®, Topamax®, Elavil®, and Doxepin®. Although Inderal XL can be helpful, it may aggravate fatigue, asthma, or depression. Another medication that can be helpful is Zonegran 100 mg. This is an anti-seizure medication. Begin with 100 mg a day for 2 weeks and then increase to 2 tablets a day. The maximum dose is 400 mg daily, although most of the benefit occurs at the first 200 mg. Because there have been rare occurrences of a life-threatening rash (most rashes caused by the medication are not, however), stop the medication immediately if you get a rash. Do not use this medication if you are allergic to sulfa drugs.

Fortunately, natural remedies are even more effective in preventing migraines. They may take up to 3 months to start working, however, so the above medications can be used while you're waiting for the natural preventives to take effect. Magnesium by mouth has been found to be effective for migraine prevention and is as effective as Elavil®.[18] Magnesium serves in an enormous number of functions in the body, including the relaxation of muscles and arteries. Most Americans get nowhere near the optimum amount of magnesium in their diet, getting less than 250 mg a day as opposed to the 650 mg that the average Chinese diet supplies. Blood testing to check magnesium levels are horribly unreliable and may not detect magnesium deficiency until it is severe.

A leading authority on natural prevention of migraine headaches is Dr. Alexander Mauskop, author of *What Your Doctor May Not Tell You about Migraines.* As discussed above, in 1995 Dr. Mauskop published a study showing that intravenous magnesium could abort a migraine headache.[19] He also found that intravenous magnesium could knock out other types of headaches as well.[20] This powerful data spurred researchers to see whether magnesium could also prevent migraines. As noted above, the answer was yes. In one German placebo-controlled study patients were given 600 mg of magnesium daily for 12 weeks or a placebo; there was a significant drop in migraine frequency in the magnesium group.[21] Another study shows similar effects in women with menstrual migraines (see below).[22] It is a good idea for most migraine patients to take 150 to 200 mg of magnesium in the morning (present in the vitamin powder) and again with dinner or at bedtime (less if diarrhea is a problem).

Riboflavin (vitamin B2) assists in the production of energy. In one study, migraine patients were given riboflavin 400 mg with breakfast every day for at least 3 months. By the end of the study they had a 67 percent decrease in migraine attacks as well as a decrease in attack severity. This was later repeated in a placebo-controlled study.[23] Note that it can take 3 months for the riboflavin to start working.

Vitamin B12 can also decrease migraine frequency. In one study in which patients received 1000 micrograms a day as a nasal spray, migraine frequencies decreased by an average of 43 percent after 3 months (the vitamin powder/B-complex contains 500 micrograms a day).[24]

Feverfew is another helpful herb for migraine prevention.[25] Using feverfew has resulted in a significant reduction in migraines in one-third of patients. It was also found to be very safe.[26]

Butterbur is a shrub which grows in Europe, Asia, and Africa. A standardized extract called Petadolex® was used in two double-blind studies. By the third month, those receiving active treatment with 100 mg a day had 60 percent fewer migraine attacks than the control group. Although 100 mg a day is effective, 75 mg twice a day with food may be the optimal dose.[27]

Fish oil has also been found to decrease the frequency of migraines. In two placebo-controlled studies of patients with frequent severe migraines that did not respond to medication, fish oil (see Appendix C: Resources) was found to be effective. Use 1 to 2 Tbsp a day and give the treatment 6 weeks to see the effect. Then you can decrease it to the lowest dose that maintains the benefit.[28 - 29]

Other natural compounds that may be helpful include glucosamine 1500 to 2000 mg a day (this compound was found to be helpful in a small study of 10 patients over 4 to 6 weeks). Coenzyme Q10, 150-200 mg daily, decreased the average number of migraine attacks per month from 4.8 to 2.8 in an open study.[30]

All this suggests that many, if not most, migraines can be prevented naturally. I would begin by taking the vitamin powder plus 300 mg of Vitamin B 2 in the morning, plus 200 mg of magnesium at night. If the cost is not prohibitive, I would add butterbur as well. Also check for food allergies, as noted below, and follow the advice for hormones if the migraines are predominately around your periods or associated with taking estrogen. I have seen this approach commonly eliminate frequent and horribly severe migraine problems, but remember that it may take 3 months to see the effect.

## *What Else Can I Do to Eliminate the Underlying Cause of the Migraines?*

Acupuncture is another option to consider for chronic migraine and tension headaches. It results in reduced pain, reduced frequency of headaches, and improved function, energy, and health. In two studies conducted in New York City and London, acupuncture was found to be cost-effective. In a randomized controlled study of 401 patients with chronic headaches (the majority having migraines), patients received up to 12 acupuncture treatments over a 3-month period vs. a control group that received standard care. The acupuncture patients had 22 fewer headache days per year, 15 percent fewer sick days, and 25 percent fewer visits to the doctor.[31]

Food allergies are also very important to consider. Approximately 30 to 50 percent of migraine patients get marked improvement by avoiding certain foods, and most people with migraines are not aware of what foods are triggering their headaches. This has now been demonstrated in at least four placebo-controlled studies. Food sensitivities are an even bigger problem in children with migraines.[32 - 35] To determine if foods are playing a role in causing your headache, it is helpful to do an elimination diet. This requires eating a very limited diet for five days. Eat only pears and lamb, and drink only bottled spring or distilled water. This kind of strict elimination diet will make it easier to tell if food allergies/sensitivities are present and triggering your migraines when you reintroduce foods into your diet. In one study, by avoiding the ten most common food triggers, subjects exhibited a dramatic reduction in the number of headaches per month, with 85 percent becoming headache free. Twenty-five percent of the patients with high blood pressure also had their blood pressure reduce to normal. The most common reactive foods were wheat in 78 percent of patients, oranges in 65 percent, eggs in 45 percent, tea and coffee in 40 percent each, chocolate and milk in 37 percent each, beef in 35 percent, and corn, cane sugar, and yeast in 33 percent each. Some studies also suggest that the artificial sweetener aspartame (NutraSweet®) can trigger migraines and other headaches, although this is controversial.[36 - 37] If you have severe and frequent migraines, it is definitely worth exploring food sensitivities.[38] You may find that instead of avoiding foods that trigger your migraines for the rest of your life, you can eliminate the sensitivities/allergies using a powerfully effective acupressure technique called NAET (see www.NAET.com).

## Estrogen Induced Migraines

In many women, migraines are triggered by a sudden drop in estrogen level. Because of this, migraines are often worse on the two days before or after the day the period starts. For those taking estrogen replacement or the birth control pill, the headaches may occur in the hours before the next dose of therapy is due (i.e. as the estrogen level is dropping). In these situations, the key is to prevent the dropping estrogen level. One way to do this is to use an estrogen patch for one week beginning a few days before your period is expected (e.g. a Climara® .025 patch). For those on the pill, switch to a different form of birth control if you get the headaches throughout your cycle. If you only get the headache for the week that you stop the pill, consider taking the pill every day and stopping it only one week every 5 months. For that week, use the estrogen patch noted above. Anti-inflammatory aspirin family medications like Motrin® and Aleve® may be helpful in combination with Imitrex® related medications in estrogen associated headaches.

### *What Are Some Other Common Causes of Severe Headaches?*

**Sinusitis** is another common cause of headaches. It is usually associated with pain and tenderness over the sinuses by the cheeks or above the eyes. Nasal congestion, often with yellow/green nasal mucus, is also common. Interestingly, I have found that most cases of chronic sinusitis are associated with yeast overgrowth. These fungal infections (similar to vaginal yeast infections but occurring predominantly in the bowels) cause an allergic-type reaction resulting in swelling of the nasal passages. This swelling blocks the sinuses resulting in a secondary bacterial infection (when the mucous turns yellow-green), which is very painful. You then get antibiotics from your doctor that knock out the bacterial infection but worsen the yeast/fungal infection and the nasal congestion. Things then get blocked up again, re-infected, and you are off to the doctor for another antibiotic (and more yeast problems). This is why sinusitis usually becomes chronic. I have found that when you treat the yeast overgrowth by taking Diflucan® for 6 weeks and avoiding sugar (see Chapter 5: Infections), most chronic sinusitis will go away. Adding silver nose spray (see Appendix C: Resources) is also worthwhile. It is also helpful to use a special prescription nose spray that contains antibacterials and anti-fungals. Your doctor can order it by calling Cape Apothecary at 410-757-3522 and asking for "Dr. Teitelbaum's nose spray." Use 1 to 2 sprays in each nostril twice a day. If it is irritating, then it is too concentrated for you. If this occurs, simply add a small amount of salt water. Patients find this to be enormously helpful. If fungal overgrowth is causing your chronic sinusitis, it may also be causing spastic colon, which also often resolves when you treat the yeast. Unfortunately, many doctors still consider the possibility of "yeast overgrowth" to be nonsense—just as occurred in medicine when we first began to understand about bacterial infections. Because of this, you may have to go to a holistic/complementary physician to get the treatment you need (See Appendix C: Resources and visit www.vitality101.com for information on how to find a holistic doctor).

**Caffeine withdrawal headaches** are common in people who drink coffee. It is especially common in the morning before people get their coffee "fix" and may occur approximately 18 hours after their last cup of coffee. It often begins with a feeling of fullness in one's head and may be aggravated by exercise. Slowly decreasing your caffeine intake by about 1 cup daily each week, and perhaps mixing decaf with regular coffee as part of your weaning process, can help. Other people prefer to simply go "cold turkey," tough out the headache and be done with it.

**Cluster headaches** occur as a repeating series of headaches that can each last 30 to 90 minutes and are very severe. They cause excruciating, piercing pain on one side of the head (often centered around one eye) and are much more common in men. Many medications can help. These include anti-seizure medications like Depakote® (Valproic acid) 500 to 1000 mg a day or Topamax® 50 to 100 mg a day. These often start to work in 1 to 2 weeks.[39] Lithium 300 mg 3 times a day can also prevent cluster headaches. High dose Lithium must be monitored with blood levels because it can cause an underactive thyroid, tremors, and other toxicity. The tremors and neurologic toxicity can be decreased by taking a few tsp of expeller-pressed safflower oil each day (from your local health food store).

**Trigeminal Neuralgia** affects a large cranial nerve and is characterized by excruciating attacks of stabbing, shooting pain in the lips, gums, cheek, or chin that last for a few seconds to minutes. It occurs almost exclusively in the middle-aged and elderly. It often responds well to treatment with the medications Tegretol® and/or Neurontin®.

In some headaches, there may actually be increased pressure in the brain. Some practitioners have found that using Diamox® (a diuretic) 125 to 500 mg once or twice daily decreases these headaches. Carbonated beverages will taste funny while you're on this medication.

**Jaw Joint Dysfunction (TMJ/TMD)**. Temporo Mandibular Joint Dysfunction (TMJ/TMD) is a common cause of facial pain and headaches. Although classically considered to come from the jaw joint (the area just in front of your ears), in many cases the pain is actually coming from tightness of the Masseter muscles, which can pull the jaw out of alignment. The Masseter is the very powerful muscle we use to chew our food, and I've been told it can generate 1000 pounds of pressure per square inch. TMJ can occur when this muscle goes into spasm/shortening. This can be caused by a poor bite, but also by all the other factors we discuss under fibromyalgia and myofascial pain in Chapter 9. By treating these same issues (sleep, hormonal deficiencies, infections, and nutritional support) the Masseter muscles often release and the pain goes away. Because of this, dentists often come to my pain workshops and use these treatments.

A simple way to tell if this muscle is contributing to the pain is to put your thumb into your mouth and put it between your molars (the teeth at the end) while also placing your second and third fingers about 2 inches in front of your earlobe. You will feel a muscle between your thumb and fingers. Squeeze the muscle between your thumb and fingers and see if it produces much pain/tenderness. If so, your TMJ pain may be coming from the muscle and not the joint. Zanaflex®, like other treatments for muscle pain, can be very helpful. In one study, 2 mg of Zanaflex was taken 2 times a day for 2 weeks by people with jaw muscle pain. By the end of the treatment period, all of the patients had improved; 42 patients (53.8 percent) showed absence of clinical symptoms; 18 (23.1 percent) showed a good improvement, while still presenting a low number of painful sites; 18 (23.1 percent) showed only a slight improvement.[40]

It is also important to be aware that pain and hot /cold sensitivity in your teeth can come from tight muscles in the face—despite your teeth being totally healthy. It is frightening to see how many people have had unnecessary root canals because their doctor/dentist is not familiar with these pain referral patterns. For tooth pain in the lower jaw, push on the muscles right below those teeth to see if they are tender. Pain in the upper teeth can be referred from the Masseter muscle (just in front of the ears) or the Pteregoid muscle (a large area by the temples). If these are tender and you do not have obvious tooth problems on your x-ray/exam, try the pain creams and /or Lidoderm® patches and a **gentle** massage over those tender muscles 3 times a day for a few weeks to see if you can eliminate the dental pain. These dental pain referral patterns are described at length (along with treatment) in *The Trigger Point Manual* by Dr. Janet Travell and Dr. David Simons, which is the best pain book for doctors ever written. Treating these muscles first is a lot more fun than having root canals or having your teeth pulled unnecessarily!

In some cases of jaw joint pain, the discomfort is coming from the jaw joint itself. Often, the bite is not in alignment, and this aggravates the pain. Treating the bite can help. In addition, it is helpful to be sure that you do not grind your teeth at night (bruxism) and to have your dentist give you a mouth guard if you do. Often the x-ray will show arthritis or cartilage slipping/loss in the jaw joint. Some dentists recommend surgery in these situations. I usually recommend that other measures be tried first.

Another form of dental pain is "burning mouth syndrome." This syndrome is characterized by chronic pain on the tongue and sometimes the anterior palate and lips without any visible lesions. It is most common in postmenopausal women and has characteristics suggestive of neuropathic pain. Lipoic acid is an antioxidant that has been shown to be beneficial for diabetic neuropathy. Another study showed that it was also helpful in burning mouth syndrome. In a study of 60 patients, half received 200 mg of lipoic acid 3 times a day and the other half a placebo for 2 to 5 months. Ninety-seven percent of the patients improved versus

40 percent of those in the placebo group. 13 percent had complete resolution of their pain and another 74 percent had "decided improvement," whereas none of the placebo patients had this level of improvement. Almost all of the patients showed some improvement by 2 months with 73 percent still showing benefit at the end of 12 months despite having stopped the treatment.[41] With burning mouth caused by cancer treatment (called mucositis), using a ketamine mouth rinse (from compounding pharmacists) can help. ■

### Important Points

1. **Tension Headaches** cause moderate pain on both sides of, and across, the forehead; They tend to both start and fade away gradually and are the result of muscle tightness, often coming from the sternocleidomastoid muscles in the neck.
2. Because tension headaches are muscular, the same treatments discussed in Chapter 9, which cause your muscles to relax, will often eliminate the recurrence of these headaches. Paying attention to structural factors can also help.
3. Many medications can be used to prevent chronic tension headaches. These include anti-depressants such as Remeron® 15 to 30 mg or Elavil® 10 to 50 mg at bedtime.
4. To treat the acute pain, begin with herbal remedies such as the End Pain formula, which contains willow bark, boswellia, and cherry. This can be very helpful for acute attacks as well as chronic pain. A physical therapy technique called stretch and spray, which approximately 10 percent of physical therapists are familiar with, is also an excellent and pain-free way to release your muscles and eliminate a tension headache. In addition, there are, of course, the old standbys of Tylenol® and Motrin®/Advil®. Other medications that can be quite helpful include Midrin and Ultram. I would begin with the natural therapies first, however, as I think these are more effective and safer.
5. Migraine headaches can be very severe and usually last for several days. Migraines are often preceded by an "aura," which may consist of visual disturbances such as flashing lights. The headaches are often associated with nausea, sweats, dizziness, and light and sound sensitivity.

*Continued on next page*

**Important Points** *(continued)*

6. In the U.S., medications in the Imitrex® family still remain the first choice for the treatment of acute migraines. A combination of indomethacin (a "super-aspirin"), prochlorperazine (for nausea and to enhance absorption), and caffeine in suppository form is commonly used in Italy and is even more effective (it can be made up by compounding pharmacies). Midrin®, which is a mix of three medications, can be effective. 2 capsules are taken immediately followed by 1 capsule every hour until the headache is relieved (to a maximum of 5 capsules within a 12 hour period).

7. A fascinating study can guide you on when to use Imitrex family medications vs. when to go with other therapies. 75 percent of migraine patients get painful sensitivity to normal touch (e.g. wearing eyeglasses) around their eyes. If you use Imitrex before you get the tenderness/pain around the eyes, it will knock out the migraine 93 percent of the time. If the pain/tenderness around the eyes had already set in, Imitrex only eliminated the migraine 13 percent of the time (although it still helped the throbbing). In other words, if you are one of the lucky ones who does not get pain around the eyes, the Imitrex can knock out your migraine at any time. If you are one of those who do get pain/tenderness around the eyes, it is a race against the clock to take the Imitrex before that pain starts. This means take the Imitrex early in the attack (the first 5 to 20 minutes) before the skin hypersensitivity gets established.

8. Anti-nausea medications can also be helpful. Phenergan® or Compazine® suppositories can be helpful. Another excellent alternative is ABHR cream (applied to an area of soft skin, such as the wrist). This prescription cream can be made by compounding pharmacists (who can also guide you in its proper use) and contains lorazepam, Benadryl®, Haldol®, and metoclopramide.

9. There are two natural treatments that can knock out an acute migraine. Butterbur can both prevent and eliminate migraines. Take 50 mg 3 times a day for 1 month and then 1 twice a day to prevent migraines. You can take 100 mg every 3 hours to eliminate an acute migraine. In the hospital emergency room or doctor's office, intravenous magnesium can effectively eliminate an acute migraine.

*Continued on next page*

**Important Points** *(continued)*

10. For patients with severe migraines who often need to go to the ER, and if the above treatments are not adequate, it is helpful to have a "rescue medication" for home use. ACTIQ (fentanyl lollipops) can be used at home and are as effective as intravenous morphine. The average dose needed is 800 mcg.
11. Many if not most migraines can be prevented naturally. I recommend taking the vitamin powder plus 300 mg of Vitamin B2 (Riboflavin) in the morning, plus 200 mg of magnesium at night. If the cost is not prohibitive, I would add butterbur 75 mg 2 times a day as well (you can use 100 mg once a day but it is not as effective). Natural approaches can commonly eliminate even frequent and horribly severe migraine problems, but remember that it usually takes 2 to 3 months to see the effect, so give them time to work.
12. Avoiding hidden food allergies can reduce or eliminate migraines in 30 to 85 percent of patients. In one study, the most common reactive foods were wheat in 78 percent of patients, oranges in 65 percent, eggs in 45 percent, tea and coffee in 40 percent each, chocolate and milk in 37 percent each, beef in 35 percent and corn, cane sugar, and yeast in 33 percent each. Clinical experience also suggests that the artificial sweetener aspartame (NutraSweet®) can trigger migraines and other headaches (although this is controversial). You may find that instead of avoiding foods that trigger your migraines for the rest of your life, you can eliminate the sensitivities/allergies using a powerfully effective acupressure technique called NAET (see www.NAET.com).
13. If the migraines are predominately around the time of the period or associated with taking estrogen, the key is to prevent the fluctuating estrogen level. One way to do this is to use an estrogen patch for one week beginning a few days before the period is expected (e.g. a Climara® .025 patch).
14. Prescription medications can reduce the number of headache days per month by an average of 50 percent. These include Neurontin®, beta-blockers (Inderal®—avoid this if you have asthma or fatigue), calcium channel blockers, Depakote®, Topamax®, Elavil®, and Doxepin®.

*Continued on next page*

**Important Points** *(continued)*

15. Sinusitis is another common cause of headaches. It is usually associated with pain and tenderness over the sinuses, by the cheeks, or above the eyes. Nasal congestion, often with yellow/green nasal mucus, is also common. Interestingly, I have found that most cases of chronic sinusitis are caused by fungal overgrowth in your body (especially your bowels—which can cause gas, bloating, diarrhea, or constipation). Chronic sinusitis routinely resolves when treated with Diflucan® and other treatments (yeast/anti-fungal therapies). It is also helpful to use a special prescription nose spray that contains anti-bacterials and anti-fungals. Your doctor can order it by calling Cape Apothecary at 410-757-3522. Use 1 to 2 sprays in each nostril twice a day.
16. Caffeine withdrawal headaches are common in people who drink coffee. It is especially common in the morning before people get their coffee "fix" and often occurs approximately 18 hours after the last cup of coffee. Weaning off excess caffeine is the solution.
17. Cluster headaches occur as a repeating series of headaches that can each last 30 to 90 minutes and are very severe. They cause excruciating, piercing pain on one side of the head (often centered around one eye) and are much more common in men. Many medications can help. These include anti-seizure medications like Valproic® acid 500-1000 mg a day or Topamax® 50 to 100 mg a day. These often start to work in 1 to 2 weeks.
18. Trigeminal Neuralgia is characterized by excruciating attacks of stabbing, shooting pain in the lips, gums, cheek, or chin that lasts for a few seconds to minutes. It occurs almost exclusively in the middle-aged and elderly. It often responds well to treatment with the medications Tegretol® and/or Neurontin®.
19. Temporo Mandibular Joint Dysfunction (TMJ/TMD) is a common cause of facial pain and headaches. Although classically considered to come from the jaw joint (the area just in front of your ears), in many cases the pain is actually coming from tightness of the Masseter muscles. Following the principles discussed above for myofascial/muscle pain (also see Chapter 9) will often make this pain go away.

CHAPTER 14

# Back Pain

One of the most common chronic pain conditions is back pain, which affects an estimated 36 million Americans.[1] It is the price we pay for being an upright species. Fortunately, it is also very treatable.

In understanding back pain, it is helpful to understand the anatomy of the spine. The spine is made up of a column of bones called the vertebrae. From top to bottom, these are divided into four sections:

1. The 7 neck/Cervical vertebrae (C1 – C7)
2. The 12 upper back /thoracic vertebrae (T1 – T12)
3. The 5 lower back/lumbar vertebrae (L1-L5)
4. The sacrum plus the tailbone (Coccyx) at the bottom of the spine

The bones/vertebrae of the spinal column are held together by tendons, ligaments, and muscles. Between each of the vertebra are shock absorbers called discs. These flexible pads of cartilage contain liquid. If this liquid leaks out, it can trigger inflammation and swelling, which pinches on the nerve roots causing pain. By eliminating the tissue swelling using intravenous colchicine (see below), disc pain can be eliminated approximately 70 percent of the time without surgery!

The spinal cord itself is a critical bundle of nerve cells that are inside the spinal column and protected by it. At each of the vertebrae, nerve roots come out of the front carrying information from the brain to the body. At each level, nerve roots enter the back of the spinal column, bringing information from the body to the brain. Compression of, or damage to, these nerve roots causes pain and loss of sensation.

It's always good to start with the basics. For example, in one study people with low back pain who slept on a medium firm mattress had less back pain than those who slept on a firm mattress.[2] Distraction and relaxation, such as listening to relaxing music for one half hour daily for three weeks, also reduced back pain by 40 percent.[3]

In disc disease, the nerve is being pinched as it comes out of the spine. As the vertebrae and discs (the building blocks that make up the spine) develop wear and tear, the disc, which acts as a shock absorber between the vertebrae, sometimes ruptures, and the fluid inside of the disc leaks out. As noted above, this disc fluid can cause inflammation and swelling that can compress the nerve as it enters or leaves the spine, causing pain. MRIs and x-rays are poor indicators of whether the pain is coming from disc disease (vs. tight muscles or muscle spasm pinching the nerve) as almost everyone shows normal "wear and tear" on their back x-rays. Fortunately, over 70 percent of back pain from disc disease can be eliminated without surgery by simply giving 6 intravenous injections of an old gout medicine called colchicine. Given intravenously (IV), this medicine gets into the disc space and turns off the inflammation and swelling. Relief usually occurs by the 5th to 6th dose. It is fairly safe, with the main risk being rare and severe allergic reactions (similar to the risk with penicillin) and a nasty skin burn if it leaks out of the IV (the medication **has** to stay in the vein, **not** anywhere else). This can usually be easily avoided by making sure the IV is flowing well. I usually recommend that as long as the IV is in, you also get the IV nutrients (see Myers Cocktails in Chapter 20 and Appendix F), because this helps associated muscle pain. Two studies with over 1000 patients (one study being placebo controlled) have shown the same 70 percent relief rate that I and others who use it in practice have found.[4–5] Only one study (conducted with 14 long-term workman's compensation patients who had failed all other treatments, where no treatment was likely to help) did not show benefit.

The main problem with the use of IV colchicine in disc disease is that it is too inexpensive. It costs $3 per dose for 6 doses, with the main cost being that of starting the IV. Because there is no money to be made, and it would eliminate most back surgeons' business, surgeons are understandably hesitant to look at the research. One excellent local orthopedist had a staffer who had disc disease for many years but refused surgery. When she came to our office, we treated her with the IV colchicine and the disc pain, as usual, went away. One night, my partner and I were out for dinner when the orthopedist entered the restaurant. When he came over to say hello, my partner asked the orthopedist what he thought about his staffer's pain going away without needing surgery. The orthopedist ignored the comment and kept on talking as if we had never asked the question.

Sciatica, or back pain in which the pain goes down the leg, is very common. It is simply disc disease from compression or irritation of the nerve from the foot as it enters the spine (although a tight muscle can also pinch the nerve). If you lie on the floor and lift the painful leg straight up without bending it (while keeping the other leg flat on the floor), it can stretch the nerve and worsen the pain. This is called the "straight leg raising test." It also usually goes away by treatment with intravenous colchicine.

## *What Else Can Help My Back Pain?*

It is reasonable to add glucosamine sulfate, 1500 mg a day, and Chondroitin® sulfate 2500 mg per day. Give this combination a 6 to 12 week trial. In one Russian study, 73 percent of those who took the Chondroitin had less back pain and more mobility. These compounds may help to rebuild the cartilage tissue worn away by wear and tear.[6]

Lamictal® (lamotrigine, a seizure medicine that acts as a sodium channel blocker with some calcium channel blockade) can also be helpful. In one study with patients who had severe refractory neuropathic pain (especially disc pain) and had failed at least two other treatments, there was an average 70 percent drop in pain in 14 of 21 patients using this medication.[7]

## *What if It Is Not Disc Disease?*

Most other back pain, unless it is coming from your chest or abdominal organs (which is rare and can be found by your internist) is muscular. Using the treatments in the chapter on myofascial pain (Chapter 9), and also taking care of any underlying structural/ergonomic problems (see Chapters 6 and 21) can routinely eliminate this pain. In addition, chiropractic (see Chapter 21) and mind-body approaches developed by Dr. Sarno (see Chapter 25) can also be very helpful, as can many forms of bodywork. ■

**Important Points**

1. By eliminating the tissue swelling using intravenous colchicine, disc pain can be eliminated approximately 70 percent of the time without surgery. Sciatica, or back pain in which the pain goes down the leg, is often a form of disc disease.
2. Start with the basics. Sleep on a medium firm mattress instead of a firm mattress.
3. It is also reasonable to add glucosamine sulfate 1500 mg a day and Chondroitin sulfate to the treatment regimen, 2500 mg per day. The End Pain herbal formula can also help. Give them a 6 to 12 week trial.
4. Lamictal and /or Lidoderm patches can also be helpful.
5. Most other back pain, unless it is coming from your chest or abdominal organs (which is rare and can be found by your internist), is muscular, arthritic, or from ligaments. Using the treatments described in the chapters on myofascial pain and / or arthritis, and also taking care of any underlying structural/ ergonomic problems can routinely eliminate this pain. In addition, chiropractic and mind-body approaches developed by Dr. Sarno can also be very helpful, as can many forms of bodywork.

**CHAPTER 15**

# Indigestion, Ulcers, Acid Reflux, and Gastritis—Getting Off Acid Blockers Naturally

Indigestion, ulcers, acid reflux, and gastritis are common causes of abdominal and chest pains. If the pain is coming from indigestion or acid reflux, drinking a few ounces of Maalox® or Mylanta® will usually cause the pain to ease up within a few seconds. When this happens, there's a high probability that your pain is coming from stomach acid. In this situation, it is okay to use Tagamet® or other acid blockers short-term to ease your symptoms. I do not feel that it is healthy to use these medications long-term, however, because stomach acid is necessary for healthy digestion.

When you're having indigestion/reflux, it is important to avoid coffee (including decaf), aspirin/Motrin® related products, and alcohol as all of these can aggravate indigestion. In addition, following the directions on the information sheet below, which I use in my office, can help you to effectively treat indigestion, reflux, and gastritis naturally.

## Eliminating Chronic Acid Reflux and Indigestion—Getting Off Acid Blockers Naturally!

### Do You Think Your Problem Is Too Much Stomach Acid?

If you still think your problem is too much acid, keep this in mind. The older people get the more likely they are to use antacids. This is interesting as stomach acid production decreases dramatically as people get older!

We seem to forget that having stomach acid is both necessary and normal. In fact, the body has gone to great lengths to be able to produce stomach acid without digesting the stomach itself! Your body needs to have proper nutrition, however, to make the mucous lining that protects the stomach. Instead of giving your body what it needs to heal, we sometimes make the mistake of turning off our stomach acid to solve the problem.

Most of your indigestion symptoms occur when any stomach acid refluxes (squirts) back up into the food pipe (the esophagus). Your food pipe is not made to resist stomach acid and even a little bit will

*Continued on next page*

cause it to burn. Because of this, we give medications that turn off all the stomach acid. Because there is no stomach acid, the burning stops and we get deluded into thinking the problem is too much stomach acid.

### What Happens When I Turn Off Stomach Acid?

Unfortunately, using anti-acid medications for an extended period causes 2 problems. First, with no stomach acid your body is not able to optimally digest food and you become nutritionally deficient. This makes it even harder for your stomach to make the mucous lining it needs to protect itself and can set you up for even more reflux. Second, in your body's attempt to make the stomach acid it desperately needs (when you take anti-acid medications), it makes huge amounts of a hormone called Gastrin, which stimulates stomach acid. Because of this, as soon as you stop your antacids the stomach makes massive amounts of acid, which it cannot protect against. In essence, you become addicted to the antacids. It is no surprise that Prilosec®, Nexium®, Zantac®, and other antacids are some of the biggest money making-pharmaceuticals!

### So What Can I Do?

A wonderfully effective way to resolve your reflux and indigestion is to do the following: (In mild or occasional cases, DGL licorice for a few days may be all you need. For more severe cases, use the entire program below to restore healthy digestion.)

1. Improve your digestion by taking the proper enzymes (see below) and drink sips of warm liquids instead of cold while eating (cold temperatures inhibit digestive enzyme function). Long-term use of digestive enzymes can also dramatically improve your over all health and well being!
2. Avoid coffee, aspirin products, colas, and alcohol until your stomach heals and then use them in limited amounts. Iced tea is OK but stimulates acid reflux in some people.
3. Take measures to heal your stomach lining. Using DGL licorice (it must be the DGL form because others can cause blood pressure problems—see below) can be powerfully effective in resolving your symptoms. Research shows that it is as effective as Tagamet®, but is healthy for you! Mastic gum 500 to 1000 mg twice a day for 2 months (see Appendix C: Resources) is also highly effective. Both of these can be used separately or together. Because they help to heal the stomach instead of just masking symptoms, they may take 3 to 6 weeks to work in severe cases. You can use your antacids during that time if you want.

4. In many patients, stomach infections (H. pylori) can be a major cause of long-term indigestion. Most doctors treat this with Prilosec® combined with 2 to 3 antibiotics used simultaneously! A better approach is to add Limonene® (Heartburn Free by PhytoPharmica), 1 every other day for 20 days once your indigestion has settled down a bit with the licorice and mastic gum. It may initially aggravate reflux symptoms but, by killing the infection, may give long-term relief after only one 10 capsule course! Mastic gum can also eliminate H. pylori infections.

### How Can I Come Off My Prescription Antacids?

After you have been on this treatment regimen for 1 to 2 months and are feeling much better, ask your doctor if you can stop your prescription antacids and switch to Tagamet (or stay on the DGL licorice/ mastic gum). This will decrease your stomach acid instead of totally turning it off. By doing this, your body can slowly ease back to a normal production of acid. Decrease the dose of Tagamet or DGL licorice until you are able to come off of it. After 2 months, most people can stop the licorice/mastic gum. They can be used as long as you want, however. If symptoms recur down the line, simply use the DGL licorice for a few days. If needed, you can repeat the course of DGL licorice/mastic gum (and even the Heartburn Free if the stomach infection recurs) whenever you like. Meanwhile, you'll have broken your addiction to antacids and allowed your body to have the stomach acid it needs for proper digestion!

To Summarize: Use 1,2 and 3. You may add 4 and 5 as needed.

1. **Similase® (by Tyler) or Complete GEST Enzymes**—Take 2 capsules with each meal to help digest your food properly and drink warm liquids with meals (see Appendix C). If the enzymes are irritating to the stomach, switch to GS Similase until your stomach feels better.

2. **DGL Licorice**, 380 mg (not the sugar-free one)—Chew 2 tablets 20 minutes before meals.

3. **Mastic Gum (any brand)**, 1000 mg twice a day for 2 months, then as needed.

4. **Heartburn Free** (Limonene)—Take 1 every other day for 20 days (may initially aggravate reflux, but can give long-term relief).

5. **Saventaro Cat's Claw** (use this form, as others are a mix of 2 compounds that cancel each other out)—Take 1 twice a day.

## Enzymes and Digestive Health

Unfortunately, medical schools do not give physicians much information on proper nutrition or digestive health. Yet how can your body stay healthy if it can't get the nutrition that it needs from food? Enzyme deficiencies can contribute to many conditions, including:

- Indigestion, gas, bloating, diarrhea, and constipation
- Arthritis and inflammatory disorders
- Fatigue and muscle aches
- Brain fog/dementia
- Heart attacks
- Many other conditions

Proper nutrition is important for all your body's functions. The ability to properly digest your food is critical for proper nutrition and the avoidance of toxicity.

### *Why Are Enzymes Important?*

In medical school, I was taught that the pancreas and salivary glands made all of the enzymes that you needed to digest your food. If there was a problem with the pancreas, we could always give digestive enzyme tablets made from an animal pancreas to take care of the problem. This information seems to be woefully deficient!

What goes on in real life is that most of the enzymes we need to digest the food we eat are naturally present in the food. This occurs because fruits and vegetables use enzymes to ripen. As the ripening process continues, the food breaks down to where we consider it to be rotten. From the perspective of an apple or grain, however, this is a perfect stage for the seed to use its food source so it can grow into an adult plant. These same plant enzymes work in the acid environment of your stomach, where approximately 40 percent of digestion can take place, while animal enzymes can't work until after they get past the stomach.

Decades ago, food processors realized that they could prolong the shelf life of food from days to years by destroying the enzymes present in the food. They also discovered that using salicylates (the active component of aspirin) is a very effective way to destroy enzymes. Over the last 30 years, the processing of foods has essentially eliminated most of the enzymes present in our food. This corresponds to the period of time in which we have seen a dramatic increase in degenerative diseases and indigestion. Meanwhile, your poor pancreas has had to pick up the slack and make almost all the enzymes needed for digestion. Many people realized, however, that if they juiced or ate a raw food diet (cooking can also destroy enzymes) they felt dramatically better. Food processors are learning new tricks though. By gassing fresh fruits and vegetables, they can destroy the enzymes present even in these fresh foods. This way these foods can look appealing on the grocery shelf for weeks instead of developing those little brown spots that we don't like to see. Unfortunately, although the food looks good when you destroy the enzymes, it has lost much of its nutritional value.

## *What Happens When I Don't Have Enough Enzymes?*

When you don't have enough enzymes to adequately digest your food, several things happen:

1. You become deficient in proteins, carbohydrates, and/or fats, depending on which enzymes you are missing.
2. You then crave the missing nutrient.
3. By eating excessive amounts of the nutrient you can't digest, it can build up in your colon and become toxic.
4. You absorb large chunks of proteins into your bloodstream before they are broken down to their component amino acids. Your immune system then has to treat them as outside invaders and uses up its energy completing the digestion of those foods. This can exhaust your immune system while contributing to food sensitivities. If you check you may find that your temperature goes up around 40 minutes after eating because your immune system has had to make up for a weak digestive system.
5. Your body works poorly because of the nutritional deficiencies. You feel poorly and have digestive disturbances.

All in all, you feel lousy. Your stomach hurts, and you may have specific food cravings. Sound familiar?

## *Does It Matter Which Enzymes I Use?*

As noted above, it is critical that the enzymes be from plant sources, as animal enzymes do not work in the acid environment of the stomach. They can also easily be destroyed in processing, so quality is critical. I recommend CompleteGest®, 2 with each meal. If the enzymes irritate your stomach in the beginning, as protein digesting enzymes might, begin with GS Similase first because this form is gentler on the stomach (see Appendix C: Resources). ■

**Important Points**

1. Indigestion is not caused by too much stomach acid. Instead, because of poor digestion or stomach infections, any acid can hurt. Turning off stomach acid long-term can markedly worsen digestion and overall health. Food processors now destroy the digestive enzymes present in food to prolong shelf life. This contributes dramatically to indigestion. Coffee, alcohol, and aspirin/Motrin® products can also cause indigestion and ulcers.

2. To get off acid blocker medications comfortably, do the following for 4 to 8 weeks:

   **Use plant based digestive enzymes** (e.g. CompleteGest®). Taking 2 capsules with each meal will help you digest your food properly. In addition, drink warm liquids with meals; cold temperatures inactivate your digestive enzymes. If the enzymes are irritating to the stomach, switch to a brand called GS Similase until your stomach feels better.

   **DGL Licorice**, 380mg (not the sugar-free one). Chew 2 tablets 20 minutes before meals.

   **Mastic Gum** (any brand), 1000mg. Take twice a day for 2 months, then as needed.

   **Heartburn Free®**. After your stomach is feeling better, take 1 capsule every other day for 20 days. It may initially aggravate reflux, but it can give long term relief by eliminating the stomach infection.

CHAPTER 16

# Spastic Colon

Spastic colon is when you have gas, bloating, abdominal cramps, and diarrhea and/or constipation with a negative medical workup. As we do not know what is causing your symptoms, we give you the label of "spastic colon", instead of more effectively searching for the source of the symptoms.

The most effective way to eliminate spastic colon is to treat the underlying cause. This is usually infection, and in my experience most patients' spastic colon resolves when the underlying bowel infections are treated. What is most important is to treat the Candida/fungal overgrowth in the gut. Unfortunately, most physicians still make believe that fungal or yeast overgrowth is a nonexistent entity. This is reminiscent of our early days in medicine when we first learned about, but still ridiculed, the possibility of bacterial infections. Although the research needs to be completed to demonstrate the role of fungal infections in chronic illness, a large body of clinical experience has shown this to be a major problem. Many people with yeast overgrowth also find that they have chronic sinusitis and/or nasal congestion that go away when the fungal infection is treated.

In addition, many patients have parasitic infections. For example, in my study on the effective treatment of chronic fatigue syndrome, 1 out of 6 of the study patients had a parasite present.[1] Unfortunately, many if not most labs are clueless about how to conduct a proper stool parasite exam and will miss the vast majority of these infections. Because of this, I would only do the parasitology testing by mail at the Great Smokey Mountain Labs or the Parasitology Center (see Appendix C: Resources). If your doctor will not give you a lab requisition for this test at these labs, or for any other tests you may need, you can obtain a lab requisition on my web site at no charge (www.Vitality101.com. Click on "Do the Program" and then on "Get a lab requisition"). In addition, I would recommend a stool test for Clostridium Difficile toxin. This is a toxin-producing bacteria, and this test can be done at any laboratory. For more information on treating these infections, see Chapter 5 in this book and my book *From Fatigued to Fantastic!*

While you're going after the underlying cause of a spastic colon, there are many treatments you can take for symptomatic relief. Natural therapies include peppermint oil. This must be in an enteric-coated capsule or it could be quite irritating. Take 1 to 2 capsules 3 times a day between meals (**not** with food) for spastic colon. I recommend Peppermint Plus® or Mentharil® (see Appendix C: Resources). Other natural remedies that can be helpful are Iberogast® (digestive system herbal), 20 drops 3 times a day in warm water with meals (takes 4 to 8 weeks to work) or artichoke extract, 160 mg. Take 2 capsules 3 times a day. Artichoke extract stimulates bile acid release and may help decrease the risk of gall stones. Over-the-counter simethicone (Mylicon®) can also be helpful. When chewed, this breaks big gas bubbles into little ones, decreasing the sense of bloating.

Prescription medications that can be helpful include anti-spasmodics such as Hyoscyamine® and Valium® family medications such as Librax®. These can be used on an as needed basis. If constipation is a predominant symptom, adding fiber and water plus the Energy Revitalization System vitamin powder can be very helpful. If these are not adequate, you can take the prescription medication Miralax®. In addition, you can add Zelnorm® 6 mg twice a day for both constipation and pain. ■

**Important Points**

1. The most effective way to eliminate spastic colon is to treat the underlying cause. This is usually infection, and in my experience most patients' spastic colon resolves when the underlying bowel infections are treated. What is most important is to treat the Candida/fungal overgrowth in the gut. In addition, many patients have parasitic infections.
2. Unfortunately, many if not most labs are clueless about how to do a proper stool parasite exam and will miss the vast majority of these infections. Because of this, I would only do the parasitology testing by mail at the Great Smokey Mountain Labs or the Parasitology Center. In addition, I recommend a stool test for Clostridium Difficile toxin. This is a toxin producing bacteria, and this test can be done at any laboratory.
3. For symptomatic relief while treating the underlying problems, consider peppermint oil. This must be in an enteric-coated capsule or it could be quite irritating. Take 1 to 2 capsules 3 times a day between meals (**not** with food) for spastic colon.
4. Prescription medications that can be helpful include antispasmodics such as Hyoscyamine® and Valium® family medications such as Librax®. These can be used on an "as needed" basis.
5. If constipation is a predominant symptom, adding fiber and water plus the vitamin powder (contains magnesium) can be very helpful. If these are not adequate, you can take the prescription medications Miralax® and/or Zelnorm®, 6 mg twice a day, for both constipation and pain.

CHAPTER 17

# Noncardiac Chest Pain

Once your doctor has ruled out heart or lung problems as a source of your chest pain, it most often turns out to be muscle/cartilage pain or indigestion/acid reflux.

Pain in the chest wall muscles and cartilage, also known as costochondritis, is fairly common and present in about 10 percent of the population. The diagnosis is made by examination and ruling out other problems (e.g. heart or lung problems) since lab and other studies provide little information about muscle pain.

Costochondritis pain tends to be aggravated by movement, deep breathing, or position change. It tends to be sharp, nagging, aching, or pressure-like, and it is usually fairly well localized, although the pain may radiate. It is usually along the sides of the sternum (the chest bone in the center of the chest), two inches below the left nipple, or in the pectoral muscles in the upper chest. Reproducing the chest pain by pushing on the area suggests that the pain is coming from the muscles or ligaments of the chest wall and is not dangerous. **Nonetheless, it is best to be on the safe side and have a physician make sure that the pain is not coming from the heart**.

Hot compresses and relaxing the muscles with your mind can be helpful, as can the treatments for muscle pain discussed in Chapter 9. For severe cases, Lidocaine patches can be very helpful[1], as can the pain creams. Aspirin family medications such as Motrin® can be helpful but can cause indigestion or stomach ulcers and bleeding, which can also further worsen the chest pain. I have found that ulcer/indigestion pain and costochondritis tend to aggravate each other. In other words, if your indigestion is acting up, your chest muscle pain may also.

If the pain is in your solar plexus and mid-chest and is relieved by taking a few ounces of Maalox®, Mylanta®, or other antacids, or is affected by eating, it is likely indigestion. See Chapter 15 for information on treating pain from indigestion.

The most worrisome causes of chest pain, however, are angina and heart attacks. These pains are usually associated with tightness and pain that radiates down the left arm, shortness of breath, and sweats and is made worse with walking or exercise. Everyone is different, however, and sometimes these pains can be atypical. It is always best to be on the safe side and have a family doctor check out the source of chest pain to be sure it is not coming from something dangerous. Most doctors are very good at diagnosing and treating angina and other dangerous causes of chest pain. Once these have been ruled out, I would go ahead and apply the treatment described in this chapter to help eliminate your chest pain. ■

**Important Points**

1. Once your doctor has ruled out heart or lung problems as a source of your chest pain, it most often turns out to be muscle/cartilage pain (costochondritis) or indigestion/acid reflux.
2. Costochondritis pain tends to be aggravated by movement, deep breathing, or position change. It tends to be sharp, nagging, aching, or pressure-like, and it is usually fairly well localized, although the pain may radiate. It is usually along the sides of the sternum (the chest bone in the center of the chest) two inches below the left nipple, or in the Pectoral muscles in the upper chest. Reproducing the chest pain by pushing on the area suggests that the pain is coming from the muscles or ligaments of the chest wall. Hot compresses and relaxing the muscles with your mind can be helpful, as can the rest of the treatments for muscle pain. For severe cases, lidocaine patches can be very helpful, as can the pain creams.
3. If the pain is in your solar plexus and mid-chest and relieved by taking a few ounces of Maalox®, Mylanta®, or other antacids, or is affected by eating, it is likely to be indigestion.

# CHAPTER 18 Pelvic Pain Syndromes—

## Menstrual Cramps, Vulvadynia, Interstitial Cystitis, Endometriosis, and Prostadynia

Pelvic pain can be caused by menstrual cramps, vulvadynia, interstitial cystitis, or prostadynia. In this chapter, we'll review each of these.

### *Menstrual Cramps*

For menstrual pain, NSAIDs can be very helpful. You can begin with over-the-counter pain relievers such as Advil® or Aleve®. For severe menstrual cramps, the prescription Bextra® 20 mg twice a day can be even more effective.

### *Interstitial Cystitis (IC)*

IC is a bladder problem that causes severe discomfort in approximately 500,000 Americans. Ninety percent of people affected are women, and the condition often occurs in association with other illnesses such as fibromyalgia. Onset of symptoms is often between the ages of 40 and 60. On average, people see five doctors before they find one who is able to make the diagnosis. IC is characterized by severe urinary urgency, frequency, burning, and pain. These symptoms in mild form are common in CFS, fibromyalgia, and chronic pain and are not what I am discussing here. IC is when these symptoms are your predominant problem and are often so severe that people want to have their bladder removed.

There are two main categories of IC. The more common is non-ulcerative and is most often seen in young to middle-aged women. It is associated with normal or increased bladder capacity. The cause of IC is not known, but there are many theories. In all likelihood, it is caused by a number of different problems. One possibility is that there are infectious triggers, which either irritate the bladder directly or cause an autoimmune reaction in which the body attacks itself. The autoimmune theory has recently been getting more support. For whatever reason, the protective inner lining of the bladder (called the GAG or glycosaminoglycan) gets damaged, resulting in severe bladder irritation and pain, urinary urgency and frequency, and decreased bladder capacity. **Again, it**

**is important to note that the above symptoms in mild form are very common and are not IC**. IC is often associated with vulvar pain and painful intercourse (see "Vulvodynia" below). There is no definitive test for IC, and the diagnosis is based on clinical symptoms and bladder cystoscopy (looking in the bladder with a tube). Other infections need to be ruled out, as does cancer.

Although there is currently no cure for IC, there is much that can be done to relieve the symptoms. Once bacterial infections have been ruled out, I add Elavil® 25 mg at bedtime plus Neurontin®. If these are ineffective, a trial of Sinequan® and the other anti-seizure medications are worthwhile. The medications Pyridium®, which numbs the bladder and turns the urine and sweat light orange, and Urispaz® an anti-spasmodic, can be helpful as well.

I would also treat the patient for presumptive Candida with oral Diflucan® for 3 months, which may help as well (see the anti-fungal/ anti-yeast protocol discussed in Chapter 5). Although it has not been well-studied, many physicians suspect that yeast overgrowth, like some other infections, may contribute to IC. A critical part of the anti-yeast/ anti-fungal protocol is avoiding sugar, which feeds yeast. Interestingly, Dr. Ward Dean had noted that one person's IC cleared up when she used Xylitol®, which looks and tastes like sugar, as a sugar substitute. It is not clear whether the Xylitol helped, or simply avoiding the sugar was the reason for the patient's relief. Either way, Xylitol is a good sugar substitute with multiple health benefits, including preventing cavities and osteoporosis, and is worth trying.

It is important to avoid certain foods and also to recognize that vitamins, especially the B vitamins and any that are acidic, can dramatically irritate the bladder in some patients with IC. Because of this, supplements, especially one as powerful as the Energy Revitalization System vitamin powder, should be tried in extraordinarily tiny doses (e.g. stick a finger in the powder and lick it) first to make sure they are tolerated. Then slowly increase the dose if you are able. Take any B vitamins with a large amount of water. Otherwise, they can achieve high concentrations in the bladder. In most people this causes no problem, but can be irritating in those with IC or bladder spasm. B vitamins are bright yellow and you can tell when they are concentrated in the urine.

Other treatments include avoiding foods that may aggravate symptoms. Urologists can also put different medications in the bladder, such as DMSO, Heparin®, and Elmiron®, all of which can be helpful. I recommend Elmiron; it may take 3 months to work. Take a 100 mg capsule 3 times a day with water at least 1 hour before, or 2 hours after, eating.

Dr. Stanley Jacob M.D., the physician who helped to get FDA approval for the use of DMSO (instilled into the bladder) for IC has also explored the use of Methyl Sulfonyl Methane (MSM) to treat IC patients. Although MSM takes longer to work (several months), it is better tolerated than the DMSO which is irritating and results in a garlicky body smell. Dr. Jacob estimates that 80 percent of his IC patients improve with MSM. He has his patients make a formula of 15 percent MSM in deionized sterile water and use a catheter to put the solution in their bladders (2 to 5 times a week), holding it in their bladder as long as is comfortable. He gives the MSM intravenously and by mouth (starting with 1 g a day and increasing to 18 g daily). For more information, see Dr. Jacob's book *MSM—the Definitive Guide.*

Surgery should be a very rare and final resort. Even after the bladder has been removed, half of the IC patients will continue to suffer from pain.[1] The good news is that most patients I have seen with IC have received significant relief using some combination of the above treatments.

In another study, lower morning cortisol levels were associated with increased symptoms of IC.[2] Many fibromyalgia patients get marked improvement in their IC as part of the overall improvement of their fibromyalgia. One of the treatments I often give is cortisol in very low dose.

Another natural remedy that has been shown to be helpful in IC is the amino acid L-arginine 500 mg 3 times a day for 3 months. In one study of 53 patients with IC, half were given the L-arginine and the other half a placebo. At the end of 3 months, 29 percent of the patients on arginine were feeling better with less pain and urgency as compared to 8 percent in the placebo group. L-arginine helps to make nitric oxide, which can relax the bladder muscle. The enzyme that makes nitric oxide has been shown to be low in interstitial cystitis patients. In another open study using 1500 mg of L-arginine daily a similar effect was seen. Another study using higher amounts did not show benefit, so more is not better.[3]

Some health practitioners have found that patients with interstitial cystitis often have chronic extremely alkaline urine. This can be aggravated by excessive coffee and cola intake. pH strip paper can be obtained cheaply at most pharmacies and one can test multiple urine samples at home to see if the pH is regularly over 7.0. In addition, certain enzyme therapies have been found to be very helpful. They can be obtained from my office at 410-573-5389 or from the Enzyme Formulations Company. For interstitial cystitis use the enzyme URT (enzyme product No. 24). Take 4 capsules five times a day between meals; and add the enzyme product called KDY, two capsules every 20 minutes, as needed during flares. In 2 to 4 weeks the symptoms may subside and the products can then be taken just as needed.

Although I have not yet used it for interstitial cystitis, it would be worth trying the herbal "saw palmetto," 160 mg twice a day for 6 weeks as this relaxes the bladder muscle in those with urinary retention and an enlarged prostate. Research shows that this safe herb promotes smooth muscle (i.e. the bladder muscle) cell relaxation by a number of different mechanisms. It takes 6 weeks to work.[4]

## *Vulvodynia*

Vulvodynia is defined as chronic vulvar itching, burning, and/or pain that is significantly uncomfortable. In this condition, vulvar/vaginal pain can either occur only during intercourse or be constantly present. It used to be thought that it was fairly rare. Recently, the NIH funded a study to see how common vulvodynia is. According to Dr. Harlow, associate professor of gynecology at Harvard Medical School, "The preliminary data suggests that possibly millions of women may be affected at some point during their lifetime." The International Society for the Study of Vulvovaginal Disease has proposed several names to describe the different types of vulvodynia. These are:

1. Generalized vulvar dysesthesia (VDY)—characterized by pain that can occur anywhere on the vulva.
2. Localized vulvar dysesthesia—characterized by pain that can be consistently localized by pushing on certain area(s) of the vulva.
3. Mixed dysesthesia—a combination of both of the above.

Symptoms can occur anywhere from the pubic bone to the anus. It may be present all of the time, sporadically, or only with intercourse. Many women feel like they have a chronic yeast infection. In others, it feels raw, swollen, or like they are sitting on a hard knot. Burning, electric shocks, and tingling are also often seen. If the area around the urethra (where the urine comes out) is involved, the woman may feel like she has a chronic bladder infection. She may have recurrent urinary urgency, frequency, and burning despite having negative urine cultures. Painful intercourse (dyspareunia) is common, and pain may even occur from tight slacks or panties.[5] Some patients have found that for painful intercourse, topical 0.2 percent nitroglycerine cream can give temporary relief (made by a compounding pharmacist in a base without any irritating additives).

In my experience, vulvodynia seems to occur as three main types:

1. **Neuropathic**. This pain appears to be caused by nerve irritation and is sharp, burning and or shooting (like nerve pain). In this case, apply the treatment principles in Chapter 8 on neuropathic pain. Begin with tricyclic anti-depressants (nortriptyline, desipramine, imipramine, doxepin, or Elavil®) at 25 to 150 mg each night and/ or Neurontin® (100 mg to 3600 mg daily), and proceed from there. Be sure to use a high enough dose of the medications, and give them enough time to work, which may take 3 months. In addition, topical lidocaine (Novocain®) gel can be helpful (e.g. EMLA cream). In severe cases, opiates may be necessary.

2. **Inflammatory**. This pain is associated with local inflammation/irritation. In this situation, I would avoid topical creams, etc., especially if they contain parabens, propylene glycol, fragrance, or sorbic acid. Also, do not use topical anti-fungals or over the counter creams. Instead, I routinely give at least a 3 month trial of oral Diflucan® 200 mg a day to be sure any chronic vaginal yeast is eliminated. Occasionally, long-term Diflucan treatment is needed. In this case, check liver blood tests occasionally, because this medicine can cause liver inflammation. Some patients find that avoiding oxalates can help decrease symptoms. In a small subset of patients, one can see a narrow ring of tissue that is inflamed and which reproduces the pain when touched (e.g. with a Q-tip). In these patients, surgically removing that small area of tissue is reasonable.

3. **Muscle pain**. If the pain is deep-seated and not triggered by touching the outer vagina, it may be coming from spasm of the deep pelvic muscles. In this situation, the pain may occur or be accentuated during the deep thrusting of intercourse. For this pain, the general principles for treating muscle pain apply. In addition, EMG biofeedback of the pelvic floor muscles may help. Muscles that are often involved include the Obturator Internus and Pubococcygeus. The sacroiliac joint and disc/spine disease (see "treatment of disc disease with IV colchicine" in Chapter 14) also refer pain to the pelvic and rectal areas. Any injury or condition affecting these can trigger pelvic pain.

In general, it is good for patients with vulvodynia to take certain precautions. As noted above, these include avoiding any direct chemical contacts that can irritate the vulva such as sprays, creams, or mini-pads. In addition, it is a good idea to wear loose comfortable clothes and to avoid thong underwear and biking. Sitz baths can also be helpful. Menopausal women should use topical **natural** estrogen (e.g. estradiol) to prevent atrophy.

Many of my patients with fibromyalgia also have vulvadynia. Like IC, it seems that symptoms of vulvodynia often resolve as their fibromyalgia resolves. I put almost all women with pelvic pain on tricyclics such as Elavil® or nortriptyline combined with Neurontin®.

## Endometriosis

Endometriosis is a complex disorder affecting females during their reproductive years. In this disorder, the tissue that lines the inside of the uterus and sheds each month during the menstrual cycle (called the endometrium) escapes the uterus and attaches to inappropriate areas within the pelvis and abdomen. These growths then respond to changes in estrogen just like tissue within the uterus. Because of this, women will often get pelvic and abdominal pains that are worse around their periods. These pains are usually worse than menstrual cramps. In addition to pain, women with endometriosis often experience a myriad of other symptoms similar to fibromyalgia (e.g. – fatigue, insomnia, widespread achiness, etc. – see Chapter 9) as well as allergies, asthma, and autoimmune problems. Although the cause of endometriosis is unknown, there are many theories.

Most doctors forget to consider this diagnosis in evaluating abdominal and pelvic pain. The diagnosis is made by laparoscopy. During this surgical procedure, the surgeon makes a small incision and inserts a tube through which he can see the internal organs to evaluate for endometrial implants. If these implants are seen, the diagnosis is made and treatment is given with hormonal therapies that attempt to stop ovulation. In addition, other pain medications are given as well. Pregnancy often causes a temporary remission of symptoms. Many alternative therapies are also available.

Although this condition is too complex to be dealt with thoroughly in this book, I recommend a book called *Endometriosis* by Mary Lou Ballweg and the Endometriosis Association. This organization is located in Milwaukee, Wisconsin and is dedicated to helping women with endometriosis.

## Prostatitis and Prostadynia

Even in the absence of a full blown attack of prostatitis, which is usually not subtle and is easily diagnosed and treated, prostate pain is fairly common in men. When no infection is found, it is called prostadynia. It is also known as chronic nonbacterial prostatitis, or chronic pelvic pain syndrome (CPPS). Unfortunately, when doctors do not know what is causing a problem, we often presume it must be psychological (i.e. "I don't know what's wrong with you, so you must be crazy!"). This is what has occurred with prostadynia.

I suspect that prostadynia often occurs because of subtle infections that do not grow on our culture media. These commonly include fungal infections and/or other slow growing antibiotic sensitive infections. In the latter case, the prostate is mildly boggy (indents like a ripe fruit) instead of firm and is tender on examination; to the patient without prostate problems it normally feels like one has to pee, but the prostate is not tender/painful when pressed on. Unfortunately, most doctors consider such an exam normal despite your having prostate symptoms. These symptoms include urinary urgency, without there necessarily being much urine present, and burning on urination. The discomfort is often felt on the tip of the penis. Because the infection is not overt, most doctors offer no treatment.

My suspicion is that this is indeed an infectious problem in many cases. This suspicion is bolstered by a recent study showing that Mepartricin® (40 mg per day for 2 months), an antibiotic with anti-fungal and anti-parasitic properties, decreased symptoms by 60 percent in these patients.[6] The study does not totally support infection as the cause, however, because the medication also lowers estrogen levels in the prostate and can work in that way as well. In the study, the authors theorized that lowering estrogen caused the improvement. My experience, however, shows that patients also improve with antibiotics and anti-fungals that do not lower estrogen. Treatment needs to be given for many months, since anti-infectious agents have difficulty getting into the prostate.

The bioflavonoid vitamin Quercetin 500 mg twice a day also decreases prostate symptoms in both prostadynia and prostatitis. In one study, 30 men with severe prostadynia lasting an average of 11 years were treated with either Quercetin 500 mg twice a day or a placebo for 1 month. There was an average 37 percent decrease in symptoms with over two thirds of patients feeling they gained a meaningful benefit.[7] Quercetin 500 mg is present in the Energy Revitalization System vitamin powder. ■

**Important Points**

1. For menstrual pain, begin with over-the-counter Advil® or Aleve®. For severe menstrual cramps, the prescription medication Bextra® 20 mg twice a day can be even more effective.
2. Interstitial Cystitis (IC) is a bladder problem characterized by **severe** urinary urgency, frequency, burning, and pain. Once bacterial infections have been ruled out, I add Elavil® 25 mg at bedtime plus Neurontin® 300 to 900 mg at bedtime and perhaps during the day as well. If these are ineffective after 6 weeks, a trial of Sinequan® and the other anti-seizure medications is worthwhile. Pyridium, which numbs the bladder (and turns the urine and sweat light orange) and Urispaz® (an anti-spasmodic) can be helpful as well. I then also treat the patient for presumptive Candida with oral Diflucan® for 3 months.
3. It is important to avoid certain foods that aggravate symptoms and to recognize that any vitamins, especially the B vitamins, and any that are acidic (including the vitamin powder), can dramatically irritate the bladder in some patients with IC.
4. Some health practitioners have found that patients with interstitial cystitis often have chronic highly alkaline urine. This can be aggravated by excessive coffee and cola intake. pH strip paper can be obtained cheaply at most pharmacies and one can test multiple urine samples at home to see if the pH is regularly over 7.0. Also take the enzyme product URT (enzyme product No. 24) at a dose of 4 capsules five times a day between meals. During flare-ups add the enzyme product called Kdy, two capsules every 20 minutes as needed. In 2 to 4 weeks symptoms may subside and the products can then be taken as needed. These products are available from 410-573-5389. If these treatments do not work, try Elmiron®. Take a 100 mg capsule 3 times a day with water at least 1 hour before, or 2 hours after, eating. In addition, I recommend adding MSM (Methyl Sulfonyl Methane) at a dose of 6 to 18 grams a day, L arginine 500 mg 3 times day, and the herbal "saw palmetto," 160 mg twice a day. These may all take 3 months to work.

*Continued on next page*

**Important Points** *(continued)*

5. Vulvodynia is defined as chronic vulvar itching, burning, and/or pain that is significantly uncomfortable. In this condition, vulvar/vaginal pain can either occur only during intercourse or be constantly present. I put almost all women with pelvic pain on tricyclics such as Elavil® or nortriptyline combined with Neurontin®. In my experience, vulvodynia seems to occur as three main types: neuropathic, inflammatory, and muscle pain.

   Neuropathic pain appears to be caused by nerve irritation and is sharp, burning, and/or shooting (like nerve pain). In this case, apply the treatment principles in Chapter 8 on neuropathic pain. Begin with tricyclic anti-depressants (nortriptyline, desipramine, imipramine, doxepin, or Elavil®) at 25 to 150 mg each night and/or Neurontin (100 mg to 3600 mg daily), and proceed from there.

   Inflammatory pain is associated with local inflammation/irritation. In this situation, I would avoid topical creams. I routinely give at least a 3 month trial of oral Diflucan® 200 mg a day.

   Muscle pain—if the pain is deep-seated and not triggered by touching the outer vagina, it may be coming from spasm of the deep pelvic muscles. In this situation, the pain may occur or be accentuated during the deep thrusting of intercourse. For this pain, the general principles for treating muscle pain apply.

6. Prostate pain is fairly common in men. When no infection is found, it is called prostadynia. I suspect that prostadynia often occurs because of subtle infections and usually improves when these are treated. The bioflavonoid Quercetin 500 mg twice a day also decreases prostate symptoms in both prostadynia and prostatitis.

7. Endometriosis is characterized by abdominal and pelvic pain that is usually worse around the muscle cycle. It is often associated with other symptoms suggestive of chronic fatigue syndrome and fibromyalgia such as fatigue, achiness, cognitive dysfunction, and insomnia. For more information read the book *Endometriosis* by Mary Lou Ballweg and the Endometriosis Association.

# Chapter 19 Wrist, Hand, Shoulder, Leg, and Foot Pains

Pain in the arms and legs are discussed in this chapter, including carpal tunnel syndrome, tendonitis, frozen shoulder, leg cramps, plantar fasciitis, and Morton's neuroma.

## *Carpal Tunnel Syndrome*

Carpal tunnel syndrome is characterized by pain, numbness, and tingling that occurs in one or both hands. It often wakes people from their sleep, leaving them feeling like they have to "shake their hands out" to make the pain and symptoms go away.

This syndrome is caused by the compression of a nerve (the median nerve) as it goes through a narrow tunnel in the wrist formed by the carpal bone, hence the name carpal tunnel syndrome. According to the American Academy of Neurology, 10 percent of the population suffers from the syndrome. It also affects up to 50 percent of industrial workers.[1] All too often the syndrome is treated by surgery. Although this can be effective, it is also expensive and can leave people with residual problems due to the formation of scar tissue that can occur after surgery.

Fortunately, unless people are continuing to stress the wrist with repetitive stress injuries (e.g. handling heavy equipment or doing large amounts of typing), carpal tunnel syndrome can almost always be relieved without surgery. In almost all of my patients, their carpal tunnel syndromes have resolved by simply using vitamin B6 (250 mg daily), Armour thyroid hormone (see information in Chapter 8 on thyroid for how to adjust the dose), and a wrist splint for six weeks. When your hand gets into funny positions while you are sleeping, it stretches and strains the nerve as it goes through your wrist. This is why you wake up in the night with numbness or tingling. The type of wrist splint to use is called a "cock up" wrist splint. It keeps your hand in the neutral position (i.e. the position your hand is in while holding a glass of water), which takes the stress off the nerve. Be sure to wear the splint for at least 6 weeks while you're sleeping. During that period, also wear it during the day when you can.

Although the treatment above generally takes care of carpal tunnel syndrome, it is worth being aware of a new treatment as well. A portable wrist traction device combines neutral wrist position and stretching to decompress the carpal tunnel. It is used 10 minutes twice a day for 1 month, followed by 10 minutes once a day for a second month. It can be used at home or at work, making it very convenient. At the end of a study of 30 patients, most had normalization or near normalization of the nerve function.[2] Other conservative measures can also be effective, including acupuncture, osteopathic manipulation, chiropractic manipulation, and myofascial release. Unfortunately, your doctor may be totally unfamiliar with these conservative therapies; in today's medicine only expensive treatments tend to get attention. If surgery is recommended, ask your physician if you can try these conservative measures instead for 6 to 12 weeks.

## Thumb Tendonitis

Thumb tendonitis is characterized by pain along the side of your hand going from the thumb joint towards the wrist. If you feel around, you may find a "ropy" cord (the tendon) that hurts, with the pain worsening when you push on it. The pain gels/creams can work very well for this (see Appendix C: Resources—give these medications several weeks to work). Steroid injections locally are also reasonable (not to be injected into the tendon).

## Shoulder Problems

Frozen shoulder has many causes, including tendon inflammation, bursitis, and injury. Anything that causes pain on motion can trigger it. This occurs as the patient stops moving the shoulder because of the pain. The shoulder gradually loses mobility and scar tissue can form around the shoulder joint causing it to become frozen. Rotator cuff tears are a common cause. If you have shoulder pain and find that you can only lift your arm up to shoulder level (i.e. a 90 degree angle) to the side, a rotator cuff tear is likely.

The usual treatments include NSAIDs and physical therapy (heat, ultrasound, and range of motion exercises). Cortisone® injections can also be given. If these treatments fail after 6 to 12 months, surgery to repair the joint may sometimes be necessary.

When doing range of motion exercises, increase the joint movement up to the point where it causes mild pain, but do not push through pain as this can further injure the joint. Several good stretches for the shoulder include using your other hand to lift your hand up to the top of a door (so that your hand holds onto the top of the door) and then gently squatting down to stretch the shoulder. After this, put your arm behind your back and use your other hand to gently pull on it and stretch it. This can also be done with your arm over your head. It is good to be sure that you maintain range of motion of your shoulder anytime you have shoulder pain to prevent a frozen shoulder.

## *Leg Pain*

A. **Leg Cramps**. In some people, the calf and other leg muscles go into spasm while they are sleeping. A number of treatments can prevent this. Begin by taking the Energy Revitalization System vitamin powder (take the vitamin B-complex capsule in the morning and the powder at night). In addition, take calcium 500 to 1000 mg at bedtime and increase the potassium in your diet (e.g. bananas, V8®, or tomato juice). Stretch your calf muscles before you go to sleep. This can be done by pulling your toes towards you when you're sitting on your bed. Wearing socks at night can also help because cold feet will sometimes be a trigger. Quinine can be helpful for nighttime leg cramps as well.[3] For most of my patients, the nutritional support I recommend plus quinine has done an excellent job in relieving pain from leg cramps. Interestingly, several readers of Dr. Peter Gott's medical column have noted that leaving a bar of soap under their bed sheet stopped their leg cramps. It seems odd, but it is cheap, safe, and easy to try.

B. **Plantar Fasciitis**. This is the most common cause of pain along the entire bottom of your foot. It occurs when you have a tightness/irritation of the muscles and tissues that form the "suspension bridge" on the bottom of your foot. This is very common in my fibromyalgia patients and routinely goes away with the overall treatment protocol. (See Chapter 9 on muscle pain). In addition, a podiatrist or chiropractor familiar with the technique can tape the bottom of your foot. This was another wonderful trick that Dr. Huse taught me. This tape then takes over the role of the suspension support and may ease the pain immediately.

C. **Morton's Neuroma**. This is an irritated nerve bundle in the web between two toes. It hurts when you squeeze that area, reproducing the pain. This is best treated by a podiatrist. ■

**Important Points**

1. Carpal tunnel syndrome is characterized by pain, numbness, and tingling that occurs in one or both hands. It often wakes people from their sleep leaving them feeling like they have to "shake their hands out" to make the pain and symptoms go away. In almost all my patients, their carpal tunnel syndrome has resolved by simply using vitamin B6 (250 mg daily), Armour thyroid hormone (see Chapter 8 on thyroid for how to adjust the dose), and a "cock up" wrist splint at night for 6 weeks.
2. Thumb tendonitis is characterized by pain along the side of your hand going from the thumb joint towards the wrist. The pain gels/creams can work very well for this type of pain (See Appendix C: Resources—give these medications several weeks to work).
3. If you get a shoulder injury or pain, be sure to maintain range of motion to prevent frozen shoulder.
4. For nighttime leg cramps, begin by taking the Energy Revitalization System vitamin powder (take the B-complex capsule in the morning and the powder at night). In addition, take calcium 500 to 1000 mg at bedtime and increase the potassium in your diet (e.g. bananas, V8, or tomato juice). Stretch your calf muscles before you go to sleep. This can be done by pulling your toes towards you when you're sitting on your bed. Wearing socks at night can also help because cold feet will sometimes be a trigger. Quinine can be very helpful for nighttime leg cramps as well.

# Section 5

# *A Review of Effective Therapies*

CHAPTER 20

# Natural Therapies

## Herbal Pain Remedies

As discussed throughout this book, natural remedies can be powerful tools in relieving pain. Because of this, there is often much to be gained from working with Naturopaths—practitioners trained in natural medicine. Unfortunately, most medical doctors have a strong bias against natural remedies. As one goes into academic centers, this only increases. Although many physicians think that their bias is based on lack of scientific evidence supporting natural therapies (what they like to call "evidence-based medicine"), it is actually simply based on a lack of awareness of the scientific data.

In addition, money strongly colors drug research; there is much more money to be made on patentable drugs than on non-patentable natural remedies. In fact, research done by Cary Gross at Yale [1] shows that studies funded by a drug company are 3.6 times as likely to have a result favorable to the sponsor. A quarter of biomedical researchers have financial ties to the companies whose products they are studying. Drug companies fund approximately 60 percent of the biomedical research done in the U.S., spending over $30 billion yearly on research and development. In addition, because universities can patent and license the results of positive research, there is a further incentive to skew the data on drug therapies over natural, non-patentable treatments.

Many physicians refuse to objectively look at studies that support natural medicine. The people in charge of the grants will rarely give money to study natural therapies. All too often, journal reviewers look for any excuse they can not to publish findings, and many doctors refuse to look at a positive study on natural therapies once it is published. Thus physicians can honestly say that they have not seen any data supporting natural remedies. On the other hand, any data against natural remedies seems to get published—no matter how poorly done the study was and how unreliable the data is.

I have repeatedly seen this in action, and this is not just my own impression. A study was conducted in which two identical study reports were submitted for publication. The only difference was that in one study the treatment was an "unconventional" therapy while the other was a "conventional" treatment. A total of 398 reviewers were recruited and did not know that they were part of a study. They simply thought they were reviewing the study reports to see whether they should be published. Although the study reports were exactly the same (except for the treatment), the studies using conventional therapies were much more likely to be recommended for publication, suggesting that a strong prejudice exists against "alternative" interventions. This makes it much harder for such studies to get published and also suggests that it would be more difficult to get research funding for studies supporting natural therapies.

## *Why Does This Bias Exist?*

A curious thing happened during the rigorous process I went through to become a physician. By the time I completed my formal training, I presumed that if an important treatment existed for an illness, I would have been taught about it. I understood that physicians need to keep reading to stay abreast of new information. But I **knew** that if someone claimed he or she could effectively treat a non-treatable disease, that person was a quack. If such a treatment existed, I would surely have been taught about it in medical school. I was wrong.

Dr. Werner Barth, my rheumatology instructor, taught me many things. The most important thing he taught me though, was to spend an hour a day reading the scientific literature. This practice has gotten me into all kinds of trouble.

When I first started my medical practice, patients would ask me if I knew about certain herbal or nutritional treatments for illnesses. One patient asked me if I had ever heard about using vitamin B6 for carpal tunnel syndrome. "That's nonsense," I answered. "If B6 cures carpal tunnel syndrome, don't you think I would have been taught to use that instead of surgery?" I said that I would look into it, however.

Joyce Miller, the Anne Arundel Medical Center librarian, has always been happy to obtain studies for me (and she has obtained many thousands over the years). When she did a literature search for vitamin B6 and carpal tunnel syndrome, she found a number of studies showing that 250 mg of the vitamin per day for 3 months, combined with wrist splints, often cures carpal tunnel syndrome. I thought that was curious. Over the months, this scene was played out again and again. I decided to keep notes on these rare "pearls" in a thirty-page spiral notebook. My notes are now over 1000 pages long.

After a while, I began to comprehend that, indeed, my professors had not taught me everything in medical school. As I continued my research, I realized that although our modern allopathic medical system might be the best in the world, it has its weaknesses. These days, it is rare (albeit wonderful) for a major medical development to come out of a doctor's office instead of a research center. This stems from a critical drawback in our economic system (and all systems have their drawbacks). In our current system, a treatment must be very profitable to be promoted. Experts estimate that it costs over $400,000,000 to develop a single new treatment and get it through the Food and Drug Administration (FDA) approval process. Unless a medication or supplement is put through the FDA approval process, its manufacturer is banned from making any medical claims for the product. However, if a product is inexpensive and **non-patentable** (as is the case with most natural therapies), its manufacturer can not afford to pay $400,000,000 to put it through the FDA process.

Vitamin B6, when used for carpal tunnel syndrome, is an excellent example. Treating carpal tunnel syndrome with B6 costs about $9 dollars for the whole course of treatment. Vitamin B6 manufacturers would, therefore, find it impossible to recoup the cost of getting FDA approval for this treatment. Because of this, most patients instead spend between $2,000 and $4,000 to have surgery. This situation is the same for hundreds of other non-patentable, effective, inexpensive, and relatively safe treatments.

The treatment approaches that we discuss in *Pain Free 1-2-3!* are well-grounded in the scientific literature. Dr. Janet Travell, professor emeritus of internal medicine at George Washington University Medical School, was considered the world's leading expert on muscle disorders. She served as the White House physician for presidents John F. Kennedy and Lyndon B. Johnson and, along with Dr. David Simons (who is also superb), authored the over 800 page bible on treating muscle disorders, entitled *Myofascial Pain and Dysfunction: The Trigger Point Manual.* Dr. Travell and Dr. Simons investigated the perpetuating factors that keep muscles from appropriately relaxing. A large percent of these perpetuating factors are the things that we discuss in this book. In one chapter alone, Dr. Simons and Dr. Travell referenced 317 scientific studies that showed how important it is to treat these perpetuating factors. There is no lack of scientific basis for treatment, just a lack of awareness of the treatments due to their relative low-cost and non-patentability.

Unfortunately, your doctor is likely to be unfamiliar with the research on effective treatment of myofascial pain and fibromyalgia. It is possible that your doctor may even be hostile to the information presented in this book, considering it to be quackery because it was not covered in medical school. I can understand his or her feeling this way, because I felt the same way before I extensively reviewed the medical literature. Because of this, I have referenced many of the sources of the information given so that your doctor can have the scientific basis needed to be comfortable with the recommendations I make.

It is possible that your doctor may choose to disregard the information, and that is OK. It simply says that he or she is not interested in this area of pain management. On the other hand, your doctor might be open-minded (though reasonably skeptical) and interested in effective treatment of pain and, therefore, may choose to explore the subject in more depth. If this last possibility is the case, the information and references in this book will give your doctor the scientific basis necessary to manage and optimize your treatment.

### *What Natural Therapies Can Help Me?*

Many natural therapies can be very helpful for pain. My three favorite pain-relieving herbals are willow bark, boswellia, and tart cherry. All three can be found in combination in the End Pain formula by Enzymatic Therapy. Begin with 2 tablets 2 to 3 times a day, as needed, until maximum benefit is achieved (approximately 4 to 6 weeks) and then you can use the lowest effective dose. Let's look more closely at these three herbals.

### *Willow Bark*

Willow bark is the original source of aspirin, but when used as the entire herb it has been found to be **much** safer than aspirin and quite effective. The active ingredient is salicin, and willow bark has been shown to be effective in both osteoarthritis and back pain. People who are severely allergic to aspirin (e.g. those with aspirin-induced asthma or anaphylaxes, which is very unusual) should not use willow bark. Like aspirin and Celebrex®, it acts as a COX (Cyclooxygenase enzyme) inhibitor, decreasing inflammation. There is clearly a combination of other elements in willow bark that markedly enhance its effectiveness and safety—which can be a major benefit over aspirin and NSAIDs (e.g. Motrin®). Unfortunately aspirin and NSAIDs cause an enormous amount of gastritis and ulcer bleeding to the extent of killing 15,000 to 20,000 Americans yearly! The studies on willow bark are quite consistent in showing its effectiveness in reducing pain. Let's look at some of the research.

In one study, 210 patients with severe chronic low back pain were randomly assigned to receive an oral willow bark extract, with either 120 mg (low-dose) or 240 mg (high-dose) of salicin, or a placebo, in a 4-week blinded trial. In the last week of treatment, 39 percent of the group receiving high-dose extract **were pain free**; 21 percent of the group receiving low-dose extract were pain free; and only 6 percent of the placebo group were pain free ($P < 0.001$). The response in the high-dose group was evident after only 1 week of treatment.[2] Researchers then studied 451 patients who came in with low back pain in an open study, using salicin 240 mg, 120 mg, or standard orthopedic/NSAID care for 4 weeks. Forty percent of the patients in the 240 mg group and 19 percent in the 120 mg group were pain free after four weeks. In the standard treatment group, using standard medications, only 18 percent were pain free. The study showed that willow bark was not only far more effective and safer than standard prescription therapies, it also decreased the cost of care by approximately 40 percent![3]

Another review found that willow bark extract has comparable anti-inflammatory activities as higher doses of acetylsalicylic acid/aspirin (ASS) and it reduces pain and fever as well. In pharmacologically active doses, no adverse effects on the stomach lining (e.g. indigestion, ulcers, etc) were observed, in contrast to aspirin.

A daily dose of willow bark extract standardized to 240 mg salicin per day was also significantly superior to placebo in patients with osteoarthritis of the hip and the knee. In two open studies against standard active treatments as controls, willow bark extract exhibited advantages compared to NSAIDs and was about as effective as Vioxx [4] (but much safer). Another placebo-controlled study found that willow bark (salicin 240 mg/day) was more effective than placebo in treating arthritis (the normal wear and tear type called osteoarthritis) after only 2 weeks of therapy.[5] Other references are also available for those of you who would like more information on willow bark.[6-9]

All of this makes willow bark a wonderful natural pain medicine. It is safe and effective for arthritis, back pain, and likely many other types of pain. I recommend beginning with enough to get 240 mg of Salicin a day until maximum benefit is seen. At that point, you may be able to lower the dose to 120 mg, or less, a day, or take it as needed.

## Boswellia

Boswellia Serrata, also known as Frankincense, has been used in traditional Ayurvedic medicine for centuries. Boswellia has been found to be quite helpful in treating inflammation and pain[10-15], and it does this without causing ulcers like aspirin family medications.[16] It has been shown in studies to be helpful for both rheumatoid arthritis[17] and osteoarthritis.[18]

In the latter study, 30 patients with osteoarthritis of the knee were given 1000 mg of either an extract of boswellia or a placebo for 8 weeks; the groups were then switched for the next 8 weeks. All of the patients on the boswellia showed significantly decreased pain and improved ability to walk. In fact, the improvement was quite remarkable, with the

**pain index falling by 90 percent after 8 weeks** and a similarly dramatic increase in function. This was recently discussed in more length in the wonderful patient-oriented newsletter *Nutrition and Healing* by Jonathan Wright, M.D.—a physician that I have great respect for (see www.wrightnewsletter.com). The article was written by Kerry Bone.

Boswellia has also been demonstrated to have significant anti-inflammatory properties, inhibiting leukotriene synthesis by inhibiting 5-lipooxygenase activity. It also decreases the activity of human leukocyte elastase (HLE). Unique to Boswellia is that it blocks two inflammatory chemicals that are increased simultaneously in a variety of human diseases.[19] This results in its being helpful in asthma and colitis, as well as pain. In one study of asthmatics, 40 patients were treated with 300 mg 3 times day for 6 weeks. Seventy percent of the asthma patients showed improvement in symptoms and lung function and a decrease in allergic blood cells (eosinophils).[20] Boswellia also helped in the treatment of ulcerative colitis. In one study of 20 patients in which Boswellia, 300 mg 3 times a day, was given for 6 weeks, 14 went into remission, while with sulfasalazine (the standard prescription treatment), the remission rate was 4 out of 10.[21] Test tube studies suggest that Boswellia also markedly inhibits cancer.[22 – 23]

Boswellia does not appear to have any major side effects that resulted in people withdrawing from the studies and it rarely causes minor gastrointestinal disturbances or rash. A common dose is 150 to 350 mg 3 times a day.

## *Cherry Fruit (Prunus Cerasus)*

Although there are not as many human studies on the use of tart cherries, they also contain compounds that inhibit COX (inflammation) as effectively as ibuprofen.[24] Tart cherries also possess both antioxidant and anti-inflammatory properties. In addition, research suggests that tart cherries may also inhibit colon and perhaps other cancers.[25] Cherries and other colored berries are very high in many antioxidants. As with eating cherries, taking cherry fruit extract is quite safe. Many people find that eating 10 to 20 cherries a day helps their arthritis considerably. 2000 mg of cherry fruit extract (present in 6 tablets of the End Pain formula) contains the active components present in 10 cherries or 32 oz of cherry juice. Early research, as well as how many people come back for more after they have tried it, which to me is a significant indicator of effectiveness, suggests that cherry fruit extract holds a lot of promise![26 – 28]

The good news is that all of these excellent and natural pain treatments can now be found in the End Pain formula (See Appendix C).

## *These Herbs Sound Like a Great Way to Treat My Pain! What Else Can I Do to Help Healing and Get Rid of Pain?*

The great thing about comprehensive medicine, which combines holistic and pharmaceutical treatments, is that you have a full tool kit to help with your problems. Otherwise, using allopathic medicine alone is like going into a shoe store and having only one pair of shoes to try on. Using comprehensive medicine, almost everyone can find "a shoe that fits" so you can get your life and health back!

As we discussed earlier, pain is often your body's way of telling you that it desperately needs something—and what it needs is usually natural and not chemical. Let's review the key things your body needs and how you can give it what it needs naturally.

## *Sounds Good! What's First?*

First you need to give your body the nutritional building blocks it needs to heal. Otherwise, your body cannot even begin to get well. As you've noticed, I've talked about the Energy Revitalization System vitamin powder and B-complex at length. This is because this formula has over 50 key nutrients that serve an enormous number of needs. Many people have told me that using the formula by itself eliminated their chronic pain!

Next, although the vitamin powder has most of what your body needs, joints require other specific nutrients for healing, in addition to what's in the vitamin powder. So if you have arthritis or back pain from arthritis of the spine bones (vertebrae), get Glucosamine **sulfate** (500 mg 3 times a day), and consider MSM (1.5-3 grams a day for 2 to 5 months) and Chondroitin (although this one is less important). MSM supplies the sulfur amino acids needed for healing in general. Although most of the studies on MSM and arthritis have not been placebo-controlled, one study showed an 80 percent decrease in arthritis pain after 6 weeks using 1500 mg in the morning and 750 mg at lunchtime.[29]

Glucosamine sulfate is a cartilage building compound that has been found to be helpful in arthritis in many studies. Although its exact mechanism of action is not yet fully understood, it is a major component of the cartilage that is damaged in arthritic joints. Glucosamine taken by mouth is incorporated in the molecules that make up this cartilage, likely contributing to the healing of arthritis. I recommend the sulfate form (as opposed to Glucosamine hydrochloride) because the sulfate can also help with wound/joint healing.

Unlike aspirin/NSAIDs that do not slow down destruction of joints in arthritis, Glucosamine has been shown to actually help stabilize and often heal the joints on x-ray. Doses of less than 1000 mg a day do not have an effect on symptoms; therefore, the standard dose is 500 mg 3 times a day. It can also be taken as 1500 mg once a day. It can be taken with or without food and has no more side effects than placebo.[30] Chondroitin sulfate is sometimes added to Glucosamine or taken by itself. Its benefits are modest as less than 10 percent of it is absorbed as compared to 90 percent of the absorption of glucosamine sulfate.[31] Because of this, I rarely use Chondroitin. On the other hand, 1200 mg a day can be helpful in slowing down arthritis and is worth trying if you do not get adequate relief with the other treatments. Chondroitin can be taken all at once or 400 mg 3 times a day with equal effectiveness.

Other nutrients are also critical for nerve healing. One such element is lipoic acid (not in the vitamin powder), 300 to 1000 mg per day (see Chapter 8). Alpha lipoic acid is an antioxidant which has been shown to be beneficial for diabetic neuropathy. Another study showed that it was also helpful in relieving "burning mouth syndrome." This syndrome is characterized by chronic pain on the tongue and sometimes the anterior palate and lips without any visible lesions. It is most often seen in postmenopausal women and has characteristics of being neuropathic pain. In a study of 60 patients, half received 200 mg of lipoic acid 3 times a day or a placebo for 2 to 5 months. Ninety-seven percent of the patients improved as compared to 40 percent of those in the placebo group. Thirteen percent had complete resolution of their pain, and another 74 percent had "decided improvement," whereas none of the placebo patients had this level of improvement. Almost all the patients showed some improvement by 2 months, with 73 percent still showing benefit at the end of 12 months despite having stopped the treatment.[32] The fact that lipoic acid helps in several kinds of neuropathies suggests it is worth trying in others as well, especially since it is quite benign and not very expensive.

SAM-e is a nutrient produced from trimethylglycine (betaine) in combination with multiple nutrients, including B vitamins, folate, and inositol. It was initially tested and found to be effective in treating depression. Researchers also noted, as an aside, that it improved patients' arthritis as effectively as anti-inflammatory medications (NSAIDs). A number of studies were conducted including one that gave patients 600 mg a day for 2 weeks followed by 400 mg daily for 2 years. Pain and stiffness decreased within one week and the improvement continued throughout the two-year trial.[33] A study that reviewed seven other studies was inconclusive. A major problem with SAM-e is that it is not stable and breaks down easily, with many products not really delivering what they claim. In addition, it is quite expensive. A better alternative is to use the nutrients needed to make SAM-e in your body. Taking the nutrients found in the vitamin powder and B-complex can increase blood levels of SAM-e similar to levels found in those taking 400 to 800 mg of SAM-e daily.

## *I'll Give My Body the Nutrients It Needs for Healing. What's Next?*

Your repair cycle occurs during sleep and your body needs 8 to 9 hours of sleep a night for optimal healing. This is discussed in Chapter 3. Unfortunately, insomnia often accompanies pain. The good news is that many natural remedies that are very effective for sleep also directly help pain. My favorites are:

- **Wild Lettuce**—traditionally, wild lettuce has been found to be wonderful for anxiety and insomnia, as well as for headaches, muscles, and joint pain. Wild lettuce also helps to calm restlessness and reduce anxiety.
- **Jamaican Dogwood**—the extract acts as a muscle relaxant and also helps people to fall asleep while calming them.[34] According to tradition, Jamaican dogwood was used by Jamaican fishermen. Large amounts were thrown in the water. The fish would then be sedated and easy to net.
- **Hops**—this is a member of the hemp family, and the female flowers are used in beer making. It also stimulates some hormonal activity; can suppress breast, colon, and ovarian cancer in test tube studies; and has been reported to reduce hot flashes in menopausal women. It also is associated with antibiotic and anti-fungal activity. It has a long history of being used as a mild sedative for anxiety and insomnia. A study using 120 mg of hops combined with 500 mg of valerian showed an improvement in insomnia with effectiveness similar to Valium® family medications. It is considered to be very safe.[35]
- **Passionflower** (Passiflora)—this excellent herb is used throughout South America as a calming agent and is even present in sodas. In fact, when one is anxious, it is not uncommon for their friends to tell them "why don't you go get a passion flower drink." In addition to being used in the treatment of muscle spasms, herbalists have also used it to treat colic, dysentery, diarrhea, anxiety, and menstrual pain. A number of studies support its having a calming effect. Early data also suggests that it may increase men's libidos. The active component is in the leaves.[36] Passionflower has other pain management benefits as well. In one animal study, it was shown to decrease morphine tolerance and withdrawal, thereby improving morphine's effectiveness and safety.[37]
- **Valerian**—this is commonly used as a remedy for insomnia. One placebo-controlled study showed that people taking valerian (400 mg of extract each night for 2 weeks) fell asleep quicker and had better sleep quality without next-day sedation. Another

placebo-controlled study using 450 and 900 mg doses for just 1 night also showed improved sleep, but there was some hangover with the higher dose. A number of other studies also show benefit, including an improvement in deep sleep. The benefits were most pronounced when people used it for extended periods as opposed to simply taking it for 1 night. Another study showed it to be as effective as a Valium family medication (Oxazepam®). A review of multiple studies found that "valerian is a safe herbal choice for the treatment of mild insomnia and has good tolerance...Most studies suggest that it is more effective when used continuously rather than as an acute sleep aid."[38]

- **Theanine**—this comes from green tea and has been shown to improve deep sleep and to also help people maintain calm alertness during the day. Green tea also is helpful as an immune stimulant and has many other benefits.

Because I have found all six of these herbals to be dramatically helpful in patients with disordered sleep, anxiety, and/or chronic pain, I had them all combined in the Revitalizing Sleep Formula. 1 to 4 capsules can be taken at bedtime to help sleep, or an hour before bedtime if the main problem is falling asleep. It can also be used during the day for anxiety and pain. Although the bottle says to take up to 4 capsules a day, one could take up to 8 capsules, or more, each day, as it is very safe. As I noted earlier, 100 percent of my royalties for products I make go to charity. The vitamin powder, sleep herbal, and the other natural products discussed in this book are available in most health food stores or from www.vitality101.com.

### *Excellent! Now I Have a Natural Pain Formula and an Herbal Sleep Formula That Also Helps Pain. What Other Natural Remedies Can Help Me?*

Many other natural therapies can be powerfully effective in the treatment of pain while also being safe and relatively inexpensive. Although we do not have space to review all of them, let's look at a few that are worth being aware of.

I am a big fan of using topical therapies (see Chapter 22). By applying these gels directly to a targeted area of pain, you get a high dose to where it's needed without saturating your whole body as you do with tablets. A promising product for the relief of muscle and arthritis pain does just that. Joint Gel® by NF Formulas is an over-the-counter natural pain reliever that is applied directly on the skin. It contains menthol, MSM (Methyl Sulfonyl Methane), white willow, pine bark, and botanical oils that provide relief of aches and pains. Joint Gel also can relieve the pain of backaches, muscle sprains, and strains. Its roll-on design delivers the gel directly onto the skin and does not leave an oily or sticky feeling. As you massage the Joint Gel over the painful joint or muscle until absorbed, you'll initially feel the menthol. The active ingredient in peppermint is menthol, which serves as a counterirritant, stimulating the nerves that perceive cold while simultaneously depressing those for pain. Joint Gel's aloe leaf, white willow bark, and MSM are also well known (see above) for their natural pain relieving properties. Pine bark also provides unique antioxidants known to play a role in the stabilization of joints and muscles. Because of the eucalyptus, rosemary, and ginger botanical oils, Joint Gel also smells good. You can use Joint Gel 3 to 4 times daily.

Another wonderful treatment for inflammation is the use of **oral enzymes**. For those looking for a gentle, natural, and fairly side effect free method of reducing inflammation, digestive enzymes can be very helpful. When taken with food, enzymes help digest fats, proteins, and carbohydrates. When taken in between meals, digestive enzymes are absorbed into the bloodstream and are active throughout the body, not just in the digestive tract. This allows them to perform other functions such as combating inflammation. My favorite enzyme supplements for pain and inflammation are MegaZyme and Ultrazyme. They contain pancreatic enzymes (Protease, Amylase, and Lipase), Trypsin, Papain, Bromelain, Lysozyme, and Chymotrypsin.

Enzymes in high doses may "digest" inflammation by removing fibrin from inflamed areas, thereby restoring drainage and reducing swelling. This speeds wound healing. For example, one study used Bromelain, an enzyme derived from the stem of the pineapple plant, in 146 boxers with multiple face bruises and black and blue marks after a boxing match. Half the boxers received the real thing and half received placebo. All signs of bruising disappeared within 4 days in 78 percent of the boxers receiving Bromelain as compared to only 14 percent of those on a placebo.[39]

Some physicians are under the misconception that enzymes taken by mouth would simply be digested and not absorbed into the body. This is not the case when they are taken on an empty stomach. In this situation enzymes are well-absorbed, raising their levels in the blood.[40]

In addition to decreasing inflammation, taking enzymes may help improve function in other ways. Enzymes are necessary for many reactions to take place within your body's cells, such as assisting with rejuvenation and healing. For example, studies showed that taking large doses of pancreatic enzymes could help people with pancreatic cancer to live longer. Research by Dr. Gonzalez has shown this to be the case, and a larger scale study using this enzyme treatment in pancreatic cancer is now being funded by the National Cancer Institute. Many people have found that taking enzymes can markedly help decrease inflammatory pain. For example, in one study of muscle soreness after downhill running, subjects were either given enzymes or a placebo. In the enzyme group, muscle soreness was much less than the placebo group.[41]

Although I strongly recommend that people use **plant** based enzymes for digestion, pancreatic enzymes are better for inflammation. The pancreatic enzymes in Ultrazyme and MegaZyme are very high potency. The other enzymes present are also powerfully effective. Papain is often used to relieve the inflammation and pain in sports injuries because athletes have discovered that it speeds up the healing process. Papain has also been used to reduce inflammation from wisdom tooth extractions, root canals, and other oral surgeries. Unlike prescription anti-inflammatories such as Prednisone® (a powerful, prescription-only corticosteroid medication with a long list of health risks), enzymes treat inflammation safely.

Bromelain is another anti-inflammatory enzyme. By working with your body, Bromelain is able to reduce pain and inflammation caused by numerous health problems. It can also dissolve scar tissue and improve circulation. Bromelain helps the body make its own enzymes to dissolve and clean up dead tissue and debris from the site of inflammation.

To summarize, although enzymes such as Ultrazyme and MegaZyme may be helpful in aiding **digestion of your food** when taken **with** meals, I recommend that you **take them on an empty stomach** because enzymes are most effective at reducing pain and inflammation when you take them **between** meals. For acute pain, enzymes can simply be taken for a few days as needed. For chronic pain, begin by taking either of them regularly (2 to 3 tablets 3 times a day) between meals for 6 to 12 weeks to see how much it helps or until the pain and inflammation are gone. Then you can take the enzymes as needed.

## *Excellent! What Other Natural Tricks Do You Have Up Your Sleeve?*

A major problem in chronic pain is that the areas that hurt often have decreased blood flow. That means that even when you feed your body, the areas in pain may still be starved. This is one reason why using the intravenous "Myers cocktails" nutritional therapies can be so effective. The magnesium in the IV causes the closed-down blood vessels in your muscles and brain to open widely, flooding the starved areas with nutrients and washing away toxins. Unfortunately, although very worthwhile, these IV treatments require repeat visits by a nurse and cost approximately $80 to $100 per dose. Another way to get the blood vessels to open wide is to take a B vitamin called niacin (**not** niacinamide, which does not cause flushing). This trick was taught to me by a brilliant chiropractor and pain specialist, Ron Huse, D.C. (phone 281-996-8100), in

Houston Texas. Take 100 to 500 mg of niacin 3 to 4 times a day, as needed, to cause a "flushing" feeling, which occurs within approximately 10 to 20 minutes. This can significantly help pain and is inexpensive. Try to keep the dose at 1000 mg a day or less, if this is enough to cause flushing, because higher doses can sometimes (but rarely) cause liver inflammation or unmask diabetes. This treatment also helps to lower cholesterol and is often used for this purpose. The flushing will make you feel like you are in the Florida sun and may be intense. Do not worry; it is not dangerous and can help your muscles to heal while decreasing pain.

As you can probably tell, there are many natural and prescription treatments available that can be helpful. You do not have to be in pain. There are other excellent natural therapies to consider. Let's briefly discuss some of these.

## Homeopathics

The classic homeopathic for acute tissue injuries is Arnica. This can be highly effective and is available as a cream (Traumeel® by the Heel Company). This is a product that should be in everybody's medicine cabinet. See the section on the use of homeopathics in arthritis in Chapter 10 for more information.

## Other Herbals

These include:

- **Turmeric** (Curcumin Longa) is a common ingredient in curry powder and a relative of ginger. Turmeric contains curcumin, which can inhibit platelet aggregation and prostoglandin synthesis. Turmeric and curcumin have been shown to be effective antioxidants, with curcumin being the most potent component. A study of 45 days of supplementation with curcumin showed marked decreases (60 percent ) in the level of serum lipid peroxide. It is suspected that the curcumin might therefore reduce the risk of heart disease, cancer, and other "inflammatory" conditions.[42] It may also help asthma .[43] A review of several studies suggests that curcumin has anti-inflammatory, antioxidant, anti-carcinogenic, anti-viral, and anti-infectious activities.[44] A common dose would be 500 to 1000 mg 3 times a day. Unfortunately, curcumin is poorly absorbed in the absence of Piperine—a compound that comes from black pepper. Piperine can increase the absorption of many different substances and medications, potentially leading to toxic blood levels, however, and should therefore be used with caution—preferably with their use being guided by a health practitioner. When used in combination with boswellia, turmeric has been shown to improve both osteoarthritis and rheumatoid arthritis.

In traditional Indian medicine, curcumin has been used to treat arthritis, inflammation, skin disease, and infections for many centuries. It contains at least 133 active compounds, and approximately 400 studies have been published on curcumin in the last several years. It has also been found to be effective in treating gastric ulcers and indigestion as well as lowering serum cholesterol.[45]

- **Ginger** acts to decrease inflammation by inhibiting two key enzymes (cyclooxygenase and lipooxygenase with secondary leukotriene inhibition).[46] Although studies suggest some benefit with arthritis, I consider the effect to be modest compared to the End Pain formula.
- **Butterbur**—development of standardized extracts of butterbur has led to a powerful new natural tool in both the prevention and treatment of migraine headaches. Two randomized placebo-controlled double-blind studies have found it to be effective. In the first study, 60 migraine patients received 50 mg of the butterbur twice a day. By the 12th week, there was a 60 percent decrease in the number of migraine attacks compared to the placebo group. A second study of 202 migraine patients, who were given 75 mg of butterbur twice a day, showed a 58 percent decrease at 3 months. The 100 mg a day group had a 42 percent decrease at 3 months. About 20 percent of people taking the Butterbur noted increased burping.[47]
- **St. John's Wort** is best known for its effectiveness in the treatment of depression. It has, however, also been found to be helpful in treating neuropathic pain. In one study using approximately 1000 mg a day of St. John's Wort for 5 weeks, approximately 20 percent of the subjects had a good response. The effect was modest however, not quite reaching statistical significance.[48] This study is a good example of the difference between clinical and statistical significance. Although there was clinical benefit that justifies trying it in some refractory and severe cases, the number of patients in the study was small enough that the effect did not reach statistical significance. Because this treatment is safe, helps depression, and is inexpensive, it is worth a try—especially if other treatments have failed. For treating neuropathies, I would recommend taking 600 mg 3 times a day for 6 weeks. At that time you can decide whether the benefits justify staying on it.
- **Marijuana**—although it may seem odd to include this as an herbal, it is an herb, and it is my job to give you the medical information regardless of the politics involved. Studies suggest that the recep-

tors that marijuana binds to can also decrease pain. In can decrease the suffering associated with pain, impro situations where weight loss is associated with pain (e and is likely much safer than many other medications gredient in marijuana, called THC, is available by prescription in a medication called Marinol®. It is, of course, much more expensive in this form and probably not as effective, but it can be helpful.

- **Capsaicin** is another cream that comes from hot chili peppers. It works by depleting the substance P pain transmitter in nerve endings, interfering with the ability to send pain signals to the brain. It can be very helpful in some situations, but I tend to avoid using it. I am uncomfortable with irritating the body so much that it depletes the pain-sending chemicals. In addition, it can make the problem worse by stimulating pain when it is first used, and it has to be taken regularly or the pain-sending chemicals have a chance to recover.

## Treat Food Allergies and Sensitivities

As discussed earlier, the best approach I have found for the elimination of food and other sensitivities/allergies is a technique called NAET (see www.NAET.com). This technique combines acupressure with applied kinesiology in a special way and is powerfully effective. It can eliminate one allergy per 20 minute treatment. It got my attention when it knocked out my lifelong hay fever in a single 20 minute visit. I recommend that you read *Say Goodbye to Pain* by Dr. Devi Nambudripad for more information.

Another food sensitivity issue to consider is that a small percent of people with arthritis suffer aggravation of their arthritis from foods in the nightshade family. These include tomatoes, potatoes, eggplant, peppers, paprika, cayenne, and tobacco. I rarely need to have people consider this, but it is worth considering if arthritis pain persists despite other treatments. Eliminate the above foods from your diet for 1 month. If you do not experience relief, reintroduce these foods to see if they affect your symptoms.

## General Lifestyle Principles and Issues

It is important not to forget that some simple general principles and lifestyle issues are critical. For example, exercise daily for at least 20 minutes if you're able. Swimming, walking, and yoga are good choices. Using a heating pad or moist heat may give relief. Only use heat for 20 minutes at a time, so you don't overheat the affected area and cause further injury. The same applies when using ice. Use the ice first for 20 minutes (this acts as an anti-inflammatory) followed by heat for 20 minutes.

. can use either of these as often as you like, as long as you wait at ̣ast 30 minutes after the treatment before repeating the cycle. Ice works best for the first 24 to 36 hours after acute injuries, or for problems where inflammation plays a role, because of its anti-inflammatory effect. Heat works best for chronic pain, or for injuries that are over 24 hours old because it increases blood flow (and therefore healing) in the area.

## Body and Energy Work

Many forms of body and energy work can be powerfully effective in treating pain. These include but are certainly not limited to acupuncture, chiropractic, osteopathy craniosacral therapy, myofascial release, Rolfing, Trager, Reiki, and many others. See the Chapter 21 for more information on structural therapies—specifically chiropractic and osteopathy—and Chapter 6 for information on other forms of body work.

## Home Remedies

The following remedy is inexpensive and easy to try. Please let me know how it works for you! You can send me messages or questions at www.vitality101.com.

> Purple Pectin for Pain (especially arthritis): Purchase Certo® in the canning section of your local grocery. It is the thickening agent used to make jams and jellies. Certo contains pectin, a natural ingredient found in the cell walls of plants. Use 1 to 3 Tbsp of Certo in 8 ounces of grape juice 1 to 2 times daily. If it's going to help, you'll likely know in 7 to 14 days. You can lower the dose as you feel better.

## Hypnosis and Magnets

Although a detailed discussion of these therapies is outside the scope of this book, they can both be very helpful. The type of magnet used is important, because the strength and field configuration can be critical. Nikkan Company magnets seem to be fairly reliable (see Appendix C: Resources).

Hypnosis can also be helpful for pain. I have seen it decrease the intensity of pain, change its location, decrease the suffering associated with pain, and change the sensation so that it feels like warmth or softness instead of pain.

These are simply a sampling of some natural remedies that are available. In the next chapter, I discuss chiropractic and osteopathic treatment therapies, which are two very effective structural therapies. ■

**Important Points**

1. Natural remedies can be powerful tools when treating pain. Unfortunately, most medical doctors have a strong bias against natural remedies. Although they think that this bias is based on lack of scientific evidence (what they like to call "evidence-based medicine"), it is actually simply based on a lack of awareness of the scientific data.
2. Three excellent pain relieving herbals are willow bark, boswellia, and tart cherry. All three of these can be found in combination in the End Pain formula. Begin with 2 tablets 2 to 3 times a day, as needed, until maximum benefit is achieved (approximately 4 to 6 weeks) and then you can use the lowest effective dose.
3. Take the Energy Revitalization System vitamin powder, which has many nutrients that help pain, and add sleep herbals, if needed, for 8 hours sleep a night (see Section 1 General Principles of Pain Relief). The sleep herbals in the Revitalizing Sleep Formula decrease pain as well.
4. If you have arthritis, or back pain from arthritis of the spine bones (vertebrae), take Glucosamine **Sulfate** (500 mg 3 times day—takes six weeks to work), and consider MSM (3 grams a day for 2 to 5 months).
5. If you have nerve pain, take lipoic acid 200 to 300 mg 3 times a day (takes weeks to months to help).
6. Joint Gel® is an over-the-counter natural pain reliever that is applied directly on the skin. Joint Gel contains many different natural products that provide relief of aches and pains.
7. Digestive enzymes can actually digest away inflammation. High potency forms aid in **digestion of your food** when taken **with** meals. I recommend that you **take the high potency enzymes on an empty stomach,** however, because these types of enzymes are most effective at reducing pain and inflammation when you take them between meals. For acute pain, enzymes can be taken for a few days as needed. For chronic pain, begin by taking either the enzymes regularly (e.g. 2 to 3 tablets 3 times a day for Ultrazyme) between meals for 6 to 12 weeks to see how much it helps, or until the pain

*Continued on next page*

**Important Points** *(continued)*

and inflammation are gone. Then you can take the enzymes as needed.

8. A major problem in chronic pain is that the areas that hurt often have decreased blood flow. This is one reason why using the intravenous "Myers cocktails" nutritional therapies can be so effective. A less expensive way to get the blood vessels to open wide is to take a B vitamin called niacin (**not** niacinamide, which does not cause flushing). Take 100 to 500 mg of niacin 3 to 4 times a day as needed to cause a "flushing" feeling, which occurs within approximately 10 to 20 minutes. This can significantly help pain and is a very inexpensive treatment. Try to keep the dose at 1000 mg a day or less if this is enough to cause flushing, because higher doses can sometimes (but rarely) cause liver inflammation or unmask diabetes. The flushing may be intense, however, it is not dangerous and can help your muscles to heal while decreasing pain.
9. Treat food allergies and sensitivities. As discussed in this book, the best approach I have found for the elimination of food and other sensitivities/allergies is a technique called NAET (see www.NAET.com).
10. Homeopathics can be helpful in treating pain (see discussion in Chapter 1).
11. Consider home remedies such as purple pectin (especially for arthritis). Purchase Certo® in the canning section of your local grocery. Certo contains pectin, a natural ingredient found in the cell walls of plants. Use 1 to 3 Tbsp in 8 ounces of grape juice 1 to 2 times daily. If it's going to help, you'll likely know in 7 to 14 days. You can lower the dose as you feel better.
12. Consider hypnosis and/or magnets for pain treatment.

CHAPTER 21

# Structural Therapies—Chiropractic and Osteopathic Medicine

## Osteopathy

Osteopathy combines both pharmacologic/surgical medicine and an emphasis on the inter-relationship between structure and function in the body. It also has an appreciation of the body's ability to heal itself. There are 14 principles of osteopathic philosophy. Here are a few of them:

1. The body is a single system that includes mind and spirit as well as muscles, bones, and organs.
2. The body is capable of self-healing, self-regulation, and self maintenance.
3. The structure of parts of the body will affect the functioning of those body parts.
4. Treatment should consider the unity of the body, as well as the interactions of specific treatments, and should harness the body's self-regulatory ability to heal as much as possible.

Where in the past, osteopathy was viewed as providing more natural therapies, some osteopathic physicians are becoming more and more like MDs. Others are taking full advantage of the strength of combining osteopathic manipulation and natural remedies with prescription and surgical therapies. Pain is the most common reason why patients seek osteopathic manipulation. Although this is a marked oversimplification, osteopathic manipulative treatment (OMT) is the manual application of forces to the body to restore maximal pain-free movement of the musculoskeletal system. Osteopathy looks at restrictions in movement and asymmetry of body parts. Manipulative therapy is then used to restore balance and range of motion. Although a proper review of osteopathy could easily fill many books, it can be said that a trained osteopathic can work wonders in ways that are both safe and cost-effective.

## Chiropractic

This is a healthcare discipline that focuses on the relationship between the spine and body function (coordinated via the nervous system). Chiropractic practitioners feel that this relationship is critical in maintaining and restoring health. Spinal manipulation was used as early as 2700 B.C. in Chinese medicine, and manipulation techniques were also used by Hippocrates and Galen.

A bit over 100 years ago, David Palmer developed the principles upon which modern chiropractic is based. He felt that abnormal nerve function was a primary cause of medical problems, and he recommended adjustments to the spine to treat this. Although some physicians accepted his principles, others objected to anybody who proposed any treatments besides their own. This resulted in Palmer and other early chiropractors being arrested. This rift between chiropractors and medical doctors persisted with the AMA even saying that it was unethical for any physician to work with a chiropractor and that any doctor who did so could lose his or her license. This continued until the AMA lost an antitrust suit brought by the chiropractors.

As is the case in many fields, growth occurred in many different directions in chiropractic. The more conservative chiropractors believed that poor alignment in the spine (subluxation) was the only problem that needed to be treated. Other chiropractors recognize that multiple causes could be at play, and they work alongside physicians and other practitioners.

Chiropractors are the most commonly used health practitioners after physicians and dentists. There are over 60,000 licensed chiropractors in the U.S. Almost 80 percent of chiropractic visits are for musculoskeletal complaints, and over 40 percent are for back pain. In 1999, 11 percent of adults and over 30 percent of patients with low back pain visited a chiropractor.

As chiropractic has continued to grow, over 100 different approaches have been developed. Most fall under the following categories:

1. Manipulation to decrease joint restriction, increase range of motion, and restore vertebrae to their normal position
2. Traction
3. Massage/soft tissue mobilization directed at muscle, tendon, and other non-bony tissues
4. Electrical muscle stimulation
5. Diathermy—using electrical currents to produce heat
6. Ultrasound
7. Ice therapy

8. Heat
9. Exercise-based programs
10. Nutritional and metabolic support
11. Energy medicine

Because body manipulation requires hands-on therapy, it is very difficult to do a double-blind study. This has been used by some traditional physicians as an excuse to ignore and put down chiropractic while conveniently forgetting that surgery faces the same scientific problem. Also, because the types of chiropractic treatment vary so widely, it is difficult to compare the results of different studies. Nonetheless, it has survived because people find it to be helpful and often safer than using medications.[1]

Although I have focused mostly on osteopathy and chiropractic in this chapter, these are simply two out of dozens of different forms of body/structural/energy work that can be powerfully effective. ■

**Important Points**

1. Osteopathy combines both pharmacologic and surgical medicine with an emphasis on the interrelationship between structure and function in the body. It also has an appreciation of the body's ability to heal itself.
2. Osteopathic manipulative treatment (OMT) is the manual application of forces to the body to restore maximal pain-free movement of the musculoskeletal system. Osteopathy looks at restrictions in movement and asymmetry of body parts. Manipulative therapy is then used to restore balance and range of motion.
3. Chiropractic is a healthcare discipline that focuses on the relationship between the spine and body function (coordinated via the nervous system). Chiropractic practitioners feel that this relationship is critical in maintaining and restoring health.
4. Chiropractors are the most commonly used health practitioners after physicians and dentists. There are over 60,000 licensed chiropractors in the U.S. Almost 80 percent of chiropractic visits are for musculoskeletal complaints and, over 40 percent are for back pain.

CHAPTER 22

# Prescription Therapies—We're Way Past Aspirin!

In this chapter, we will review prescription pain medications. These include:

- Topical therapies—creams and gels that can be rubbed directly on the painful areas, can be effective, and have almost no side effects
- Oral pain medications—tablets and capsules taken by mouth
- IV medications—those that are administered intravenously

Today, on one hand we have dozens of tools that can be used to eliminate your pain. On the other hand, it can be overwhelming to have so many options. This is why I provide the pain algorithms in Appendix B: Pain Treatment Protocol. Eliminating pain is like buying shoes. You don't want to go into a shoe store that sells only one pair or you're likely to be out of luck. With so many options available to eliminate pain, it's nice to know where to start. Following the algorithms in Appendix A will tell you exactly what to try and the order in which to try them until you (or your patients) become pain-free.

As a reminder, although these medications can be helpful, it is always best to go after the underlying causes of the pain first, so that you can make it go away permanently. This is discussed in the earlier part of this book. In most cases, medications simply give symptomatic relief without eliminating the underlying cause of the pain. We began by discussing the natural therapies, as these remedies are likely to be safer, less expensive (unless you have prescription coverage), and have less side effects.

I would begin by going after the perpetuating factors involved in pain (i.e. nutritional, hormonal, and sleep deficiencies, and underlying infections), followed by adding in natural remedies (see Chapter 20). Then use the prescription pain creams. The oral and IV medications below can (and should) be added if needed, because it is unhealthy to be in pain. On the other hand, it is also reasonable to begin immediately with the prescription pain medications such as Ultram® for immediate pain relief while you're waiting for the other treatments to take effect.

Keep in mind the following general principles before beginning pain medications:

A. Do not get pregnant while on any medication.

B. Some medications are expensive. Most often, a generic medication is as effective as a brand name, but much less expensive. Some patients like to get 10 to 30 tablets of the brand-name medication first, so they can see what it does, and then switch to the generic. If there is a difference between the brand name and generic medications, you would be able to tell. Unfortunately, some pharmacies are drastically marking up the cost of generics, keeping the savings for themselves. To see what a generic medication really should cost, go to Costco pharmacies (or visit them online at www.Costco.com). They have a policy of marking up the price to a set amount over their cost, passing the savings on to the customer. You do not have to be a Costco member to use the pharmacy. If you go to one of their stores, simply tell the person at the door that you are going to the pharmacy.

C. Most medications are much less expensive in higher dose tablets. For example, a 40 mg dose tablet may cost the same as a 20 mg dose tablet. You can save 50 percent by getting a higher strength tablet and breaking it in half.

D. The price of the same medication can vary dramatically from pharmacy to pharmacy. It pays to call around and check prices. An excellent mail order pharmacy is Consumers Discount Drug Company (phone 1- 323-461-3606). If you can find a reliable Canadian pharmacy, I recommend ordering from them directly.

E. For some medications, you are likely to get more benefit relative to the side effects at a lower dose. As you push the higher doses, you get more side effects for less benefit. In addition, people sometimes get the full benefit without side effects at a small fraction of the "standard" starting dose—a fact that most doctors are not aware of. Because of this, if you have a medication that helps but causes side effects, try lowering the dose to even a fraction of the starting dose. Find the dose that gives the most benefit relative to side effects. This said, some medications do require a high dose before you see the effect.

F. Doctors are often taught to give one medication, raise it to the maximum tolerated dose, and then switch to another medication if an adequate effect is not seen. They avoid combining medications because of the risk of drug interactions. In treating chronic pain or insomnia, however, I have found that patients are more likely to get excellent results with fewer side effects if they mix low doses of several medications instead of taking a high dose of a single medicine. As noted previously, this is because most people get more benefit and fewer side effects at lower doses of a medication. This is especially true with medications that can be sedating. Mixing medications from different categories (see below) is more likely to help than combining medicines within a category. The exception is if a medication greatly helps, but you cannot get an adequate dose without unacceptable side effects. In that situation, trying other medications within the same category is a good idea.

G. Do not drive while on any medication that is sedating. You may not always be aware of the sedation. In addition, some of these medications interact poorly with alcohol. Some people will (I think reasonably) try having a drink at home when on a steady dose of the medications to see if it causes any reactions. Legally, I must tell you not to take any alcohol with these medications.

H. It takes less medication to prevent than to knock out pain when it is severe.

I. Many people are afraid to take the amount of pain medication they need because of side effects, addiction, or because they consider it a sign of weakness to take medication. For those of you who have these concerns, I would like to make several points:

  1. As noted above, you'll use less medicine in preventing pain than in trying to eliminate it once it is severe. This means that if the pain comes back every 6 hours after you take the pain medicine, take the medicine every 5 hours—even if you're not in pain when you take the medicine.
  2. The stress of pain takes a toll on your body that is not healthy. Pain is simply meant to tell you that there's something wrong that you need to pay attention to. Once you do this, the pain is no longer healthy and should be eliminated.
  3. I suspect that you get no bonus points in heaven for having suffered through the pain instead of taking the medications needed to be comfortable. I often tell my patients the story about the pious man who lived in Johnstown during the Johnstown flood. The National Guard came into the city and told everyone they had to evacuate or they would drown. This man refused to leave, saying that he had faith in God and that God would protect him. The floodwaters came and soon the Coast Guard boat arrived, floating by his second story window. They beseeched him to

climb in the boat and be saved but he refused, once again saying that he had faith in God to protect him. Pretty soon he was up on the top of his roof and a helicopter came by and yelled at him to get in. Once again he refused—and the man drowned. He went to heaven, and God came by. The man was very angry at God and said, "I had full faith in you and you let me drown!" God said, "What are you talking about? I sent the National Guard, the Coast Guard, and a helicopter!" The medications are like the National Guard, the Coast Guard, and the helicopter. It's okay to use them!

## *The Anatomy of Pain Transmission*

For background about how the pain medications work, it is helpful to look at how pain is transmitted in the body. However, it is not critical to know the details and, once again, feel free to skip this section.

In most cases, the sensation of pain is generated in nerve fibers in the skin or joints. It is then sent to the spine, and from there to the brain. In the brain, the pain signal is either ignored, modified, or amplified. The pain signal can be disrupted or modified anywhere along this pathway.

There are an immense number of receptors along this route, and researchers are finding more all the time. To list and discuss them all would be a mind-numbing adventure that is not necessary for you to understand to make your pain go away. But, for those who are interested, I will mention a few of the key ones.

The key receptors in the central nervous system (brain) for moderating pain are the NMDA (N-Methyl-D-aspartate) receptors. These receptors can be stimulated by glutamate, which is one reason why some people are so sensitive to the MSG (mono sodium Glutamate) in Chinese or other foods. When these receptors are stimulated, pain is increased. Other chemicals then become involved. These include substance P (a major chemical that transmits pain), alpha agonists (enhancers included in medications such as Clonidine® and Zanaflex®), and antagonists (blockers such as minipress), and GABA (gamma-amino butyric acid), which settles down the pain signal. For all of these to work, we need adequate minerals such as calcium, magnesium, potassium, and sodium, which travel through channels. Modifying these channels can also impact pain. Different medications impact a different mix of receptors. One is more likely to see an effect by trying or combining medicines that work on different parts of the system, than by combining two medicines with the same type of action.

For example, the anti-seizure medicine Neurontin® (which also blocks glutamate) and the calcium channel blocker Procardia® can both be effective for nerve pain. Both suppress NMDA reactivity by different mechanisms, thereby muting the pain signal. Catapres®, which is a calcium channel blocker, stimulates alpha receptors and blocks the release of norepinephrine. In cases where adrenaline is stimulating pain, this can settle down the discomfort. Like most medications, however, it has multiple actions. Catapres also enhances the opioid (narcotic) receptors, decreasing substance P, which also decreases pain. Blocking the calcium channels also relaxes the blood vessels and gets more blood flowing into the tissues, which is another way that pain is decreased. Although both Catapres and Procardia are calcium channel blockers, only the Catapres also stimulates the opioid receptors.

Zanaflex® is an alpha stimulator that also relaxes muscles. In addition, it decreases reflex activity within the spine, reducing the release of glutamate and substance P and thereby decreasing NMDA activity. Lidocaine® and Novocaine® are anesthetics that work topically by blocking sodium channel activity.

These are just a few examples of how different medications can be combined, taking advantage of their different effects. It's really not necessary to understand or follow any thing in this section, except to remember that it can help to combine medications that work by different mechanisms. It is not a clear-cut issue however, as most medications work through a number of different mechanisms—many of which we may not even be aware of. In the section below in which oral medications are reviewed, the treatments are discussed and categorized by their general mechanisms. Again, it is not necessary to understand these mechanisms to treat pain. It is reasonable to simply try the medications to see what works.

## Topical Medications

The use of topical delivery systems for pain medications is a major leap forward in pain management. It allows high doses of multiple medications that get right to your area of pain—usually with no side effects. One of the many common "recipes" for the pain gel is the following combined in a PLO gel:

- Ketamine®, 10 percent
- Lidocaine®, 15 percent
- Baclofen®, 4 percent,
- Amitriptyline®, 2 percent,
- Clonidine®, 0.2 percent,
- Ketoprofen®, 10 percent
- Ibuprofen, 10 percent

Rub a large pea sized amount into a silver dollar sized area at the center of a painful area 3 times a day. Give it 2 weeks to work.

There are over a dozen medications that can be combined in these topical gels. Although they are administered by prescription, compounding pharmacists are usually happy to guide your physician in their use. (See Appendix C: Resources.)

Some gels and creams can markedly enhance the penetration of medications through your skin. Medications go directly to the area of pain in high concentrations while the rest of your body (which does not need the medication) receives very low levels. This is why side effects are usually nonexistent despite the creams being highly effective. These creams need to be put together by compounding pharmacists, who can sometimes tailor the dosing to your case. Because of the time and work involved in mixing these medications, most drug companies and pharmacists are not willing to mix them. Although the creams require a prescription, many prescription plans will not cover them. I recommend paying for the first tube of the cream yourself (approximately $50 to $100 for a 1 to 3 months supply). If it helps you and allows you to lower your dose of other pain medications, or keeps your doctor from having to prescribe the new very expensive medications, you'll often find that you can talk your insurance company into covering the cost.

For those of you who are getting benefit from a NSAID (e.g. Motrin®) for treating a small area of pain, at least four studies have now shown that they can also be effective (and much safer) when used in a topical cream. In one double-blind study using a topical cream for knee arthritis without swelling, patients rubbed a 5 percent ibuprofen (Motrin) cream (containing 200 mg of ibuprofen) into the knee 3 times a day. The cream started to work by the fourth day, and by the eighth day there was an average 45 percent decrease in pain. All patients were helped and 40 percent considered the treatment to be "very good." No side effects were seen.[1]

To get an even more powerful, yet safe, effect from these creams and gels, there are many medications that can be combined, and selecting the correct combination is an art. Some pharmacists and physicians prefer to begin with just few medications (e.g. ketoprofen 10 percent and Flexeril® 2 percent applied 3 times a day locally for trigger point pain). Others would begin with ketoprofen 15 percent, Flexeril® 3 percent, and Lidocaine® 5 percent. I often begin with a mixture of 5 or more medications as this can enhance the effectiveness—usually without any side effects. Give the creams at least 1 to 2 weeks to work, and be willing to continue adjusting the mix until you find what works. Below is a list of just some of the medications that can be added to the creams:

- Ketoprofen®, Piroxicam, Diclofenac, or Ibuprofen (these four are NSAID anti-inflammatories)
- Neurontin®
- Clonidine
- Amitriptyline
- Cyclobenzaprine®
- Baclofen®
- Ketamine
- Lidocaine
- Guaifenesin
- Capsaicin
- Cortisone and/or Sarapin®

Fortunately, even though topical medications are in the "baby stages" of development, researchers and the pharmaceutical companies are beginning to recognize their power. Dr. Stephen Hersh M.D., Clinical Professor at George Washington University School of Medicine and a member of the American Pain Society has found compounded pain creams to be very helpful. For his RSD patients, he uses a combination of gabapentin and clonidine cream, which is applied to the affected area 2 to 3 times a day. He notes, "instant relief [using pain creams] has not been my goal nor has it been my experience...unless a patient is allergic to one of the compounds in the topical medication, these are interventions that, unlike many in the treatment of chronic pain, truly do no harm."[2] If your physician is not familiar with compounded pain creams, the pharmacist at Cape Apothecary (Tom @ 410-757-3522) can help guide your physician and can mail you the cream if prescribed.

## Patches

If you have a prescription plan, you may want to begin with the Lidocaine® patch. This Novocain-like patch is applied directly over the area of maximum pain. It can be cut to fit the area, and up to 4 patches can be used at a time (although the package insert says to use only 3). It is left on for 12 hours and then removed for 12 hours each 24-hour period, although recent reports have suggested that they can be left on for 18 to 24 hours and still be safe and effective.[3] Results will usually be seen within two weeks. Because the effect is local, side effects are minimal. The most common side effect is a mild skin rash from the patch. It should not be used if you have an allergy to Novocain®/Lidocaine®.

The patches are most likely to be helpful if the pain is localized to a moderately sized area. Even in a large area however, patches can be used on the most uncomfortable spots. The main downside of the patches is that they are expensive. If you have prescription insurance however, they will usually be covered. I suspect that, overall, patches will be more effective than the creams by themselves, because putting a medication "under occlusion" (i.e. with the patch over it) drives medication through the skin more effectively.

## Oral Pain Medications

Although I have organized the medications by "category," it is not at all important that you understand what these categories mean (the information here is mostly for your physician). The chapters in which we discussed the different kinds of pain (e.g. neuropathic, muscular, arthritic, etc.) and the summary sections on these chapters (see Appendix A) give the order in which to try the pain medications. If you are not clear on the source/type of your pain, there are many reasonable sequences in which to try the medications. One way to try them is in the order below. When there are several medications on the same line, if the first medication helped but was not tolerated because of side effects, go to the next medication on the same line. If that medication does not help significantly, go to the next line. If you get partial benefit from a medication, continue it and add another medication as needed to get pain-free. Here is the order:

1. Lidocaine® patches and/or gels for localized area of pain
2. Tylenol®
3. Motrin®, Voltaren®, or Daypro® (your insurance company prefers that these be tried before Celebrex® because of cost). Long-term use is associated with significant risks and side effects, and other medications may be better for non-arthritis pain. If you try any two NSAID medications (e.g. Motrin and Naprosyn®) and your doctor notes on the medical record that you had side effects such as acid stomach from both of them, your insurance company is much more likely to cover the Celebrex.
4. Celebrex
5. Skelaxin® (for muscle pain/achiness)
6. Ultram® (like narcotics, it is good for overall pain relief and is a reasonable medication to begin with as well)
7. Neurontin®, Gabitril®, and/or Pregabalin®
8. Flexeril® (for muscle pain/achiness)
9. Elavil®, Doxepin®, Desipramine® (norpramin), or nortriptyline (Pamelor®)

10. Zanaflex®
11. Effexor®
12. Baclofen® (for muscle pain/achiness)
13. Klonopin® (for muscle pain/achiness)
14. Topamax®
15. Lamictal®
16. Keppra®
17. Narcotics

This is not a complete list of medications discussed in this chapter. There are many treatments that can help. Appendix B: Pain Treatment Protocol gives the directions on how to use each medication.

## *Aspirin and NSAIDs (Non Steroidal Anti-inflammatory Drugs)*

NSAIDs block inflammation by inhibiting hormones called prostaglandins (PGE). This family of hormones comes from special fats/oils in our diet (essential fatty acids). The prostaglandin that causes inflammation is called PGE2. This hormone is made from animal fats (arachadonic acid). Other oils (especially fish oil, flaxseed oil, and borage oil) make different prostaglandin hormones (PGE1 and PGE3) that inhibit inflammation. In addition, these prostaglandins protect your stomach from developing ulcers. Aspirin/NSAID family medications block all of these prostaglandins, resulting in approximately 1 percent of chronic users per year developing ulcers or other serious gastrointestinal complications.[4] This is why approximately 15,000 to 20,000 Americans die each year from these medications (mostly from bleeding ulcers). In fact, NSAIDs are the most common cause of prescription drug adverse reactions, accounting for over 107,000 U.S .hospitalizations and 16,500 U.S. deaths annually. Over $2.5 billion dollars a year is spent on the purchase of these drugs with another 4 billion dollars being spent to manage their side effects.[5–6] Using fish oil and cutting down on animal fats is a safer way to get much of these medications' benefits. In addition, willow bark and other natural remedies (see Chapter 20) can be effective, and are much safer than NSAIDs.

NSAIDs are rarely beneficial in fibromyalgia (a muscle pain disorder). In one study, NSAIDs were no more effective than a placebo.[7] There are many different categories of NSAIDs. As your physician is likely familiar with this family of medications, and as I am not thrilled with their being used for long-term treatment because of side effects, I'm not going to talk about them at great depth. Let's review the key points, however.

It is important to be aware that NSAIDs can belong to different families (chemical structures), and therefore all NSAIDs do not behave the same. If you do not get better with an NSAID in one family, do not try another in the same family. Instead go to one in a different family.

Families of NSAIDs:

1. Propionic—includes ibuprofen (Motrin® and Advil®), naproxen (Naprosyn® and Aleve®), Oxaprozin® (Daypro®), and ketoprofen
2. Acetic—includes diclofenac (Voltaren®), indomethacin (Indocin®), Tolmetin®, and Sulindac® (Clinoral®)
3. Salicylic (carboxylic)—includes aspirin and diflunisal (Dolobid®)
4. Anthranilic (enolic)—piroxicam (Feldene®)
5. Pyrrolopyrroles—etodolac and Ketorolac® (Toradol®)

For example, you may not respond to ibuprofen, but may respond well to Voltaren®. The important thing is that if you try ibuprofen, don't try naproxen next because you're just adding a chemically similar agent. If you use one type of NSAID and it does not work, change to another family altogether if you're going to try another NSAID. This applies not just to effectiveness, but also to tolerability.

I recommend beginning with Motrin® (Advil®, ibuprofen) or Daypro®, followed by Voltaren® (which seems to be easier on the stomach). If these do not work, I recommend switching to a COX-2 inhibitor (i.e.- Celebrex®, see below). Although NSAIDs can be very good for inflammatory pain, they usually work poorly for muscle/myofascial pain. Based on its mechanism of action, one would expect that Celebrex would not work for muscle pain either. Nonetheless, my patients taught me that this medication can be highly effective for muscle pain that is not helped by NSAIDs. We still have a lot to learn.

## *Selective COX-2 Inhibitors*

These medications inhibit certain inflammatory pathways more specifically than the NSAIDs, inhibiting those involved in inflammation, while not affecting those that protect the stomach lining. Because of this, they're considered less likely to cause stomach bleeding and irritation In my experience, patients have found Celebrex (100 to 200 mg 1 to 2 times a day) and Bextra (20 mg 1 to 2 times daily) to be far more effective for fibromyalgia and muscle pain than the NSAIDs, which only seem to help in 10 to 15 percent of patients. They are also much easier on the stomach.

In one study conducted over a period of 12 weeks, stomach ulcers were seen in 7 percent of patients given a placebo, approximately 7 percent of patients on a Cox-2 medication, and 29 percent of patients on Motrin (800 mg 3 times a day).[8] Unfortunately, Cox-2 medications are expensive (costing about $75 to $100 a month) and many insurance companies will not pay for them unless you have tried two NSAIDs and they either did not work or you were not able to tolerate them because of stomach pain. Many of you have already tried Advil® and Naprosyn (Aleve®). If these did not help or caused indigestion, you can then request that your insurance company pay for the Celebrex. Vioxx® has been removed from the market as it may increase rates of heart attack and stroke. In addition, it may result in high blood pressure. Researchers at the Arthritis Research Center Foundation in Wichita, Kansas, examined data on 8538 patients who were taking rofecoxib (Vioxx), celecoxib (Celebrex), or other NSAIDs. They determined that taking Vioxx also increased the risk of lower leg swelling (a symptom often linked to hypertension and other cardiac diseases) by 23 percent and increased blood pressure by 21 percent compared to other NSAID use.[9]

Overall, I prefer to use Celebrex over Bextra. Patients, who are allergic to sulfa antibiotics cannot take Celebrex, however, but can consider Bextra (although some cross sensitivity in sulfa allergic patients may still occur). In addition, for severe menstrual cramps, Bextra (20 mg twice a day) can be very effective.

## *Acetaminophen/Tylenol®*

For many people, acetaminophen can be a safe and effective pain medication. Simply be aware that chronic use at too high of a dose can cause liver and sometimes kidney problems. Do not take over 4000 mg a day, and for chronic use it is best to stay under 2000 to 3000 mg daily. If you are taking more than 1000 mg a day on a regular basis, you are probably depleting a critical antioxidant called glutathione. This can result in many other problems. Taking the Energy Revitalization System vitamin powder can help restore your glutathione levels by supplying vitamin C, NAC, and other key amino acids. Unfortunately taking glutathione by mouth is not effective. If you are taking over 1500 mg of acetaminophen a day on a regular basis, get an extra 500 to 650 mg of NAC from your health food store (or www.vitality101.com) and take it each day along with the vitamin powder.

A common problem is that people often take several different medications that contain acetaminophen. In addition to Tylenol®, it can also be found in many prescription and over-the-counter cold, sleep, pain, and other remedies. Please check to see how much acetaminophen is in each medication you are taking, so that you can be sure that you're not getting toxic amounts. This has become a significant concern with an alarming number of patients suffering from serious side effects associated with accidental overdosing of acetaminophen. This results in over

56,000 hospital emergency room visits and 100 deaths a year according to the FDA.[10] This risk is especially alarming when you realize that acetaminophen is only modestly superior to a placebo for treating arthritis. At higher doses of acetaminophen (over 2 g a day), the risk of gastrointestinal bleeding increases 3.6 fold. At doses of over 3600 mg, the risk was equivalent to that of aspirin and NSAIDs. In addition, kidney failure and death from liver failure was more common in people taking acetaminophen for pain than in those who overdosed.[11]

Although I consider acetaminophen to be an excellent drug for short-term or intermittent use, especially at doses under 2000 mg a day, other medications may be safer for long-term and chronic use—and will likely be more effective.

## *Muscle Relaxants*

Some muscle relaxants work directly on the brain, causing less muscle weakness. One excellent medication is Skelaxin® (800 mg 3 to 4 times a day), which is low in side effects. In some people it works wonderfully and in others it does nothing. For muscle pain, give it a few weeks to see the effect. This is a medication I use frequently because it is not sedating.

Other medications work directly on the muscles to cause relaxation instead of working at the level of brain or nerve function. Because of this, they are also not likely to cause sedation or confusion, but they are more likely to cause muscle weakness.

One such medication is Dantrolene® (Dantrium®), which works directly on the muscle causing it to relax (by blocking the release of calcium from the sarcoplasmic reticulum and inhibiting muscle contraction). The usual dose is 25 to 100 mg given 3 to 4 times daily. The main problem with using this medication is that it can cause liver damage in about 1 percent of patients who use it, and liver blood tests may need to be monitored.

## *GABA-augmenting Medications*

GABA is a chemical compound in the brain that tends to settle down excess stimulation. Historically, GABA-augmenting medications have been used to treat muscle spasm. The medication Baclofen® has been used for almost 40 years, and has been found to be safe and effective and is considered a key first-line therapy for spasticity.

Unlike some medications, Baclofen® can be used over a wide range of dosing. Although a common dose is 10 to 20 mg 2 to 4 times a day, doses as low as 5 mg or as high as 200 mg a day can be used. Its main limiting side effects are sedation and, at higher doses, muscle weakness.

In addition, withdrawal spasms and other side effects ca medication is stopped abruptly. Because of this, if you ha Baclofen® for an extended time and you want to stop, yo weaned off the medication slowly. This medication may a for post traumatic stress disorder.[12]

I found that newer medications that affect GABA are m... effective than Baclofen® and work on many different kinds of pain. These include:

1. **Neurontin**® (gabapentin). This seizure medication can help a wide variety of pain patients. Although it is related to the GABA neurotransmitters, how it works is unclear. It does stimulate GABA receptors in ways that are different from Baclofen®. Although it causes sedation and other neurologic side effects in some patients, overall it is very safe and well-tolerated. It has been proven to be effective in both diabetic neuropathy and post herpetic neuralgia (shingles pain). Begin with 300 mg at bedtime. Patients who are very sensitive to medications should begin with only 100 mg. If tolerated, you can increase the dose to 600 mg the 2nd night and 900 mg the 3rd night. You can then increase the neurontin dose by 300 mg once or twice weekly (or more quickly if side effects are not a problem). When taking over 900 mg a day, divide the total amount into 3 daily doses. If there is no effect at 2400 mg a day, the medication is not likely to help. If you have been on the medication for more than a few months, it should be tapered off over several weeks. Although it is rare, withdrawal can occur if this medication is stopped suddenly. If only partial relief is seen at 2400 mg a day, the dose can be raised as high as 4800+ mg daily. The medication may not be absorbed as effectively if taken within a few hours of magnesium (or aluminum antacids). Therefore, if it's convenient, take the vitamin powder, which contains magnesium, a few hours away from the Neurontin® dose.

2. **Gabitril**®. As noted in Section 3 on neuropathic pain (see Chapter 8), Gabitril® (tiagabine) is an anti-seizure medication that has also been shown to increase GABA by inhibiting reuptake (the same way that Prozac® raises serotonin). Although not FDA approved for sleep, studies have found that, in addition to decreasing pain, the medication can also can improve deep sleep.[13] The main side effects are sedation, dizziness, irritability, and gastric upset. It is best to take Gabitril® with food. The most common effective dose of the Gabitril® is 16 mg a day (range 10 to 24 mg a day)

   In one study, Gabitril® was given at a dose of 2 mg twice a day and increased by up to 4 mgs daily each week to a maximum of 24 mg a day. Other patients received Neurontin, beginning at 100 mg

..ce daily and increasing by 300 mg a day each week to a maximum of 2400 mg a day. The 91 patients participating all had chronic pain of different types. Gabitril® decreased pain by approximately 30 percent and decreased sleep problems by approximately 40 percent. Similar albeit smaller improvements were seen with Neurontin®. Especially important is the finding that the amount of time spent in deep, restorative sleep was increased.[14]

3. **Pregabalin®**. This drug is related to neurontin, and was supposed to be released at the end of 2004, although safety concerns may prevent this. This is the first drug that may have FDA approval for use in fibromyalgia, so insurers will more likely pay for it. It may also be approved for epilepsy, neuropathic pain, and anxiety. A multi-center drug study showed that Pregabalin was helpful with both pain and increasing deep sleep in patients with fibromyalgia. It also reduced restless leg syndrome, a very common problem in fibromyalgia. The main side effects are dizziness and drowsiness, which tend to decrease over time. Unfortunately, it also has the side effect of causing weight gain, ranging between 2 to 5 pounds per month (less with lower doses).
4. **Topamax®** (topiramate). This is another anti-seizure medication that can be very helpful for pain. Although it acts as a GABA agent, it has other effects that contribute, sometimes dramatically, to its effectiveness. These include being a sodium channel blocker. Begin with 25 to 50 mg daily and increase it by 25 to 50 mg a week until you get the desired effect. This medication is usually given twice a day at a total daily dose of 50 to 100 mg per day for migraines and 200 to 300 mg a day for nerve pain, although lower doses can be effective. This is a medication that I have seen work wonderfully in patients who failed numerous other treatments, and it sometimes starts working in less than one week. If you get side effects, decrease the dose and perhaps later increase it more slowly until you get the desired effect. The most common side effects are diarrhea (11 percent), loss of appetite (11 percent ), sedation (10 percent ), and nausea (10 percent ). The side effects often go away after 2 to 3 months. Along with pain relief, it also has the benefit of causing weight loss. Besides sedation, its most worrisome, albeit unusual, side effect is that it can make your body very acidic—to the point where it is dangerous. Because of this, it is reasonable to check a blood bicarbonate level every so often (especially if you start developing symptoms such as fatigue) and make sure that the level is over 17.

## *Anti-depressants*

Anti-depressants can be very helpful in alleviating pain even if the person is not depressed.[15] Do not presume that your pain specialist thinks that you have a psychological problem if you're offered an anti-depressant for pain. The following types of anti-depressants have been found useful in alleviating pain:

1. **Tricyclic anti-depressants** (e.g. Elavil®/amitriptyline, doxepin, etc.) can be dramatically beneficial (even at very low doses) for neuropathic pain. They also improve the sleep problems caused by the pain. Where the anti-depressant dose of Elavil® is approximately 200 to 250 mg a day, the neuropathic dose is usually about 10 to 25 mg at bedtime. In addition to neuropathic pain, tricyclic anti-depressants have also been found to be effective for fibromyalgia.[16 - 17] Tricyclics have also been found to be effective for headaches and vulvadynia/pelvic pain syndromes. They also can markedly enhance the effect of narcotic pain medications.[18] Their main side effects include dry mouth, sedation, weight gain, constipation, low blood pressure, and palpitations. In addition, these medications can cause a worsening of glaucoma and urinary retention. Desipramine® (norpramin—use 25 to 150 mg at bedtime) or nortriptyline (Pamelor®—use 10 to 25 mg at bedtime) cause less sedation and fewer side effects than Elavil®, and may be as effective. If sedation is still a problem, consider switching to doxepin (10 to 40 mg at bedtime).

   **Flexeril**® (cyclobenzaprine) is a muscle relaxant in the tricyclic family. Unlike Elavil®, which is more effective for nerve pain, Flexeril is mostly effective for muscle pain and sleep problems. In my experience, it is better tolerated than Elavil, and is worth trying even if the other tricyclics were ineffective or poorly tolerated. In one fibromyalgia study, Flexeril was far more effective than a placebo.[19 - 20]

   Flexeril can be sedating and many people choose only to take it at night, using 10 to 20 mg at bedtime. It can also be taken 5 to 10 mg 3 times a day instead. Recent studies have found, however, that a 5 mg dose is almost as effective as 10 mg with much less drowsiness. In one study of patients with muscle spasm, most patients experienced moderate to complete symptom relief within 48 hours of starting Flexeril (5 mg, 3 times a day). Only 29 percent were sedated at the lower dose and in most cases, sedation was mild with only 2 percent of patients reporting severe sedation.[21] As an aside, the generic form is much less expensive. If it is not available in the 5 mg generic size, simply get the 10 mg tablet and break it in half.

2. **SSRI anti-depressants such as Prozac®, Effexor®, and Celexa®** can also be highly effective for pain. These medications raise serotonin, which lowers levels of a major pain messenger (substance P). Substance P levels can be increased by 300 percent in the brains of patients with fibromyalgia and is elevated in other pain states as well. One third of fibromyalgia patients find that SSRIs help their pain significantly. Interestingly, people may feel horrible with one SSRI and wonderful with another, so it is worth trying several sequentially to find one that "fits." Being off-patent, Prozac has the benefit of being less expensive. Celexa causes fewer side effects than other anti-depressants. In my experience however, Effexor is the most effective anti-depressant for decreasing the pain and other symptoms of fibromyalgia patients, so it is a reasonable medication to try first. This may occur because the medication raises both serotonin and norepinephrine—an excellent combination in pain management. It can be helpful in neuropathic pain and headache as well, especially in patients with associated depression and/or anxiety.[22] Dr. Argo, a pain specialist at the Pain Management Center at Columbia Rose Medical Center, Denver, has found that Paxil® can be very helpful for reflex sympathetic dystrophy where other SSRIs are not.[23]
3. A new family of medications is very promising. **Cymbalta®** (duloxetine) is a norepinephrine and serotonin reuptake inhibitor. It has fewer side effects and does not cause weight gain. It has been shown to be very helpful in many FMS pain patients and will likely be an excellent addition to the pain armamentarium. It is scheduled to be released in the latter part of 2004.
4. If sleep is a problem, consider adding Trazodone (**Desyrel®**) at bedtime. This novel anti-depressant is very good for sleep (use a low-dose such as 25 to 75 mg at bedtime) and anxiety. As noted in previous chapters, good sleep is critical for pain relief!

One of the most troublesome side effects of anti-depressants is sexual dysfunction. This especially manifests as delayed orgasm. As one of my female patients said "an orgasm delayed is an orgasm lost." Many treatments are available to help with this type of sexual dysfunction. I recommend beginning with the herb ginkgo biloba, 120 mg 2 times daily. This higher dose is necessary to counteract the loss of libido from anti-depressants, as the usual dose (60 mg twice daily) was not effective in a recent study. It takes 6 weeks to see the effect on the libido.

Medications that can be helpful for anti-depressant induced sexual dysfunction include Cyproheptadine (Periactin®), 2 to 16 mg daily—average dose 8 mg. It can be taken 1 to 2 hours before intercourse on an "as needed" basis, or it can be taken every day. Its main side effect is sedation, and it will sometimes reverse the effectiveness of the anti-depressant—so taking it on an "as needed" basis may be the best approach. Buspar (Buspirone®), a medication used to treat anxiety, has also been shown to help. It is best taken every day when used for sexual dysfunction. The anti-depressant Serzone®, 150 mg taken 1 hour before intercourse, completely reversed the sexual dysfunction caused by Zoloft®. Stimulants such as a Dexedrine® and Ritalin®, 5 to 25 mg daily, are also effective. Other medications that raise dopamine, such as amantadine (symmetral), 100 mg twice daily, or the anti-depressant Wellbutrin®, have also been shown to be effective. Although most of the studies on these medications were conducted in a small number of patients (except for ginkgo biloba, which was a larger trial), there are plenty of options available so that you can have your Prozac® and your sex life too![24]

## *Alpha2-adrenergic Agonists (Enhancers)*

Zanaflex® (tizanidine) and Catapres® are two key medications in the category of enhancers. The former appears to be more effective for pain management and has fewer side effects. Like GABA agents, these medications tend to settle things down (they depress polysynaptic reflexes and reduce excitatory amino acid release and the release of substance P). Unlike Baclofen®, however, Catapres® has the benefit of not causing muscle weakness.

The main side effect of Zanaflex is sedation, but this can also be a benefit. In most patients, I recommend that they take 2 to 8 mg at bedtime. This helps sleep and also helps both nighttime and next-day pain. Dry mouth is sometimes seen with this medication. If sedation is not a problem, Zanaflex® can be taken 3 to 4 times a day as needed, with a maximum dose of 36 mg a day. Most patients find that 4 mg at bedtime works just fine. If Zanaflex is too expensive, try Catapres® instead.

## *NMDA Receptor Antagonists*

NMDA receptors are highly involved in triggering pain and can cause "irritation" that results in the persistence of pain. Because of this, medications that settle down this "NMDA" irritation can be very helpful. These include:

1. **Ketamine®** is a general anesthetic that has traditionally been given IV. Because it works by blocking a critical pain mechanism (the NMDA receptor) that is missed by other therapies, it holds promise in the treatment of refractory pain, especially neuropathic, myofascial, post amputation pain, and reflex sympathetic dystrophy.

It has been used clinically for over 25 years for anesthesia. In addition, pain relief often persists long after the medication has worn off. This suggests that Ketamine® may actually be "breaking the pain cycle" (when the pain itself triggers more pain) in some conditions.

In the section below on IV therapies, I briefly discuss the role of IV Ketamine. Because this is an anesthetic and can cause hallucinations and a feeling of unreality, the side effects by necessity limit its use on a regular basis. Nonetheless, it can be very helpful in certain refractory cases—especially with nerve/neuropathic pain and reflex sympathetic dystrophy. Side effects tend to decrease with continued use and can be decreased by adding other medications (e.g. Haldol® or midazolam). A number of reports on the use of oral Ketamine can be found in the medical literature. One patient with severe post herpetic neuralgia, who did not respond to conventional treatments, improved dramatically with oral Ketamine, 200 mg, 5 times a day.[25] In a placebo-controlled study of eight patients with severe long-standing neuropathic pain who had responded to IV Ketamine, oral Ketamine was also used (1/2 mg per kg body weight each 6 hours). Pain relief began 15 minutes after a dose, lasted for 6 to 8 hours, and was much more effective than placebo.[26] Because of IV and oral Ketamine's psychological side effects, these forms of Ketamine are best prescribed by those physicians who have more experience with pain management. It can be very helpful (and side effect free) in gel form applied to the pain, taking 1 to 2 weeks to see the effect.

2. **Klonopin®** (clonazepam) is in the Valium® family but I find it to be much more effective and safer than Valium for a number of reasons. Klonopin acts as an NMDA receptor antagonist. It also acts as a muscle relaxant and can be very helpful for sleep (unlike Valium, which actually interferes with restorative sleep, keeping people in light stage 2 sleep). Like Valium, it can be addictive. In my experience, addiction has been rare at doses under 1 ½ mg a day. Its main side effect is sedation, so I mostly have patients take it at nighttime. It can also be very helpful for anxiety and restless leg syndrome (where your legs are rhythmically moving all night—your sleep is not very restful if you're running a marathon all night).

   Patients often come to my office that have been on benzodiazepines (Valium family medications) for many years and are often addicted. If the medication is not interfering with their life and is helping their symptoms, I do not consider getting them off the medication to be a high-priority. For those who want to wean off

Valium family medications, it must be done under a physician's supervision as withdrawal is common. Neurontin® (e.g. 200 mg 3 times a day) can help make it easier to wean off Valium and other related medications.[27]

3. **Dextromethorphan**® is not usually very effective on its own in treating pain, but when added to narcotics, it helps to keep the narcotics effective.[28] It has also been shown to be helpful for post herpetic neuralgia.[29] Only a small percent of fibromyalgia patients (less than 18 percent), however, received significant benefit from the dextromethorphan (a 51 percent decrease in pain at an average dose of 50 mg, 3 times a day). For most patients, the side effects—dizziness, mental fog, nausea, and fatigue—at these doses are prohibitive. But if you have persistent pain, Dextromethorphan is worth trying by starting at 50 mg a day and slowly increasing the dose as tolerated.[30] Although this medication is over-the-counter, it is usually found mixed with other medications. It can be obtained in pure form from compounding pharmacists.

## *Sodium Channel Blockers*

Except for lidocaine, this family of medications tends to be high in side effects. Because of this, I usually use other medications first. Nonetheless, in some patients these medications can be a godsend.

1. **Lidocaine**®. This medication is discussed in the section below on IV pain medications.

2. **Dilantin**® (phenytoin). This is one of the oldest seizure medications and is underused. I was amazed about 20 years ago when I received a book on the uses of Dilantin in the mail. A millionaire was given Dilantin for a severe chronic problem with almost miraculous results. He researched the benefits of Dilantin use, put them in a book, and sent a free copy of the book to every physician in the country. Since he derived no benefit except helping others from this expensive action, I was impressed enough to explore the use of this medication further. Although it is old and fairly inexpensive, it can be very helpful. It is useful for nerve pain of several types, including times when cancer is infiltrating into nerve bundles. The recommended dose is 300 to 400 mg daily.

   Dilantin does have more side effects than most of the other medications we are using, and therefore I rarely use it as a first line treatment, saving it for cases that do not respond to other therapies. Check Dilantin blood levels to make sure they do not go too high.

Dilantin can also cause birth defects if one gets pregnant while taking it. Otherwise, its main side effects include dizziness, sedation, and nausea. It can also cause unwanted hair growth (sometimes on the ears in females) and overgrowth of gum tissue. The latter side effect can actually be beneficial in those who have receding gums. Dilantin can be given as a topical cream applied to the gums for this purpose.

3. **Tegretol®** (carbamazepine). This anti-seizure medication is most often used for trigeminal neuralgia, peripheral neuropathy, and post herpetic neuralgia (post shingles pain). Begin with 100 mg, 3 times a day and increase the dose to 200 mg 3 times a day after 1 week. If no benefit is seen at 1200 mg a day for 1 month, the patient should be weaned off the medication. Check a baseline blood count before treatment. When you are on the medication, check the blood level and blood count every two weeks while the dose is being increased, then check each month for 6 months, then every 6 months while on the medication. The main side effects include sedation, tremor, and difficulty with speech. A drop in white blood cell count can occur in 10 percent of patients, but this sometimes resolves after 4 months. If blood counts go too low or there is lymph node enlargement, stop the medication. This medication can also cause birth defects if one gets pregnant while taking it. As you can tell, this medication has many more side effects than most of the others that I use, and therefore I rarely use it.

## Other Medications

Other types of oral medications for pain include:

1. **Ultram (Tramadol®)** is an excellent medication for almost any kind of pain. Although not addictive or a narcotic, it does work on the "codeine receptors" and also raises serotonin and norepinephrine. Although it can be taken up to 100 mg 4 times a day, many people find they get nausea and sedation at doses over 200 mg a day. Rarely is this a problem at a low-dose, so only take 50 mg for the first dose. If 4 to 6 hours later nausea is not a problem, feel free to increase the dose to a maximum of 100 mg twice a day the first day. If nausea is still not a problem at this dose, you can continue to increase the dose to the maximum above. The medication can also be taken on an "as needed" basis.

2. **Lamictal** (Lamotrigine®) can also be effective for many kinds of pain, including nerve pain from AIDS and central brain pain from strokes. In early studies where lower doses of 200 mg a day or less

were used, the effects were marginal. Doses of 200 to 400 mg a day, divided through the day, are more effective for some kinds of pain. You can start with a low dose and increase by 25 mg a week to decrease the probability of side effects. The most worrisome side effect is a rare rash (called Stevens-Johnson syndrome), which can be fatal. If you develop a rash, stop the medication immediately and let your doctor know. The vast majority of the time it will not be this dangerous type of rash, but better safe than sorry.

3. **Keppra® (levetiracetam)** is another new anti-seizure medication that we are just starting to explore. It has been effective when other treatments have not helped. The recommended dose is 500 to 1500 mg twice daily.

4. **Trileptal®** (oxcarbazepine) is a cousin to the medication Tegretol®, and both of these medications are helpful for trigeminal neuralgia. The dose is 150mg 2 times a day, although one can go as high as 600 mg 2 times a day. The side effects (sedation, blurred vision) decrease after the initial 3 weeks of treatment.

5. **Lithium** is a natural mineral that is available by prescription for the treatment of manic-depressive disorders. It has many other properties including being antiviral. Interestingly, several case reports have noted that debilitating chronic pain, which has been refractory to other treatments will sometimes improve dramatically with lithium. Sometimes this can be achieved with doses as low as 300 mg 1 to 2 times daily.

## *Narcotics*

Some physicians consider narcotics to be a pain reliever of last resort—only to be used with terminally ill cancer patients. The use of narcotics for chronic pain continues to be controversial and has become highly politicized. Fortunately, the vast majority of chronic pain cases can now be treated effectively without narcotics. Nonetheless, there are cases in which they are necessary. Sometimes, the toxicity of the pain dramatically outweighs the toxicity of the medication.

Data suggests that longer-acting narcotics are less likely to cause addictive behavior than short acting-narcotics. In addition, for severe chronic pain, giving the medication on a regular basis (e.g. 2 to 3 times a day) to **prevent** pain is more effective than waiting for the pain to occur before taking the medication—with the result that less medication is needed.

When treating with narcotics, it is helpful to be aware that different narcotics can work on several different types of opioids receptors. This means that combining different narcotics may result in their having a synergistic effect (i.e. a lower dose of two different types such as oxycodone and morphine may work much better than a higher dose of one of them). In addition, if one is developing resistance to one narcotic, rotating to others may result in improved effectiveness. Some narcotics also have multiple effects. For example, methadone affects the opioids receptors while also blocking NMDA receptors.[31]

The main **side effects** of narcotics are constipation and sedation. The magnesium in the vitamin powder can be very helpful for the constipation, and other treatments can also help. I recommend using the following as many other constipation treatments can be addictive. Adjust as needed for one soft bowel movement a day. Increase water, fiber (e.g. 1 bowl of whole grain cereal in the morning) and magnesium intake. Other natural over-the-counter treatments for constipation include prunes and/or prune juice. Although we often forget about these, they have been used for centuries and can be quite helpful. If prunes and prune juice are not adequate, prescription treatments can help. These include Miralax® laxative (comes in 14 oz. and 26 oz bottles)—take 1 heaping Tbsp a day in 8 oz. of water; Sorbitol® 70 percent—take 1 to 3 tsp 3 times a day as needed; and Lactulose® liquid as needed.

A new medication called Provigil® can be very helpful for narcotic induced fatigue. Aricept® (donepezil), a medication for Alzheimer's disease that increases acetylcholine levels, has also been found to be helpful for this problem. In one study of cancer patients receiving massive doses of morphine (approximately 844 mg/a day), 73 percent improved on Aricept. Patients were started on 5 mg a day, and the average patient needed approximately 9 mg daily. After 3 weeks on the medication, sedation decreased markedly, and pain also decreased somewhat as well.[32]

I would note that there is also a small subset (approximately 2 to 5 percent) of fibromyalgia patients who experience dramatic clearing of exhaustion and fatigue (associated with their pain) with narcotic pain medications. They state that (and I've heard this statement many times) they "feel like healthy normal human beings" when they are taking the narcotic medication. Although I have not yet figured out the biochemistry of this effect, in the future I hope to have non-narcotic alternatives that will give the same benefit.

Another important side effect of using opioids in men is that the narcotics will routinely drop the patients' testosterone levels (often by elevating a hormone called prolactin), resulting in loss of libido and sometimes difficulty with erections. Because of this, it is reasonable to have a patient's testosterone level checked before beginning chronic opioids. If symptoms of low testosterone occur, and the testosterone level has decreased on treatment with opioids, it is reasonable to treat with testosterone cream as well.

Oxycontin® has been associated with vitamin B2 (riboflavin) deficiency, which will sometimes cause the corners of the mouth to crack. This is called angular stomatitis, cheilitis, or perleche. In one study of 22 patients receiving OxyContin, 20 of them were found to have this problem. High-dose vitamin B2 (present in the Energy Revitalization System) eliminated the problem in almost all patients within a few days.[33]

There are a number of different long-acting narcotic pain medications. These include methadone (Dolophine®), sustained-release morphine (e.g. MS Contin®), and sustained-release oxycodone (OxyContin®), which may be preferable to short acting combinations of codeine with acetaminophen, oxycodone, or hydrocodone. The longer-acting medications maintain a steady blood level so there is less of a euphoric effect (and therefore less drug craving) and more consistent relief of pain. In addition, **not combining** the medication with acetaminophen allows one to safely use higher doses, as needed. Using more than 3000 to 4000 mg of acetaminophen (Tylenol®) daily can be toxic to the liver and immune system (see above).

Methadone is one of the oldest, longer-acting narcotics and has many benefits. It is inexpensive, long-acting, effective, and usually well-tolerated. It also may have some activity as an NMDA receptor antagonist, making the medication useful in neuropathic pain as well. Unfortunately, I do not use methadone in my practice despite its being an excellent pain medication. The regulatory and bureaucratic risks and hassles associated with its use are simply too great. This has also been the experience of many other pain specialists.

Fortunately, there are other longer-acting narcotics available. One of the best known is Oxycontin® (timed-release oxycodone), which can be very safe and effective when used orally as directed. Sadly, it can be illegally diverted and used illicitly. Therefore, it has also become dangerous for physicians to prescribe Oxycontin, even appropriately, because the federal government will sometimes put a physician in jail for doing so.

An alternative is the use of **timed-release morphine**. This can be given every 12 hours, although in some patients it needs to be given 3 times a day. Another alternative is non timed-release oxycodone (e.g. Percocet® and Roxicet®), which is stronger and less sedating than morphine. Although not as safe (they are more addictive) as the timed-release form (Oxycontin), they're still highly effective and physicians are less likely to be arrested or lose their licenses for prescribing them. Again, be aware that many of these medications are combined with acetaminophen (Tylenol®) and that many pain patients are getting acetaminophen from many sources. It is worth repeating that chronic use of more than 3000 to 4000 mg of acetaminophen a day can cause severe liver damage. **Please check everything that you are taking to make**

**sure that you do not take more than this amount of acetaminophen daily**.

As noted previously, Dr. Argo, a pain specialists at the Pain Management Center at Columbia Rose Medical Center, Denver, has found that adding low dose Elavil® can markedly enhance the effect of narcotic pain medications.[34] In addition, taking dextromethorphan (25 mg 2 times a day) can decrease the tolerance that people develop to a narcotic's effectiveness.[35] Because of this, it is reasonable that anyone on narcotic pain medications should also take dextromethorphan.

Experience and the scientific literature have shown that opioids are very unlikely to cause addiction when used properly for treatment of pain. Addiction needs to be contrasted to a physical dependence and tolerance. Addiction is an uncontrolled compulsive use of the drug even though it is harming the user. Clinical experience and medical literature suggest that this is a very **uncommon** situation when opioids are used for chronic pain in non-drug addicts. Habituation and physical dependence, however, are common with this family of medication as well as with anti-depressants, anti-seizure medications, and many other medications. All this means is that you do not want to stop the medication suddenly, as you might go through withdrawal. Instead, the medication should be tapered off over time. Physical dependence does not become a problem in the clinical setting unless the medication is stopped suddenly, or the dose is reduced substantially without tapering it.

## Cannabinoids

The medical components found in marijuana can be helpful in a number of painful conditions, especially when anxiety and/or loss of appetite (e.g. due to cancer) are also problematic. In most studies, pharmaceutical fractions are studied (e.g. THC in the medication Marinol®) instead of whole marijuana. Studies have found marijuana to be effective for cancer, neuropathic, and spasticity pain.[36 - 37] Unfortunately, the more expensive synthetic pharmaceutical forms of marijuana may not be as effective.[38]

Current evidence suggests that there are brain receptors for cannabis just as there are receptors for opioids, and that migraine headaches, fibromyalgia, and irritable bowel syndrome may all display an underlying deficiency of the body's own "cannabis production." Especially in cases where the brain has been sensitized to pain (called a central sensitization state with secondary hyperalgesia) such as occurs in fibromyalgia, the data suggests that cannabis therapies could be helpful.[39] Unfortunately, the politics surrounding drug policy precludes these treatments from currently being used—despite their being safer, more effective, and certainly less expensive than many other treatments.

## Intravenous Pain Medications

In severe cases of persistent pain, the use of intravenous pain therapies can be powerfully effective. Anytime IV pain medications are used, it is worth giving intravenous nutritional support at the same time. This can contribute powerfully to healing the underlying problem, and a series of these treatments can help you feel better and may actually eliminate the source of the pain. These IV nutritional therapies are called Myers cocktails, and the details for using them are in Appendix F.

In a study of 86 patients with chronic muscle pain, including myofascial pain and fibromyalgia, a series of injections with IV or IM magnesium with other nutrients, including B vitamins, calcium, and vitamin C, were given. Seventy-four percent of the patients improved with 64 percent requiring 4 or less injections to see optimal results. Some patients required long-term treatments to maintain the effect. Side effects leading to discontinuation of therapy occurred in 4 percent of the patients. The need for prescriptions for anti-inflammatory medications and muscle relaxants was decreased markedly.[40] In addition, (as noted in Chapter 13), intravenous magnesium has also been shown to be very helpful for acute migraine headaches.

A second highly effective intravenous pain therapy is the use of Lidocaine®. I have found this to be very effective in a large number of patients with widespread pain. In my practice, I give a 60 mg test dose during a time period of approximately 45 minutes. This is to screen for patients who tend to drop their blood pressure or have other side effects. If the initial treatment is well-tolerated, an additional 40 to 60 mg can be given the first day (this low dose is unlikely to result in much pain relief). For follow-up treatments, I usually give 75 mg of Lidocaine over a time period of approximately 10 to 20 minutes, followed by 2 mg per minute (i.e. 120 mg per hour) for a total of 200 to 300 mg. This can be repeated once or twice a week as needed, and pain relief tends to be more sustained after the first 3 to 6 treatments. Using this treatment approach without heart monitoring is controversial because there's a possible risk of abnormal heart rhythms with Lidocaine use. These abnormal rhythms occur predominantly in patients who are in intensive care units for acute heart attacks. I have never seen heart rhythm problems and do not use monitoring because this can increase the patient's cost from $80 to $700 per dose. One study using high-dose Lidocaine (up to approximately 500 mg per day over 6 hours for 6 days) showed marked pain improvement, but two of the patients did have cardiac side effects that were transient but significant. This suggests that caution be used when administering Lidocaine in patients with heart problems.[41]

In one study of 18 fibromyalgia patients,[42] Lidocaine was given at a dose of 5 mg per kilogram of body weight over 30 minutes. This is a much higher dose/speed than I recommend; it is safer to give it slower. Ketamine® and morphine (each at 3/10 mg/kilogram IV administered over a one half-hour time period) and a salt water placebo were also given with each of these 4 treatments a week apart. Fifteen of the 18 patients improved with one or more of these medications. Half of the patients improved with Lidocaine, with pain decreasing by an average of over 60 percent. Similar effects were seen for Ketamine and morphine. Most patients developed a very comfortable sedation. Although patients felt numbness around the lips with Lidocaine and "spacey" with the Ketamine, the treatments were found to be effective and were well tolerated. Pain relief lasted several days in over half the patients. The fact that different patients responded to different medications in this study shows the importance of tailoring treatments to each patient.

Other studies of Lidocaine have shown similar effects. In one study, 10 patients with fibromyalgia were given 250 to 500 mg of Lidocaine each day for 6 days (each dose was given over 6 hours). There was a 50 percent decrease in pain, with most of this benefit persisting when patients were checked 30 days later.[43] Another study was conducted with 11 fibromyalgia patients, who were give 240 mg of Lidocaine over a one half-hour time span each week (as noted above I think this is too fast a speed to give this dose) for 4 weeks. Six of the 11 patients had complete resolution of their fibromyalgia, and 8 of the 11 felt that they were better overall. On a zero to 10 scale, pain dropped from 7.2 to 2.0 on average. Despite the high-dose being given fairly quickly, no abnormal heart rhythms were seen. A friend of mine, Jay Goldstein M.D., has used intravenous Lidocaine in hundreds of fibromyalgia patients. He finds that the treatment improves not only the pain but also the fatigue, spastic colon, and cognitive dysfunction. In his experience, the treatments increase in effectiveness with each dose up until about the fifth dose at which point the effect levels out. Some people have no effect until they receive the fourth or fifth dose. He has never seen anyone suffer any serious reactions from the IV Lidocaine.

Other studies have also found IV Ketamine (at a dose of 3/10 mg per kilogram over one half hour) to be helpful.[44] Because of the sometimes uncomfortable spaciness/mental changes that can occur during the IV infusion, IV Ketamine is used less often than Lidocaine. Its main promise may be in the treatment of those with reflex sympathetic dystrophy/regional complex pain syndrome and others with severe refractory pain (see Chapter 8).

Despite the intoxicated/disassociative feelings that can routinely occur with Ketamine in higher dosing, it can be powerfully effective in very difficult pain syndromes. In another small study at an Irish Hospice, Ketamine given subcutaneously was very helpful for 10 patients with narcotic resistant chronic cancer and non cancer pain. Seventy percent of these severe pain patients had no pain after Ketamine treatment, and all had some pain relief. Patients were treated for an average of 42 days, and some were able to switch to Ketamine by mouth. The only significant adverse reaction was inflammation at the site of injection, which ranged from mild redness to tissue necrosis. Hydrocortisone cream did help settle down some of the inflammation, but four patients still needed to stop the injections because of this. Most patients noted benefit at a dose of approximately 300 mg subcutaneously daily.[45] Any uncomfortable (most often they are not) psychological side effects of Ketamine can be decreased by giving the patient Klonopin® and having them sleep right after the injection.

It is interesting to note that patients with fibromyalgia and other pain syndromes respond well to one medication but not another that works by a different mechanism. This demonstrates that there is not a single cause to many pain problems. This is why looking for the single "magic bullet" approach to pain management does not work as well as the "try a combination of therapies until you see what works" (i.e. Integrative or Comprehensive Medicine). Of course, this approach works better if you have more options to choose from than only Tylenol® or Motrin®/aspirin family medications! ■

**Important Points**

1. The use of topical delivery systems for pain medications is a major leap forward in pain management. It allows high doses of multiple medications to get right to your area of pain—usually with no side effects.
2. Begin by going after the perpetuating factors (i.e. nutritional, hormonal, and sleep deficiencies, and underlying infections) followed by adding in natural remedies. Then use the prescription pain creams. The oral followed by IV medications can (and should) then be added if needed, because it is unhealthy to be in pain. On the other hand, it is also reasonable to begin immediately with the prescription pain medications like Ultram® for immediate pain relief while you're waiting for the other treatments to take effect.
3. Give the creams at least 1 to 2 weeks to work, and be willing to continue adjusting the mix until you find what works. Here are some of the medications that can be added to the creams: Ketoprofen®, piroxicam, diclofenac, or ibuprofen (these four are NSAID anti-inflammatories); Neurontin®, clonidine, amitriptyline, Cyclobenzaprine®, Baclofen®, Ketamine®, Lidocaine®, guaifenesin, capsaicin, cortisone, and/or Sarapin®.
4. Your physician may not be familiar with compounded pain creams; the pharmacist at Cape Apothecary (phone 410-757-3522) can help guide your physician and will mail you the cream if your doctor prescribes it.
5. The chapters in which we discussed the different kinds of pain (e.g. neuropathic, muscular, arthritic, etc.) and the summary sections on these chapters give the order in which to try the various medications for pain. If you are not clear about the source/type of your pain, there are many reasonable sequences in which to try the medications (see the order sequence below). When there are several medications on the same line, if the first medication helped but was not tolerated because of side effects, go to the next medication on the same line. If it did not help significantly, go to the next line. If you get partial benefit from a medication, continue it and add

*Continued on next page*

**Important Points** *(continued)*

the next medication as needed to get pain-free. Here is the sequence:

1. Lidocaine® patches or gels for localized area of pain
2. Tylenol®
3. Motrin®, Voltaren®, or Daypro® (your insurance company prefers that these be tried before Celebrex® because of cost)
4. Celebrex®
5. Skelaxin® (for muscle pain/achiness)
6. Ultram®
7. Neurontin®, Gabitril®, and/or Pregabalin®
8. Flexeril® (for muscle pain/achiness
9. Elavil®, Doxepin®, Desipramine® (norpramin), or nortriptyline (Pamelor®
10. Zanaflex®
11. Effexor®
12. Baclofen® (for muscle pain/achiness)
13. Klonopin® (for muscle pain/achiness)
14. Topamax
15. Lamicta®
16. Keppra
17. Narcotics

Appendix B: Pain Treatment Protocol gives directions on how to use each of these medications.

**6.** For refractory pain consider IV nutrients (see Appendix F: Myers Cocktails), IV Lidocaine® or Ketamine®, or Prolotherapy (see Chapter 23).

CHAPTER 23

# Prolothery

*The following chapter on Prolotherapy was written by two wonderful pain specialists from Texas. In addition to helping you understand a very powerful tool, it also offers a broader perspective on how many different effective approaches there are to pain management. If you'd like, it's okay to simply skip over the technical details, and leave those to the physicians, who will administer the Prolotherapy injections. Many people receive benefit from the technique discussed in this chapter. I think you'll enjoy reading it.*

## Prolotherapy: An Orphaned Medical Intervention Repairing Connective Tissue Weakness to Resolve Chronic Musculoskeletal Pain

**by Brad Fullerton, M.D. and David Harris, M.D.**

Prolotherapy is a proven, safe, cost-effective treatment that can eliminate chronic pain in approximately 80 to 90 percent of sufferers, yet it has been ignored by mainstream medicine for almost 70 years. C. Everett Koop, M.D., former U.S. Surgeon General, credits Prolotherapy with curing his chronic low back pain in the late 1950s. After receiving training in the technique, he practiced Prolotherapy in his office at the University of Pennsylvania for 20 years and has publicly expressed that Prolotherapy should have a prominent place in the modern treatment of musculoskeletal pain. By the end of this chapter, we hope that you understand why Prolotherapy (or "Prolo") was orphaned in the first half of the 20th century and why it is now on the leading edge of a revolution in medicine.

The conventional model of pain management has the underlying belief that inflammation is at the root of almost all pain problems. This core belief is so well-established that almost no one bothers to question it any longer. It has become part of the common language that we all use. Patients come into our offices almost everyday complaining of "inflammation" rather than pain. We ask, "Where do you feel the pain?" Patients reply, "Well, my elbow is really inflamed." or "The inflammation started in my low back, now it's going down my leg." They have already decided that what they feel is inflammation, not pain. Often, when they describe "swelling," this is actually a muscle in spasm.

When new diseases were being identified in the 19th and early 20th centuries, the first clue to the problem often came when doctors would look at tissue under a microscope. They would identify "inflammatory cells" in the tissue; these were often the bodies own white blood cells responding to a virus or bacteria. So, if the infection and thus the inflammation were found in the liver, the disease would be called "hepatitis," meaning inflammation of the liver. If these inflammatory cells were found in the stomach, the disease was initially called "gastritis" or inflammation of the stomach. But of course, the problem wasn't really the inflammation, it was the infection. The body's **response** to the infection was what the researchers were seeing under the microscope.

In the musculoskeletal system, names like "tendonitis," "bursitis," and "arthritis" imply that the problem is inflammation in the tendon, bursa, or joint. However, the most common problem in all these tissues is a degeneration or slow breakdown of the tissue over time. If the body does not adequately respond to this degeneration by making new tissue, we get pain and disability that progresses over a lifetime. Our modern medical model is solely focused on the concept of calming inflammation. There are entire shelves of name-brand and store-brand anti-inflammatory medications waiting for you at your local grocer, drug or variety store. If those don't work, you can respond to the latest pharmaceutical industry ads and "ask your doctor" about the newest name-brand prescription anti-inflammatory, such as Celebrex®, Mobic®, or Bextra®. Or you can go to your family practice, sports medicine, or pain management physician for any of a variety of steroid injections, such as cortisone. Most of us accept these treatments gladly, because they seem to work so well. They temporarily take away the pain; they stop the inflammation.

Yet, we have an epidemic of chronic pain and degenerative arthritis. There is growing dissatisfaction with the current approach because it only works temporarily. We have to come back again and again for the latest anti-inflammatory prescription or another injection of steroids. Or we are offered a lifetime of treatment with anti-depressants, anti-seizure medications, muscle-relaxants, or slow release opiate medications, such as Oxycontin® or Methadone. These medications have their use but have potential side effects, including tolerance, addiction, stomach irritation, kidney damage, and liver damage. Anti-inflammatory medications have become a standard medical treatment, but many studies have demonstrated that these medications actually inhibit the healing process and eventually weaken tissues in the body.

If you are fortunate, your doctor is willing to refer you to a competent and skilled manual/massage therapist, acupuncturist, or chiropractor. Many of these therapies have grown out of a grass roots response to mainstream failures in treating musculoskeletal pain. As these attempts to control pain begin to fail, the next phase of treatment tends to progress towards destructive, expensive, and riskier procedures, such as surgery, implantation of morphine pumps, implantation of stimulating devices to block the sensation of pain, and procedures to destroy the nerves that conduct the sensation of pain. Surgical procedures such as these have their place, but often may be used before attempts have been made to promote a more natural healing and strengthening process for the underlying tissue weakness and injury that is often causing the pain. Many destructive procedures are performed with minimal recognition of the actual source of the pain. The justification for destructive procedures is "there is nothing else that can be done," a statement usually made by a physician who has never heard of Prolotherapy or who is not skilled in connective tissue repair with Prolotherapy.

## What Is Prolotherapy?

A form of Prolotherapy was performed by Hippocrates 2500 years ago, in which an athlete's shoulder instability was treated by a red-hot needle, initiating healing through inflammation and strengthening of the capsule of the shoulder, and allowing him to ultimately return to his athletic activities. Injections of irritant solutions were performed in the late 1800s to repair hernias and in the early 1900s for TMJ dysfunction before surgery became available. These early attempts at promoting healing were called "sclerotherapy," implying formation of scar. Older doctors sometimes ask why we would want to create scar tissue around a degenerated spine or joint. The answer is that we don't. Sclerotherapy is an outdated and inaccurate term. George Hackett, M.D., a surgeon in Ohio, refined the technique and named it Prolotherapy. Over the years it has developed the nickname Prolo. Prolo is short for proliferation, thus Prolotherapy is a series of injections to stimulate proliferation of **normal** tissue. Since Dr. Hackett's original work in the 1940s, studies in animals and humans have shown normal tissue formation after Prolotherapy, **not scar**. High resolution imaging with ultrasound is now confirming Dr.

Hackett's work; the tissue that is regenerated is organized, normal fibrous tissue.

Prolotherapy stimulates the body to repair painful areas. Its effectiveness is wide-ranging and includes pain associated with the back, the neck, all joints throughout the body, arthritis, migraine headaches, fibromyalgia, sciatica, herniated discs, and Temporo Mandibular Joint Dysfunction (TMJ). Chronic musculoskeletal pain is often due to weakness of ligaments and tendons. Joints, such as the knee and shoulder, often develop instability as well as weakening of the internal cartilage surfaces, and these are often improved by intra-articular (inside the joint) injections of dextrose and other irritant solutions.

Prolotherapy involves the injection of a natural solution (something as simple as a sugar or salt solution, cod liver oil, or herbal extract) into the area where the ligaments have either been weakened or damaged through injury or strain. Milder solutions of dextrose (corn syrup, essentially sugar), Lidocaine® (a local anesthetic), and Sarapin® (an herbal extract of the pitcher plant) are often used for the first several sessions. If the response is sluggish, stronger irritants may be used, such as mild concentrations of glucosamine, phenol (an alcohol), glycerin, or cod liver oil extract (known as sodium morrhuate).

The injection is given at the point where the ligament or tendon connects to the bone. Many points may require injection. The injection causes the body to heal itself through the process of controlled inflammation and production of growth factors. In the case of weakened or torn fibrous tissue, this repair results in as much as 30 to 40 percent strengthening of the attachment points.

Prolotherapy treatment sessions are generally given every 3 to 6 weeks to allow time for the growth of the new connective tissue. Patients usually require 4 to 6 treatment sessions for complete recovery, although some experience more immediate results. Many studies over the last fifty years show at least an 80 percent success rate.

## *Connective Tissue Weakness, Myofascial Pain, Arthritis, and Referred Pain*

Pain that fails to respond to the traditional approaches is often caused by an injury to fibrous connective tissues, such as tendons and ligaments. Ligaments connect bone to bone, while tendons connect muscle to bone. Both ligaments and tendons may be damaged by major trauma, or may be exposed to minor repetitive trauma. In most people, these injuries tend to heal over 4 to 8 weeks. However, sometimes the tissue damage is too great, and the repair is not complete. These tissues have poor blood supply and are known to heal poorly compared to other tissues such as muscle. In other cases, patients with conditions such as fibromyalgia and chronic fatigue syndrome have underlying metabolic deficiencies that impair the healing process. These patients will often demonstrate pain and tenderness at the connections of their ligaments and tendons, with referral patterns of pain, numbness, tingling, and other abnormal sensations.

The joints are connected by strong taut ligament tissue, and cartilage lines the joint space. Laxity in the ligament structures may allow too much "play" in the joint, which results in muscle tension as the body attempts to stabilize the weak or loose structures. The muscles become fatigued after a period of time, resulting in myofascial pain. "Myo" refers to muscle; "fascia" is the fibrous tissue that surrounds, supports, and defines muscle and other tissue layers. The muscle may develop small regions of hyperactivity, which on examination show the clinical findings of trigger points and taut bands in the muscle bellies. These trigger points are thought to be neuromuscular junctions, where the smallest nerve fibers connect to the smallest muscle fibers. Normally, the neuromuscular junction is a highly regulated and balanced electrical connection that turns on and off with great precision. However, when trigger points are present, this connection is out of balance as if the neuromuscular junction has a short circuit. So, our muscles go into spasm and/or feel weak. In myofascial pain, some muscles become inhibited from achieving their full strength and become weak. This tends to happen with muscles that move the limbs through space, further away from the center of the body. The muscles closer to the spine whose purpose is to stabilize the body while limb motion is taking place tend to react more with tension and spasm. Thus, it is common to see a combination of weakness and tension in a region of the body, depending on the extent of injury and strain.

In lax joints over time, the body grows larger bony surfaces to support the increased stress and strain, creating the findings of arthritis that the physician notes on x-ray studies. Calcium is deposited in the weakened ligaments. Strengthening the supporting ligaments with Prolotherapy around an arthritic joint does appear to protect the remaining cartilage from further decline in current studies. There is some evidence that cartilage may even be thickened or strengthened, but that is not conclusive. Many physicians believe, and their patients are told, that arthritis is inevitable and irreversible. However, studies show that with Prolotherapy, the supporting ligaments and tendons can be repaired, thus potentially reversing or at least halting this "inevitable" decline.

Myofascial pain also develops from strain at the junction of the muscle tendon where it connects to the bone. There are extensive nerve connections on the outer surface of the bone (the periosteum) where the tendons and ligaments attach, and a strain on the damaged connection points may thus be extremely painful. These nerves provide information to the body regarding the position of the parts of the body, known as proprioception. Pain may be perceived distant from the actual source of the pain, producing the phenomenon of "Referred Pain." Such pain may not demonstrate abnormalities with nerve testing or any other technique, such as MRI, CT, X-Ray studies, etc., and thus the source of the pain may be difficult to resolve. In such cases, the diagnosis of Reflex Sympathetic Dystrophy (RSD) is often given, when in fact there is a very treatable pain generator in the ligament, tendon, or joint pain generator.

## Studies Supporting Prolotherapy

Placebo-controlled, randomized, double-blind studies on Prolotherapy performed with standard techniques have shown statistically significant improvement in pain reduction, stability, increased cartilage growth, improved "arthritic changes" on x-rays, increased range of motion, and greater overall function. It is estimated that over 1,500,000 patients have tried Prolotherapy over the past 70 years, with an extremely low risk and complication rate. Retrospective reviews of large numbers of patients verify a success rate of greater than 80 percent, with success defined as at least an improvement of 50 percent pain reduction. The bibliography attached provides a listing of studies and publications for further review.[1]

## Guidelines for Determining Whether Prolotherapy May Be Useful

- Recurrent swelling or fullness involving a joint or muscular region
- Popping, clicking, grinding, or catching sensations with movement
- A sensation of the "leg giving way" with associated back pain
- Temporary benefit from chiropractic manipulation or manual mobilization that fails to ultimately resolve the pain
- Distinct tender points along the bone at tendon or ligament attachments
- Numbness, tingling, aching, or burning referred into an upper or lower extremity
- Recurrent headache, face pain, jaw pain, ear pain
- Chest pain with tenderness along the rib attachments on the spine or along the front of the chest
- Spine pain that does not respond to surgery or whose origin is not clear from MRI, CT, X-Ray, Myelogram, or other similar studies

## Specific Regions Benefiting from Prolotherapy

### *Spine Pain (Neck, Mid Back, Low Back)*

Most back and neck pain results when weak ligaments and tendons cause the spine to become "unstable." Vertebrae begin to slip, move, and rotate from their proper position, causing the disks to take on the additional load and producing the familiar "disk bulge" or "disk herniation." The disk is simply a specialized ligament tissue with the same characteristics as other ligamentous tissues. The disk may be the primary source of pain as well, especially with moderate to severe trauma, which may cause an acute tear; this can be very painful and may cause nerve compression. Disk herniations may require treatment with medication, epidural steroid injections, therapy, or surgery, and may not respond well to Prolotherapy. However, the majority of spine pain does not originate in the disks, and thus a focus on disks as the sole source of pain reduces a physician's "batting average" to far less than 50 percent long-term success. Because current diagnostic studies, such as MRI scans, CT scans, x-rays, bone scans, and myelograms do not reveal abnormalities of the numerous small ligaments, the typical and often unsuccessful focus is on the larger and more noticeable disk structures.

In summary, the disk is one of many potential sources of pain in the spine; however, successful treatment of spine pain requires a practitioner to recognize the numerous other pain generators as well.

Structures frequently treated in the spine and pelvis include the supraspinous ligament, the interspinous ligament, intertransverse process ligaments, facet joint capsules, sacroiliac ligament, sacrotuberous ligament, sacrospinous ligament, sacrococcygeal ligament, among many others.

Prolotherapy strengthens the connections along the spine, providing stability to reduce strain on the other structures. Over 3 to 6 months of treatment, muscle spasm and tenderness resolve, as well as the localized and referred pain. Strengthening the neck segments frequently reduces spasm and pain in the shoulder blade regions. Success often requires injections along the upper and inner aspects of the shoulder blades as well, where the trapezius, levator scapulae, rhomboid, and subscapularis muscles attach.

### *Headaches*

Most headaches originate at weaknesses of the attachments of the suboccipital muscle tendons and fascia at the base of the back of the skull. This form of headache is referred to as tension, suboccipital, or cervicogenic and often refers to the eye, forehead, ear, or temple. The Greater and Lesser Occipital nerves run through this fibrous tissue and appear to contribute to the sensation of headache. Trauma, such as a motor vehicle accident, often causes a "whiplash" injury, creating small tears in this fibrous tissue. Although migraine headaches are thought to have a vascular (blood supply) origin, they are often triggered by the same tissue weaknesses as for tension headaches. Prolotherapy strengthens these tissue attachment weaknesses and usually greatly reduces the intensity and frequency of headaches.

## *Temporo Mandibular Joint Dysfunction (TMJ)*

Popping, clicking, locking, and pain commonly occur in the joints of the lower jaw known as the TMJ. This can occur on one or both sides. The TMJ has been successfully treated for over 75 years with Prolotherapy; it remains the most successful and safest treatment available. Unfortunately, many patients have undergone various unproven surgeries over the last 25 years without attempting, or even being informed, about Prolotherapy first. Most of those surgical procedures are no longer practiced because of widespread failure. Prolotherapy for the TMJ usually involves 3 to 4 intra-articular (inside the joint) injections.

## *Shoulder, Elbow, Wrist and Hand*

The shoulder, elbow, wrist, and hand have numerous ligament and tendon structures. Cartilage within these joints also may become damaged or torn. Repetitive motion of the upper extremity often results in laxity of the supporting joint capsules and ligaments, as well as a weakening of the tendon attachments. Intense athletic activities, such as pitching, golf, or tennis often result in shoulder and elbow pain. Many physicians will often be confused regarding the source of pain, often attributing numbness, tingling, swelling, and burning or achy pain to a nerve injury, which in fact, is fairly uncommon. There are painful conditions involving nerve compression that require surgery, but this is much less common than many believe. The vast majority of such injuries do not require surgery and are treated with very specific Prolotherapy injections into each localized connective tissue attachment and also inside each involved joint.

Instability of the shoulder joint is relatively easy to resolve with Prolotherapy and very difficult and inconsistent to cure with any other technique. Other causes of shoulder pain include: weakened attachments of the trapezius muscles all along the upper border of the shoulder blade and clavicle (collarbone); the attachments of the deltoid muscle tendon at the outer border of the shoulder and also the distal attachment along the outer upper arm; laxity of the acromioclavicular joint; and tears of the rotator cuff tendons. "Tennis elbow" and other elbow pain is usually caused by injury to the annular ligament, the elbow joint, and to the tendon and fascia attachments at the epicondyles, all of which respond well to strengthening with Prolotherapy injections. Wrist pain is frequently the result of ligament tears, cartilage tears, and joint capsular weakness and often is successfully resolved with Prolotherapy. The diagnosis of "Carpal Tunnel Syndrome" is commonly made for generalized wrist pain, when in fact classically this diagnosis should be reserved for true nerve entrapment of the Median nerve. Often, nerve studies, MRI, CT, and X-Rays reveal no clear abnormality, and surgery is contemplated because "there's nothing else to do." Although true "Carpal Tunnel Syndrome" may require surgery to decompress the nerve, surgery infrequently improves pain at the wrist, especially if studies do not reveal a significant abnormality of the nerve. All of the above respond very well to Prolotherapy injections to stimulate repair of the injured structures.

## *Hip, Knee, Ankle, and Foot*

Hip and knee pain often are the result of joint capsule or ligamentous laxity, which ultimately may lead to degenerative arthritis if not corrected. Numerous ligaments surround the hip, knee, ankle, and foot, any of which may produce debilitating pain. Another source of pain is the tendon insertions, especially along the head of the femur (thighbone) and at the inner aspect of the knee ("Pes Anserinus"), where the hamstring muscles attach. Young men often develop "Osgood-Schlatter Disease" where the tendon from the patella (kneecap) weakens at the attachment to the tibia bone. Cartilage injury, muscle misalignment, and quadriceps weakness cause pain in the knee and under the kneecap, known as Patellofemoral Syndrome, or Chondromalacia Patellae. Recurrent ankle sprains result in weakness and lengthening of the supporting ligaments of the ankle, and may also cause cartilage injury inside the complex ankle joint. Pain also may occur with chronic tears in the Achilles tendon and in the anterior tibialis attachment on the tibia ("shin splints"). Heel pain commonly occurs along the sole of the foot, originating where the Plantar Fascia connects to the undersurface of the heel, resulting in Plantar Fasciitis. Pain in the forefoot occurs at the toe joints, the metatarsal bones, at bunions, and between the toes with tears of the transmetatarsal ligaments (commonly called "Morton's Neuroma" or Metatarsalgia).

All of the above structures respond extremely well, permanently, to Prolotherapy, with injections given either inside the involved joints, or into the tendon and ligament attachments outside the joints. Traditional medical practice (medication, steroid injections, surgery, joint replacement) has a fair chance of resolving these problems, but at much greater risk and expense. Surgery may be justified if other less invasive techniques fail to resolve the painful structure. Usually, 4 to 6 treatments with Prolotherapy are required for each of these problems.

### *Chest Wall and Rib Pain*

Obviously, chest pain can be serious. Assuming a more severe problem, such as cancer, heart disease, or lung disease has been ruled out, the primary causes of chest wall pain can be successfully treated with Prolotherapy. The pain is frequently associated with tears or weakness at the rib-breastbone (sternum) attachments, the muscle tendon attachments all along the rim of the ribs, the rib-vertebrae attachments, or the junction of the clavicle (collarbone) at the sternum. Prolotherapy will often reduce or resolve pain from these sites.

### *Groin, Vaginal, Testicular, or Rectal Pain*

Numerous pelvic structures produce pain in these regions. A careful, thorough, and respectful examination of these structures will usually lead to a correct diagnosis and successful treatment. Structures may include the suprapubic joint, inguinal ligament attachments on the anterior pelvis, anterior hip capsule ligaments, sacrococcygeal ligament, iliolumbar ligament, and many others. Cramping during menstruation and back pain during pregnancy are often caused by ligamentous laxity in the pelvic region and can be greatly reduced with Prolotherapy. Prolotherapy often provides permanent relief of the pain over 4 to 6 visits.

## Adopting the Orphaned Medical Intervention

To even consider Prolotherapy as an option, your physician has to question whether inflammation is always at the root of pain, or could the problem sometimes be inadequate inflammation? Health is always an act of balance. When our body is in a state of good health, the body is inflaming in a controlled way to fight off intruders and to repair damage from trauma, disease, or the wear and tear of facing gravity over a lifetime. Currently, we are taught that when we sprain our ankle, we must take anti-inflammatory medication as soon as possible. From the perspective of natural healing, this is essentially treating our body's response to a trauma as if that response were a disease.

As doctors, if we only anti-inflame in response to pain, we are like the captain of a ship who believes the only way to steer a ship across the ocean is to always turn the wheel in one direction. If we appear off course, we just need to turn the wheel farther. But, of course, this will only lead us in circles and we will never reach our patient's goal of health. Our present way of thinking is very much like the way we used to "care" for forests. For decades, or even centuries, we believed that we must fight all forest fires. As the bigger picture became clearer, we realized that suppressing every fire caused an overgrowth of unhealthy trees and underbrush that actually increased the chance of a devastating forest fire. By trying to help, we were creating imbalance in the ecosystem. Realizing that fires are a healthy event in the life of a forest, the forest service now thinks before acting. Sometimes it is best to suppress a certain fire, sometimes to allow a wildfire to burn itself out, and sometimes it is best to actually start a "prescribed fire." After a prescribed fire, the unhealthy overgrowth is gone; vibrant, healthy growth begins anew. Then, the entire forest can return to balanced health.

As our health care system has moved toward integrative, complementary medicine, patients are seeking and demanding interventions that help our body do what it is naturally doing for itself. Prolotherapy is just such an intervention; it's time for adoption has finally arrived. ■

---

*Brad Fullerton, MD*
*The Patient-Physician Partnership*
*2714 Bee Cave Rd, Suite 106*
*Austin, TX 78746*
*(512)347-7246*
*(512)347-7245 FAX*
*http://www.proloaustin.com/*

*Dr. Brad Fullerton received his medical degree from the University of Texas, Southwestern Medical School in Dallas. He completed his internship and one year of psychiatric training at the University of Connecticut, then residency training in Physical Medicine and Rehabilitation at the Graduate Hospital of the University of Pennsylvania in Philadelphia. He currently serves as medical director for the Spasticity Clinic at Children's Hospital of Austin, while maintaining his private practice specializing in the treatment of chronic pain and sports injuries. His research interests include diagnostic musculoskeletal ultrasound imaging in Orthopedic Medicine and its use with Prolotherapy. Dr. Fullerton enjoys hiking along Austin's beautiful spring-fed creeks and swimming holes with his wife and two daughters.*

*David K. Harris, MD*
*The Lakewood Clinic*
*7307 Creekbluff Drive*
*Austin, Texas 78750*
*512-454-1234*
*Fax 512-476-0850*
*www.lakewoodclinic.com*

*Dr. David Harris specializes in Physical Medicine and Rehabilitation in Austin, Texas. He primarily manages patients with sports and spine injuries at the Lakewood Clinic and at SpineAustin. He has used Dr. Teitelbaum's approach with his chronic fatigue and fibromyalgia patients with great success, and this has led to the use of many of these techniques with his less "metabolically involved" patients. He has a BS in Electrical Engineering from The University of Texas, is on faculty at the University of Texas, and teaches regularly for the Texas Medical Association. He and his Physical Therapist wife, Michele, have two boys, A.J. and Kyle. He enjoys the outdoors and playing guitar with his local Austin band, Natural Causes.*

*To find qualified physicians who have been trained in Prolotherapy, please refer to http://www.aaomed.org (American Association of Orthopedic Medicine) and http://www.getprolo.com.*

### Important Points

1. Prolotherapy is a series of injections of a natural solution (something as simple as a sugar or salt solution, cod liver oil, known as sodium morrhuate, or herbal extract) into the area where the ligaments have either been weakened or damaged through injury or strain. This stimulates proliferation of **normal** tissue, which helps the body to repair painful areas.
2. Its effectiveness is wide-ranging and includes pain associated with the back, the neck, all joints throughout the body, arthritis, migraine headaches, fibromyalgia, sciatica, herniated discs, and Temporo Mandibular Joint Dysfunction (TMJ).
3. Chronic musculoskeletal pain is often due to weakness of ligaments and tendons. The injection is given at the point where the ligament or tendon connects to the bone. Many points may require injection. The injection causes the body to heal itself through the processes of controlled inflammation and production of growth factors.

CHAPTER 24

# *Traditional Chinese Medicine—* Acupuncture for Coordinated Wellness-Care

**by Peter Marinakis, Ph.D.**

*This chapter on acupuncture is written by Peter Marinakis. He gives an overview of this system of treatment, describes its benefits, and gives details on how you can best use this ancient form of Chinese medicine to treat pain.*

Acupuncture is one of the oldest, most commonly used medical procedures in the world. Originating in China more than 3,000 years ago, acupuncture began to become better known in the United States in 1971, when New York Times reporter James Reston wrote about how doctors in China had used needles to ease his abdominal pain after surgery. Research shows that acupuncture is beneficial in treating a variety of health conditions.

The term acupuncture describes a family of procedures involving stimulation of anatomical points on the body by a variety of techniques. American practices of acupuncture incorporate medical traditions from China, Japan, Korea, and other countries. The acupuncture technique that has been most studied scientifically involves penetrating the skin with thin, solid, metallic needles that are manipulated by the hands or by electrical stimulation.

In the past two decades, acupuncture has grown in popularity in the United States. A Harvard University study published in 1998 estimated that Americans made more than 5 million visits per year to acupuncture practitioners.[1] The report from a Consensus Development Conference on Acupuncture held at the National Institutes of Health (NIH) in 1997 stated that acupuncture is being "widely" practiced by thousands of physicians, dentists, acupuncturists, and other practitioners for relief or prevention of pain and for various other health conditions.[2]

NIH has funded a variety of research projects on acupuncture. These grants have been awarded by the National Center for Complementary and Alternative Medicine (NCCAM), the Office of Alternative Medicine (OAM, NCCAM's predecessor), and other NIH Institutes and Centers.

This research report provides general information about acupuncture, research summaries, and a resource section. Terms that are underlined are defined at the end of this report.

## Acupuncture Theories

Traditional Chinese medicine theorizes that there are more than 2,000 acupuncture points on the human body, and that these connect with 12 main and 8 secondary pathways called meridians. Chinese medicine practitioners believe these meridians conduct energy, or qi (pronounced "chee"), throughout the body.

Qi is believed to regulate spiritual, emotional, mental, and physical balance and to be influenced by the opposing forces of yin and yang. According to traditional Chinese medicine, when yin and yang are balanced, they work together with the natural flow of qi to help the body achieve and maintain health. Acupuncture is believed to balance yin and yang, keep the normal flow of energy unblocked, and maintain or restore health to the body and mind.

Traditional Chinese medicine practices (including acupuncture, herbs, diet, massage, and meditative physical exercise) all are intended to improve the flow of qi.[3]

Western scientists have found meridians hard to identify because meridians do not directly correspond to nerve or blood circulation pathways. Some researchers believe that meridians are located throughout the body's connective tissue;[4] others do not believe that qi exists at all.[5,6] Such differences of opinion have made acupuncture an area of scientific controversy.

## Mechanisms of Action

Several processes have been proposed to explain acupuncture's effects, primarily those on pain. Acupuncture points are believed to stimulate the central nervous system (the brain and spinal cord) to release chemicals into the muscles, spinal cord, and brain. These chemicals either change the experience of pain or release other chemicals, such as hormones, that influence the body's self-regulating systems. The biochemical changes may stimulate the body's natural healing abilities and promote physical and emotional well-being.[7] There are three main mechanisms:

1. **Conduction of electromagnetic signals**. Western scientists have found evidence that acupuncture points are strategic conductors of electromagnetic signals. Stimulating points along these pathways through acupuncture enables electromagnetic signals to be relayed

at a greater rate than under normal conditions. These signals may start the flow of pain-killing biochemicals, such as endorphins, and of immune system cells to specific sites in the body that are injured or vulnerable to disease.[8,9]

2. **Activation of opioid systems**. Research has found that several types of opioids may be released into the central nervous system during acupuncture treatment, thereby reducing pain.[10]
3. **Changes in brain chemistry, sensation, and involuntary body functions**. Studies have shown that acupuncture may alter brain chemistry by changing the release of neurotransmitters and neurohormones. Acupuncture also has been documented to affect the parts of the central nervous system related to sensation and involuntary body functions, such as immune reactions and processes whereby a person's blood pressure, blood flow, and body temperature are regulated.[3,11,12]

Preclinical studies have documented acupuncture's effects, but they have not been able to fully explain how acupuncture works within the framework of the Western system of medicine.[13, 14, 15, 16, 17, 18]

According to the NIH Consensus Statement on Acupuncture:

> "Acupuncture as a therapeutic intervention is widely practiced in the United States. While there have been many studies of its potential usefulness, many of these studies provide equivocal results because of design, sample size, and other factors. The issue is further complicated by inherent difficulties in the use of appropriate controls, such as placebos and sham acupuncture groups. However, promising results have emerged, for example, showing efficacy of acupuncture in adult postoperative and chemotherapy nausea and vomiting and in postoperative dental pain. There are other situations such as addiction, stroke rehabilitation, headache, menstrual cramps, tennis elbow, fibromyalgia, myofascial pain, osteoarthritis, low back pain, carpal tunnel syndrome, and asthma, in which acupuncture may be useful as an adjunct treatment or an acceptable alternative or be included in a comprehensive management program. Further research is likely to uncover additional areas where acupuncture interventions will be useful."[7]

Increasingly, acupuncture is complementing conventional therapies. For example, doctors may combine acupuncture and drugs to control surgery-related pain in their patients.[19] By providing both acupuncture and certain conventional anesthetic drugs, some doctors have found it possible to achieve a state of complete pain relief for some patients.[10] They also have found that using acupuncture lowers the need for conventional pain killing drugs and thus reduces the risk of side effects for patients who take the drugs.[20, 21]

Currently, one of the main reasons Americans seek acupuncture treatment is to relieve chronic pain, especially from conditions such as arthritis or lower back disorders.[22,23] Some clinical studies show that acupuncture is effective in relieving both chronic (long-lasting) and acute or sudden pain, but other research indicates that it provides no relief from chronic pain.[24] Additional research is needed to provide definitive answers.

## FDA's Role

The U.S. Food and Drug Administration (FDA) approved acupuncture needles for use by licensed practitioners in 1996. The FDA requires manufacturers of acupuncture needles to label them for single use only.[25] Relatively few complications from the use of acupuncture have been reported to the FDA when one considers the millions of people treated each year and the number of acupuncture needles used.

## Research Sponsored by NCCAM and OAM

NCCAM and OAM have supported scientific research to find out more about acupuncture. Examples of recent NCCAM-supported projects include:

- Studying the safety and effectiveness of acupuncture treatment for osteoarthritis of the knee
- Investigating whether electroacupuncture works for chronic pain and inflammation (and, if so, how)
- Finding out how acupuncture affects the nervous system by using MRI (magnetic resonance imaging) technology
- Bringing together leaders from the Oriental medicine and conventional medicine communities to collaboratively study the safety and effectiveness of acupuncture and further develop the standards for clinical trials
- Studying whether acupuncture can decrease the release of adrenalin in heart patients and improve their survival and quality of life. Adrenaline can make the heart beat faster and can thereby contribute to heart failure.
- Looking at the effectiveness of acupuncture for treating high blood pressure

- Studying the effects of acupuncture on the symptoms of advanced colorectal cancer
- Testing the safety and effectiveness of acupuncture for a type of depression called major depression

With regard to earlier findings, researchers at the University of Maryland in Baltimore, with the support of OAM, conducted a randomized controlled clinical trial and found that patients treated with acupuncture after dental surgery had less intense pain than patients who received a placebo.[26] Scientists at the university also found that older people with osteoarthritis experienced significantly more pain relief after using conventional drugs and acupuncture together than those using conventional therapy alone.[27]

OAM also funded several preliminary studies on acupuncture:

- In one small randomized controlled clinical trial, more than half of 11 women with a major depressive episode who were treated with acupuncture improved significantly.[28]
- In another controlled clinical trial, nearly half of the seven children with attention deficit hyperactivity disorder who underwent acupuncture treatment showed some improvement in their symptoms. Researchers concluded that acupuncture was a useful alternative to standard medication for some children with this condition.[29]
- In a third small controlled study, eight pregnant women were given a type of acupuncture treatment called moxibustion to reduce the rate of breech births, in which the fetus is positioned for birth feet-first instead of the normal position of head-first. Researchers found the treatment to be safe, but they were uncertain whether it was effective.[30] Then, researchers reporting in the November 11, 1998, issue of the *Journal of the American Medical Association* conducted a larger randomized controlled clinical trial using moxibustion for breech births. They found that moxibustion applied to 130 pregnant women presenting breech significantly increased the number of normal head-first births.[31]

## Acupuncture and You

The use of acupuncture, like the use of many other complementary and alternative medicine (CAM) treatments, has produced a good deal of anecdotal evidence. Much of this evidence comes from people who report their own successful use of the treatment. If a treatment appears to be safe and patients report recovery from their illness or condition after using it, others may decide to use the treatment. However, scientific research may not support the anecdotal reports. Patient outcomes continue to be one of the best forms of feedback to the practitioner, patient, and the health care industry at large. Studies done by state acupuncture societies, such as the Maryland Acupuncture Society, have reported in a January 2000 patient survey that 71 percent of the patients reporting in had a "very satisfied experience with acupuncture and had excellent results." See www.maryland-acupuncture.org for the full report.

Lifestyle, age, physiology, and other factors combine to make every person different. A treatment that works for one person may not work for another who has the very same condition. You as a health care consumer (especially if you have a preexisting medical condition) should discuss any CAM treatment, including acupuncture, with your health care practitioner. Do not rely on a diagnosis of disease by an acupuncture practitioner who does not have substantial conventional medical training. If you have received a diagnosis from a doctor and have had little or no success using conventional medicine, you may wish to ask your doctor whether acupuncture might help.

### *Finding a Licensed Acupuncture Practitioner*

Health care practitioners can be a resource for referral to practitioners of acupuncture, as more are becoming aware of this CAM therapy. More medical doctors, including neurologists, anesthesiologists, and specialists in physical medicine, are becoming familiar with acupuncture, traditional Chinese medicine, and other CAM therapies. In addition, national organizations (consult your local library or search with a Web browser) may provide referrals to practitioners, although some organizations may encourage the use of their practices.

### *Check a Practitioner's Credentials*

A practitioner who is licensed and credentialed may provide better care than one who is not. About 47 states have established training standards for acupuncture certification, but States have varied requirements for obtaining a license to practice acupuncture.[32] Although proper credentials do not ensure competency, they do indicate that the practitioner has met certain standards to treat patients through the use of acupuncture. See the addendum for a complete list of national and federal organizations.

### *Check Treatment Cost and Insurance Coverage*

A practitioner should inform you about the estimated number of treatments needed and how much each will cost. If this information is not provided, ask for it. Treatment may take place over a few days or for several weeks or more. Physician acupuncturists may charge more than nonphysician practitioners. Check with your insurer before you start treatment as to whether acupuncture will be covered for your condition, and if so, to what extent. Some plans require preauthorization for acupuncture.

### *Check Treatment Procedures*

Ask about the treatment procedures that will be used and their likelihood of success for your condition or disease. You also should make certain that the practitioner uses a new set of disposable needles in a sealed package every time. The FDA requires the use of sterile, nontoxic needles that bear a labeling statement restricting their use to qualified practitioners. The practitioner also should swab the puncture site with alcohol or another disinfectant before inserting the needle.

During your first office visit, the practitioner may ask you at length about your health condition, lifestyle, and behavior. The practitioner will want to obtain a complete picture of your treatment needs and any behaviors that may contribute to the condition. Inform the acupuncturist about all treatments or medications you are taking and all medical conditions you have.

## The Sensation of Acupuncture

Acupuncture needles are metallic, solid, and hair-thin. People experience acupuncture differently, but most feel no or minimal pain as the needles are inserted. Some people are energized by treatment, while others feel relaxed.[33] Improper needle placement, movement of the patient, or a defect in the needle can cause soreness and pain during treatment.[34] This is why it is important to seek treatment from a qualified acupuncture practitioner.

## Addendum

For a complete list of National and International Acupuncture and Oriental Medicine Organizations see the www.aomAlliance.org or www.who.org, click health topics, acupuncture, to see a list of health issues treatable with acupuncture. ■

*Peter Marinakis, PhD; Mac, is Director of Full Circle Healing Arts, a multidisciplinary well care clinic in Annapolis, Maryland. Dr. Marinakis was on the faculty of Tai Sophia for the last twenty years and is now a distinguished lecturer at the Institute. He is founder and director of the Community Health Initiative (CHI), a community relationship based drug abuse treatment and wellness care clinic with some 350 clients per day. He is the past president of the Maryland Acupuncture Society, past president of the American Association of Acupuncture and Oriental Medicine (now the AAOM), founding member of the AOM Alliance, and a past Accreditation Commissioner of the Accreditation Commission for Acupuncture and Oriental Medicine. Dr. Marinakis lectures and does workshops throughout the United States on energy medicine and emotion.*

### *I am passing this on to you because it has definitely worked for me, and at this time of year we all could use a little—calm!!!*

By following the simple advice I read in an article, I have finally found inner peace. The article read, "The way to achieve inner peace is to finish all the things you've started."

So I looked around the house to see all the things I started and hadn't finished—and before going to work this morning I finished off a bottle of red wine, a bottle of white, the Bailey's, Kahlua and Tia Maria, my Prozac, some valium, my cigarettes, and a box of chocolates.

You have no idea how freakin good I feel. You may pass this on to those you feel are in need of inner peace.

# CHAPTER 25 Sexual Dysfunction, Depression, and Mind-Body Aspects of Pain

## Sexual Dysfunction

In our study of patients with fibromyalgia, 73 percent had loss of libido.[1] Loss of sexual function in FMS was also found in a study conducted in Brazil.[2] Sexual dissatisfaction was present in 55 percent of patients, with 74 percent of women having pain with intercourse. This is also a very common problem in chronic pain as well.

Loss of libido and/or sexual function can occur from any of the multiple problems that are common in chronic pain. For example, depression, pain, and anxiety may cause loss of self-esteem and associated loss of libido in both men and women. In addition, the chronic stress of pain itself can lead to decreased production of many hormones including testosterone. Chronic opioid use has also been shown to significantly lower testosterone levels. Because of this, checking testosterone levels is appropriate in anyone, both male and female, with sexual dysfunction—especially in the presence of chronic pain. When treating for low testosterone, I strongly recommend that natural testosterone be used instead of synthetics. In men, testosterone 1 percent (Androgel®) can be applied to the skin over the chest twice daily for a total daily dose of 50 to 100 mg. Testosterone cream can also be made less expensively by compounding pharmacists. Testosterone tablets should not be used in men because the high dose can result in elevated cholesterol levels when taken by mouth. In men with low or low-normal testosterone who also had angina, high cholesterol, and/or diabetes, repeated studies have shown **decreased** angina, cholesterol, and diabetes with the addition of **natural** testosterone.[3] Sadly, this data has been largely ignored. I bring my patients' testosterone blood level up to the mid to upper part of the normal range.

Testosterone can also help loss of libido in women. For example, a recent study has demonstrated that small doses of testosterone may improve the sex lives in women who have had hysterectomies. Delivered transdermally (via the skin) by a patch applied twice a week, the testosterone raised desire and improved function in 74 percent of the study participants.[4] Even if you have not had a hysterectomy, a trial of testosterone is reasonable if your "free" testosterone level (use the results of this blood test, not the **total** testosterone) is in the lowest quarter of the normal range. In women, 2 to 6 mg of testosterone in cream or tablet form daily is usually adequate and can help pain, libido, and overall well-being.

Other factors also contribute to sexual dysfunction. These include pain caused from assuming sexual positions or marital stress from chronic pain. Anti-depressants such as Prozac® commonly cause difficulties with erections, decreased libido, and difficulty with achieving orgasms (the latter being especially important in women). If you need to continue the anti-depressants, the associated sexual dysfunction is treatable. One study showed that taking the herb ginkgo biloba 120 mg twice daily often eliminated the sexual dysfunction caused by anti-depressants after 6 weeks (this higher dose was needed, because the lower dose was not as effective). Wellbutrin®, trazodone, or Remeron® do not seem to cause the sexual dysfunction caused by other anti-depressants.

I recommend using Viagra® or Cialis® for erectile dysfunction. Viagra can be taken in doses of 25, 50, or 100 mg tablets. It is most effective when taken on an empty stomach and the higher dose is often effective if the lower dose is not. In addition, it is generally cheaper to buy a 100 mg tablet and break it in half than to buy two 50 mg tablets. Cialis is a newer medication for erectile dysfunction. It may work faster (within 10 to 15 minutes) than Viagra and the effects last for 24 hours. It comes in 10 and 20 mg strengths and can be taken with food. Both medications should not be used in conjunction with nitroglycerin, and they may cause problems in patients with heart disease. A newer medication that may not have this problem (called Vardenafil®) is being developed.

At the 2004 meeting of the American Psychiatric Association, researchers from Columbia University reported on the growing use of complimentary medicines to boost sexual function and desire. Offering even greater benefits than Viagra or the other erectile dysfunction drugs currently in use, natural sex enhancing drugs such as Rhodiola® may reduce premature ejaculation and boost sexual desire in both men and women. Rhodiola also seems to revive sexual energy, provide increased pleasure, improve erections, and intensify orgasms, allowing for more satisfying sex. The presentation also discussed the effectiveness of the herbs ginseng, ginkgo, maca, and horny goat weed in restoring sexual desire and function in both men and women.

# Pain—The Mind-Body Connection

## *Pain and Depression*

Chronic pain and depression have long been linked, and patients with chronic pain suffer a high incidence of major depressive disorders (MDD). Thomas Elliott of St. Mary's Duluth Clinic Health System set out to further characterize this link by looking for correlations among age, sex, chronic pain, and depression. He found that the prevalence of MDD was significantly higher in younger patients with chronic pain—59 percent in the 18 to 44 years age group. Furthermore, 70 percent of women with chronic pain also suffered MDD, a significantly higher percentage than the men in this sample.[5] It is understandable that anyone with a severe illness, especially one that is treated as poorly as pain, would go through periods of depression. You are not alone. With new treatments, however, you finally have the opportunity to become pain free—which is a great start at treating depression!

It is okay to acknowledge that chronic pain devastates people's lives in many ways. It can dramatically worsen the quality of your life on many levels, including physical, social, emotional, and spiritual. It can trigger depression, anxiety, and loss of independence. It also can severely interfere with your ability to work and maintain friendships and relationships. All of these issues need to be addressed and supported.

People with chronic pain, however, are often afraid to bring up these problems with their family, friends, and physicians. Although it may be appropriate not to continually bring up one's pain in personal relationships since you may find yourself getting tuned out and avoided, it is important that your doctor be made aware of persistent pain at each visit. Research has shown that patients are often hesitant to bring up their pain doctor visits for the following reasons: they're afraid of being viewed as complainers, are concerned about distracting the doctor from other medical issues, or because the patient has a fatalistic view that nothing can be done.

It is important to recognize that **it is <u>not</u> okay to be left in chronic pain**. You need to make your doctor aware of your situation if the pain is persistent and not adequately controlled. If your physician is not able or willing to take further measures to help, ask for a referral to a pain specialist (or another one if you are already seeing one). If your doctor does not feel like another physician may have any other options for you, let him or her know about the options we are discussing in this book, or go ahead and get a second opinion.

## *Besides Treating the Pain, How Can I Move Past My Depression?*

Depression can often be effectively treated using natural therapies. I recommend beginning by making sure that you have adequate levels of most nutrients, especially B vitamins (e.g. B12 and folate). The easiest way to do this is with the Energy Revitalization System powder, which also dramatically raises levels of SAM-e—another nutrient highly effective against depression.[6] Many studies show that Sam-e is as (or more) effective at treating depression than tricyclics, without the side effects. Unfortunately, SAM-e tablets are not very stable, are very expensive, and require a high dose. Because of this, the vitamin powder is likely the best approach. I recommend also adding fish oil (1/2 to 1 tbsp per day-see Appendix C) to your regimen. Several studies have shown fish oil to be very helpful in treating depression.[7-8]

St. John's Wort, 1000 to 2000 mg daily, is the next thing I would add. Use a brand (e.g. available at GNC) that's a standardized extract. Dozens of studies have found it to be as effective as prescription anti-depressants for treating moderate depression. Like most prescriptions, it is unlikely to be effective by itself for severe depression, although limited data suggests that higher doses might be effective.[9] Do not combine it with prescription anti-depressants unless OK'd by your doctor, because the combination can (very, very rarely) drive serotonin levels dangerously high. In my practice, I may combine St. John's Wort with prescription anti-depressants, because this allows for a lower dose of the anti-depressant medication and therefore fewer side effects.

5HTP, the nutrient that your body uses to make serotonin, can also be helpful for both depression and pain.[10] It also has the benefit of improving sleep and causing weight loss. The usual dose is 200 to 400 mg at bedtime. As with St. John's Wort, it raises serotonin levels, so limit the dose to 200 mg a night if taking it with other prescription anti-depressants.

Other commonsense approaches are also very important. Walking, for example, has been shown to be as effective as Prozac® in treating depression. Bright light exposure during the winter time, yoga and tai chi, spiritual healing, and other similar modalities can also be very helpful. Most important, it is essential that you get in touch with, and express, your feelings. My book *Three Steps to Happiness: Healing through Joy!* is a short book that will teach you how to do this (available online at www.Vitality101.com and at www.amazon.com).

The mineral Rubidium, 500 mg daily with food, can also help even resistant depression. It takes 1 month to work and is available without a prescription from compounding pharmacies. In studies of the mineral, participants used between 180 to 720 mg daily. Some minor side effects include constipation, diarrhea, insomnia, or agitation (do n you have manic-depressive illness). It is a good idea to eat a or take a glass of V-8 juice each day along with the Rubidiu

Emotional stress can also contribute to pain. John Sarnc Professor of Clinical Rehabilitation Medicine at New York University School of Medicine and attending physician at the Rusk Institute of Rehabilitation Medicine at New York University Medical Center. He found that the mind often decreases the blood flow to areas of the body in an attempt to distract us from uncomfortable emotions by causing pain. This occurs even though the pain is often hundreds of times more uncomfortable than the feeling our mind is trying to "protect" us from. Fortunately, although the pain caused by decreased blood flow is real and can be severe, it generally does no permanent harm. This concept may seem odd at first, but it gives us a powerful, simple, safe, natural, and inexpensive way to eliminate many kinds of pains—especially when we combine this knowledge with the physical treatments. This approach is quite simple, and I find that it works best for **localized** pain (e.g. back pain, tendonitis, and localized nerve pain).

As noted, your mind may be decreasing blood flow to muscles and other areas to distract you from uncomfortable emotional feelings. When you feel pain, tell your mind that you will repeatedly use the pain as a signal to look for and "feel" those uncomfortable emotions for 10 to 15 minutes—then do so. The pain will often leave within 6 weeks. Interestingly, this works well even for pain that began after an injury. For more information about this approach, read Dr. Sarno's current book *Healing Back Pain: the Mind Body Connection* and his earlier book, *The Mind Body Prescription* (1998).

Dr. Sarno theorizes that what is actually causing pain is not the herniated disc, or some other structural thing, but a condition of mild oxygen deprivation that is brought about by the brain simply altering the blood flow to a particular area. This mild oxygen deprivation is what causes pain in muscles, nerves, and tendons. This can result in pain anywhere in the body. He calls this tension myositis syndrome (TMS). He feels the problem is not based on inflammation but rather a decreased oxygen supply. He theorizes that this is why treatments that increase local circulation, such as deep heat in the form of ultrasound, deep massage, and active exercise can temporarily decrease pain.

Dr. Sarno explains that x-ray and MRI studies find normal changes in the area of the pain that are unrelated to the pain. He gives an example published in a 1994 research paper by Maureen Jensen and colleagues in the *New England Journal of Medicine*. They performed MRIs on about 98 people who had no history of back pain. The researchers found normal discs in only 36 percent of the people. Everyone else had ges, or herniations of various kinds and yet no pain. That's the kind of information that doctors in this country totally ignore.

## *What Kind of Emotional Factors Does Doctor Sarno Attribute Pain to?*

Dr. Sarno came to many of the same conclusions about the psychodynamic of pain that I discuss in my book *From Fatigued to Fantastic!* The difference is that he feels that the pains come entirely from the psyche without a physical cause (other than the self-induced decreased blood flow). In my experience, pain, much like other illnesses including heart attacks, cancer, etc., has both a physical and psycho-spiritual component, and I find that addressing both simultaneously results in the best outcome.

In a recent interview, Dr. Sarno discussed his experience of the psychodynamic of pain.[20] He feels that it primarily has to do with the stresses in patients' lives and the stresses that they put themselves under. Dr Sarno stated:

> "People were responding to the pressures and the stresses that they put on themselves. I came to realize that people who tend to be perfectionists—that is, hard-working, conscientious, ambitious, success-oriented, driven, and so on—that this type of personality was highly susceptible to TMS.
>
> Later, I realized that there is another kind of self-induced pressure, and that is the need to be a good person. This is the need to please people, to want to be liked, to want to be approved of. This, too, like the pressure to excel or to be a perfectionist, is a pressure and seemed to play a big role in bringing on this disorder…I realized that these self-imposed pressures were causing some difficulty inside our minds. There's a leftover child in all of us that doesn't want to be put under pressure, and indeed he can get very, very angry. It began to look as though the primary factor psychologically here was a great deal of internal anger to the point of rage…Things of this sort could contribute to a reservoir of rage that I believe we all carry around inside of us. This is part of the human condition in Western society. It's because we're all under such pressure, and so many of us are conscientious and hardworking…It turns out that the rage is the primary difficulty."

## *What Other Mind Body Issues Are Important?*

The bottom line is if you are repressing emotions, not letting go of your feelings, and you feel like a victim (which leaves you powerless), and you are not keeping your attention on what feels good when you can, you are likely to not stay healthy. This cycle of repression and lack of focus on what feels good can result in many illnesses including pain.

In addition to pain coming from decreased blood flow to the muscles, pain can also come from muscles being stuck in the shortened position. In addition to the biochemical triggers that we have discussed earlier in this book, this can occur in response to emotional stresses where we tighten our muscles as a form of "emotional armor." It can also occur in response to other physical injuries as well. The body will often tighten the muscles in the area of injury to form a kind of a splint. This helps to decrease pain initially, but can then add to pain in the long run.

Another critical point to remember is that we are only aware of 3 to 5 percent of the sensory input that comes into our brains any given time. The rest is filtered out. For example, take a moment to notice the sounds of your heating/cooling system, the buzzing of the lights, the feeling of the air on your skin, and the numerous other sensations that you do not notice until somebody points them out. Pain is a fairly loud sensory input because it is meant to get our attention. It does so to tell us many things. We are familiar with the messages to avoid something traumatic, like our hand being on a hot stove, or to pay attention to, and take care of, an injury—and we heed these messages fairly well. We are also aware of some of the less overt but equally important needs of our bodies that pain informs us of. These include the physical needs of nutritional support, sleep, hormonal support, and of eliminating infections. It also includes the psychological, and perhaps even the spiritual, needs to be true to ourselves, acknowledge our feelings, and to do what feels best to us. This may not always be what other people are expecting of us or telling us to do. Simply attending to these issues will eliminate many pains.

In other situations, there may be a malfunction in the pain system itself. Once your psyche knows that you have finally attended to those things you needed to pay attention to, a remarkable thing can happen. Your brain's "filtering system" is now able to recognize that the pain signal is no longer important and it can start to filter the signal out as it does with other sensory input presented to it. This process of muting your pain signal can be helped by the many pain treatments we've discussed in this book. At this point a fairly remarkable thing occurs. You'll find that your chronic pain becomes intermittent, then mild, then gone! ■

**Important Points**

1. Sexual dysfunction and loss of libido is common in chronic pain. Pain can cause a low testosterone level, as can treatment with codeine/narcotics. Check a free testosterone level and take natural testosterone supplements if the level is in the lowest $25^{th}$ percentile of the normal range.
2. Depression is also common in chronic pain, and it is important to be able to talk about your feelings with your doctor and family. Usually depression can be reversed naturally by taking the vitamin powder, fish oil, exercise (if able), St. John's Wort, 5-HTP, and natural hormones including Armour Thyroid and testosterone as needed. If depression persists, I recommend using anti-depressants, which can also decrease pain.
3. Anti-depressants can cause sexual dysfunction. The herb ginkgo biloba, 120 mg twice a day, can often reverse this condition after 6 weeks.
4. Work by Dr. John Sarno, M.D. has shown that emotional stress can also contribute to pain. He found that our minds often decrease the blood flow to areas of our body in an attempt to distract us from uncomfortable feelings by causing pain! To overcome this, learn to feel and express your feelings. In addition, when you feel pain, tell your mind that you will repeatedly use the pain as a signal to look for and feel uncomfortable feelings for 10 to 15 minutes—then do so. The pain will often leave within 6 weeks.
5. Read the book *Three Steps to Happiness: Healing through Joy!* It will help you get from where you are to feeling great in 144 pages.
6. By treating those things that your pain is pointing out, the pain signal decreases and often stops. In addition, the filtering system of your mind now knows that it is okay to ignore any residual pain signal.

CHAPTER 26

# Eliminating Weight Gain

*This chapter is an article on weight gain in pain related illnesses that I wrote for a magazine. I think you will find it interesting, and it will also serve as a helpful overview of many of the things we have discussed in the book.*

Weight gain can be a major problem in chronic pain and chronic stress states. For example, our study of fibromyalgia patients showed an average weight gain of 32 lbs.[1] It's bad enough to feel awful and be in chronic pain. The blow that many people feel to their physical self-image from the weight gain can add further suffering. So why is weight gain such a problem here?

For starters, we live in a society where being overweight is epidemic. It is much easier to lose weight and keep it off, however, when you understand that there are many things that contribute to this problem. Most of us are familiar with the more common ones such as:

1. **The Standard American Diet (SAD)**. Our standard diet contains excessive sugar and fat. In addition, food processing causes the loss of even more vitamins and minerals, resulting in "high calorie malnutrition." It is quite possible that this is the first time in the history of the human race that this has occurred! Being nutritionally deficient in numerous vitamins and minerals is one of many causes of excessive food cravings. Unfortunately, it is hard to get adequate nutrition out of the American diet, even if one's diet is relatively healthy.

2. **Lack of exercise**. During most of human history, people had to walk if they wanted to get somewhere. In addition, work often consisted of physical labor. This is no longer the case. In fact, we seem to even get upset if we can't get a parking space right near the entrance of the mall!

For many people, simply altering their diet and increasing their exercise is enough to let them lose weight. A large percentage of you, however, have found that it is impossible to lose weight and keep it off no matter what you do.

## *Why Is It Impossible for Me to Lose Weight and Keep It Off?*

There are a number of ways that stress, fibromyalgia, and/or chronic pain can contribute to your inability to lose weight. Fortunately, understanding these can help you overcome this problem. Both physical stresses (e.g. pain, infections, nutritional deficiencies, toxic chemical exposures) and emotional/situational stresses (having a toxic boss, working too hard without enough sleep, worrying) can result in a metabolic chain reaction that results in weight gain. Interestingly, chronic fatigue syndrome and fibromyalgia (CFS/FMS) are good models for the occurrence of weight gain during stress and chronic pain.

## *What Is Going On in CFS/FMS?*

As noted in the chapter on fibromyalgia, I do not view these syndromes as the enemy. Rather, I see them as attempts by the body to protect itself from further harm and damage in the face of many toxic situations. A simple way to look at fibromyalgia and CFS is to view them as circuit breakers. In a house, when certain systems are over-stressed, some of the circuit breakers will go off to prevent damaging the home's wiring. In the body, under normal circumstances, by supplying proper rest and nutrition, the circuit breakers can come back on and systems can return to healthy functioning. In CFS/FMS, however, it is as if the main circuit breaker (in this situation it's the hypothalamus—a master gland in the brain) has turned off. When this occurs, rest is no longer enough to restore proper functioning.

Despite the many diverse stresses that can cause these syndromes, most patients' symptoms seem to come from a common endpoint—dysfunction or suppression of the hypothalamus. This gland controls sleep, hormonal function, temperature regulation, and the autonomic nervous system (e.g. blood pressure, blood flow, and movement of food through the bowel). This is why these patients can't sleep, have low body temperatures, and, because poor sleep causes immune dysfunction, are prone to multiple and recurrent infections. The hypothalamic dysfunction by itself can cause most of the symptoms we listed above. In addition, I suspect that problems with the mitochondria (the "energy furnaces" in the cells) are also present and are what cause hypothalamic suppression.

### *How Does This Lead to Weight Gain?*

This process contributes to weight gain in several ways. The expression "getting your beauty sleep" actually has a basis in fact. Deep sleep is a major trigger for growth hormone production. Growth hormone stimulates production of muscle (which burns fat) and improves insulin sensitivity (which decreases the tendency to make fat). The other two main triggers for growth hormone production are exercise and sex. In fact, one study showed that people who have sex at least three times a week look ten years younger than those who don't. The study notes that this was because of the increase in growth hormone release. Oddly enough, getting the eight to nine hours sleep a night that the human body is meant to have can powerfully contribute to your staying young and trim!

### *Why Do You Say That the Body Is Meant to Have 8 to 9 Hours of Sleep a Night?*

100 years ago, the average American got nine hours of sleep a night. If you ask anthropologists, they will tell you that the average night's sleep 5,000 years ago was 11 to 12 hours a night. When the sun went down, it was dark, boring, and dangerous outside, so people went to sleep. They woke up at sunrise, and the average time from sunset to sunrise is 12 hours a day. As candles and torches became more common, people went down to the nine hours sleep each night. When light bulbs, followed by radios, televisions, and computers were developed, the average night's sleep went down to the current six and one half to seven hours. This is simply not adequate for health and contributes to much of the chronic pain, fatigue, and general poor vitality seen in this country! Sadly, not getting adequate sleep can then actually trigger insomnia so that people are not able to sleep.

### *How Does Stress Contribute to Weight Gain?*

As noted above, the hypothalamic "circuit breaker" that gets suppressed with stress also controls the hormone system. This results in inadequate levels of thyroid hormone (which acts as our body's gas pedal) and adrenal hormone. The blood tests that we currently use are notoriously unreliable in picking up thyroid and adrenal deficiencies. This is discussed at length in my book *From Fatigued to Fantastic!* Over the last decade, the tests for thyroid deficiencies and their normal ranges have been modified. The result was that millions of people (who previously had been told by their doctors that they were crazy or that there was nothing wrong with them) were finally diagnosed with hypothyroidism. This happened again in November 2002 when the American Academy of Clinical Endocrinology changed the normal range for the TSH blood test in a way that resulted in 13 million more Americans having hypothyroidism! As always, they think that **now** we finally have them all. Unfortunately, even with this new change, many millions of Americans who suffer with hypothyroidism still have normal blood tests. In addition, the most common medication used to treat hypothyroidism, Synthroid®, is ineffective or inadequately effective in a large percentage of patients. **As long as your thyroid function is inadequate, it will be nearly impossible for you to keep your weight down.**

## *How Can I Tell if I Need Thyroid Hormone?*

The symptoms of hypothyroidism are fatigue, weight gain, cold intolerance with low body temperature (under 98.6 degrees Fahrenheit), achiness, and poor mental function. You don't have to have all of these. Having even a few of these symptoms is enough to justify a therapeutic trial of thyroid hormone. The form that I recommend is Armour Thyroid, and it should be adjusted to the dose that **feels** best while keeping the Free T4 blood test in the normal range. I do not recommend using the TSH blood test to monitor therapy since it often results in patients being under treated. Although this approach is controversial, hundreds if not thousands of doctors are using it, because they find it to be highly effective.

## *What Other Hormone Problems Contribute to Weight Gain?*

The adrenal gland is the body's stress handler. If you think about what is called the "fight or flight reaction," in times of stress the adrenal gland releases cortisol and adrenaline. In times past this might occur every few weeks when we saw a saber tooth tiger or an enemy. Since this only occurred once in a while, our system would have plenty of time to recover. Today, however, we set off the fight or flight reaction dozens if not hundreds of times a day. This can result in exhaustion of the adrenal gland. As it is the job of the adrenal gland to maintain blood sugar levels in time of stress by making cortisol, people initially have elevated cortisol levels, which results in weight gain. Over time, adrenal exhaustion occurs that can result in episodes of hypoglycemia (low blood sugar). If you get periods where you feel like somebody better feed you **now** or you're going to kill them, you are likely hypoglycemic and would benefit from adrenal support. Other symptoms of inadequate adrenal function include crashing emotionally and physically during stress, low blood pressure, and dizziness when first standing. Unfortunately, people crave sugar and eat more than they normally would when they get hypoglycemic. This leads to further weight gain, which can occur paradoxically whether your cortisol levels are too high or too low. Whether your cortisol is high or low, treating the overall process that is causing your pain lowers the stress on your body and can help you lose weight.

## *What Else Contributes to Weight Gain?*

Clinical experience has shown that fungal (also known as Candida or yeast) overgrowth contributes powerfully to both sugar cravings and weight gain. Although doctors do not know the mechanism for this, we have repeatedly seen excess weight drop off once this overgrowth is treated and eliminated. The main causes of fungal overgrowth are excess sugar intake and antibiotic use. Yeast grows by fermenting sugar and requires an area that is warm, dark, and moist. This means that your gut is an ideal environment for fungal overgrowth. The American diet has added approximately 150 pounds of sugar per person per year beyond the diet of hundreds of years ago, so it is easy to see how this would become a problem. To look at it a bit more graphically, carbonated soda has approximately 1 spoon of sugar per ounce. Think about what happens to the yeast in their guts when people go to the local convenience store for a 64 ounce "big burp!"

The main symptoms of yeast overgrowth are chronic sinusitis and spastic colon (gas, bloating, diarrhea, and/or constipation). If you have these, you probably have fungal overgrowth. The good news is that treating this will not just help you to lose weight but can also help eliminate your spastic colon and sinusitis.

## *How Can I Lose Weight and Feel Better?*

1. Cut down on sugar and simple carbohydrates (e.g. potatoes, bread, and pasta) and increase your water intake. Do not count glasses of water—that is a very annoying way to spend the day. Instead, check in with your mouth and see if it is dry. If it is, you are thirsty and need to drink water. We sometimes confuse thirst with hunger and this leaves us eating more than we really want.

2. Get optimum nutritional support. When you are deficient in vitamins or minerals your body craves more food than you need, and your metabolism will be sluggish. To keep it simple and avoid the need to take tablets all day, I recommend that you use the Energy Revitalization System (see Appendix C: Resources) plus 500 mg two times a day Acetyl-L-Carnitine.

3. Get 8 to 9 hours of solid sleep a night. If you have insomnia, herbals can help. I recommend Revitalizing Sleep Formula, 1 to 4 capsules, 1 hour before bedtime. This is a mix of 6 herbals and is the most effective natural sleep aid available.

4. If you are overweight, tired, and have cold intolerance or achiness, ask your holistic doctor for a prescription of Armour Thyroid. Adjust to the dose that feels best while keeping the Free T4 blood test in the normal range. For instructions on adjusting the dose, see Appendix B: Treatment Protocol.

5. Exercise. Find something that is fun and feels good. It also helps to have a regularly scheduled exercise time 3 to 4 times a week in which you meet a friend to exercise with. Otherwise, human nature is to make excuses not to show up!

6. If you have chronic sinusitis or spastic colon, there is a good chance you have fungal/yeast overgrowth in your bowels. Avoid sugar (stevia is a great substitute—the best tasting one is by Body Ecology®). Take Acidophilus Pearls (healthy milk bacteria to combat yeast), 2 pearls twice a day. If you have a holistic physician, ask for a prescription for nystatin and Diflucan® anti-fungals, (or see "http://www.vitality101.com/" www.vitality101.com, click on "treatment protocol" [bottom left link] and scroll to antifungals. Other natural alternatives are also listed).

7. Pay attention to adrenal stress support, as both elevated and low adrenal cortisol levels can cause weight gain. Start by making an attitude change. Whenever you notice that you're getting anxious or worried, ask yourself the simple question "Am I in imminent danger?" The answer is almost always no, and you'll find that your adrenal glands relax as you realize this. If you have problems with relaxing or letting go of worry, my new book *Three Steps to Happiness: Healing through Joy* can help you get from where you are to a life that you love. The book is available online at www.vitality101.com and also at www.Amazon.com. If you are experiencing hypoglycemic episodes, consider taking an adrenal glandular. I recommend Adrenal Stress End, 1 to 2 capsules each morning as needed.

It is no longer necessary to be on extreme, unsustainable or unhealthy diets to lose weight and keep it off. The recommendations above will not just help you stay trim, but they will leave you healthy and full of vitality as well.

## *What Role Do Medications Play in Weight Gain and Weight Loss?*

Many medications contribute to weight gain. Lithium®, for example, has been associated with average weight gains of 8 to 13 pounds. This is similar to the amount of weight gain associated with taking Depakote® (Valproic Acid). Anti-psychotic medications are also associated with gaining an average 4 to 9 pounds. In the treatment of pain, however, the biggest culprits for weight gain are tricyclic anti-depressants (such as Elavil®). Other anti-depressants such as those related to Prozac® can cause either weight gain or weight loss depending on the individual. Medications that increase norepinephrine such as Wellbutrin® and Effexor® are less likely to cause weight gain. In most studies, Lamictal® produced little or no weight gain.

Topamax® (topiramate) causes appetite suppression, with people on average losing 9 percent of their body weight. In studies, the average weight loss was 14 pounds; people who were taking high doses (138 mg per day) lost more weight than those using low doses (70 mg a day—no weight loss). The target dose for optimum weight loss is probably 150 to 250 mg per day. Starting at a low dose and gradually increasing tends to decrease side effects. Zonegran® (zonisamide), another anti-seizure/pain medication, is also associated with weight loss averaging approximately 20 pounds.

Other medications used in pain and fatigue treatment can also be helpful with weight loss. For example, many people with fatigue associated with pain benefit from the use of Dexedrine® (related to Ritalin). In addition, using Meridia® (Sibutramine) resulted in an average 16 pound weight loss over 1 year, with the weight staying off after the medication was stopped. The main side effects were dry mouth, constipation, sweating, and headache. Its mechanism is similar to the anti-depressant Effexor®. However, it may be more potent.

One of the nice side effects of treating pain, fibromyalgia, and chronic fatigue syndrome is that in addition to feeling great you can also look great. One patient that I recently treated had lost 50 pounds by her 4-month follow-up visit—in addition she had great energy and no pain. She was thrilled. It is time for you to also be treated properly so that you can get a life you love, look great, feel great, and be thrilled. I know this is possible. I had chronic fatigue syndrome and fibromyalgia, so I understand what you have been through. I have made it to the other side and feel fantastic. I have helped thousands of patients make the same journey to health, and taught hundreds of doctors to help tens of thousands more. It's time for you to make the journey back to health. ■

**Important Points**

1. The average weight gain in fibromyalgia/chronic pain is 32 pounds.
2. Several factors contribute to the weight gain. These include inadequate thyroid and adrenal function, poor sleep, yeast overgrowth, and sometimes decreased ability to exercise because of the pain.
3. Treating these problems can result in marked weight loss.

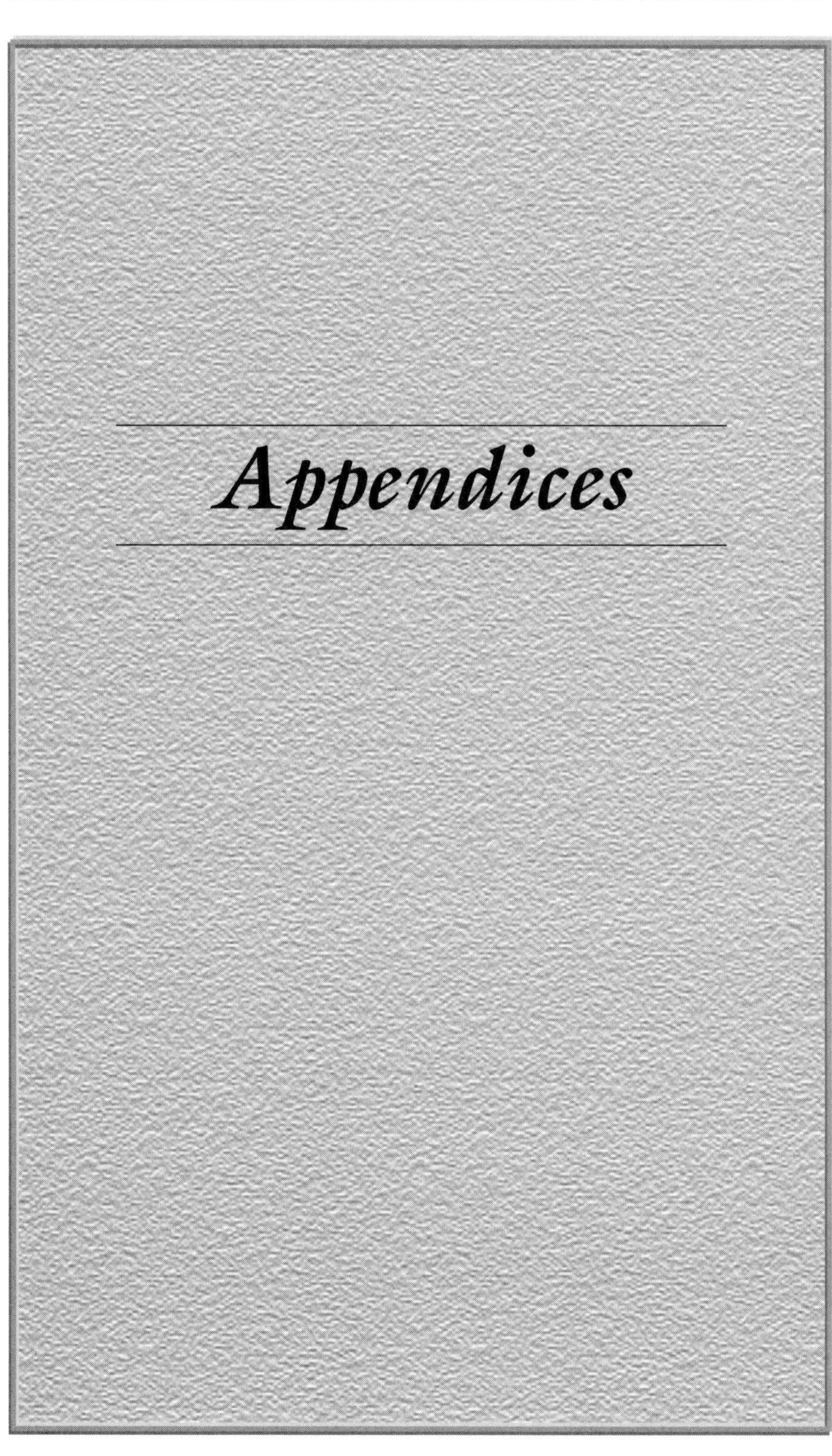

# Appendices

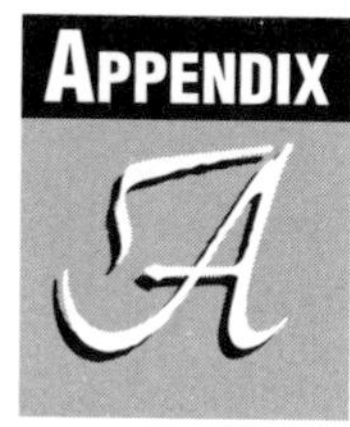

# Summary (like "Cliff Notes") and Flowcharts for Quickly Evaluating Your Pain and Determining How to Treat It

## Read Section 1 The Basics, then:

| Go to Section: | For information on: |
|---|---|
| 2 | Neuropathic pain characterized by pain that is burning, shooting (often to distant areas), or stabbing. It also has an "electric" quality to it. |
| 3 | Widespread achiness with insomnia (fibromyalgia) and/or muscle pain |
| 4 | Arthritis |
| 5 | Inflammatory pain—anything else that ends in the letters "itis" |
| 6 | Osteoporosis and bone pain/fractures |
| 7 | Cancer pain |
| 8 | Headaches |
| 9 | Back pain |
| 10 | Indigestion (heart burn/solar plexus pain) |
| 11 | Spastic colon |
| 12 | Non cardiac chest pain |
| 13 | Pelvic pain—menstrual, bladder, vulvar, and prostate |
| 14 | Wrist, Carpal tunnel syndrome, hand, shoulder, leg and foot pains |
| 15 | Natural therapies |
| 16 | Prescription therapies |
| 17 | Prolotheraphy |
| 18 | Sexual dysfunction, depression, and mind-body aspects of pain |
| 19 | Eliminating weight gain |

## Section 1 The Basics

Start with the basics. **Pain is often your body's way of saying it needs something**. Begin with three key areas for all types of pain (see Appendix C for information on these treatments/products):

1. **Nutrition**. Your body needs dozens of critical nutrients to heal and eliminate pain, and the American diet is awful. The easiest way to begin is:

   A. Use the Energy Revitalization System powder and B-Complex (see pages 9, 323).
   B. If inflammation is present, add Eskimo 3 Fish Oil (see pages 15, 326).
   C. If your mouth or lips are dry, you are dehydrated. Drink more good quality water (e.g. Dasani or use a multi-pure water filter. See pages 15, 322).
   D. Cut down on sugar, except for chocolate. (Russell Stover® makes excellent sugar free chocolates so you can have yummy treats and stay healthy.) Substitute stevia in place of sugar. (Use Body Ecology® or Stevita® brands—these taste great. Many others are bitter.) Saccharin® (the pink packet), Inositol®, and Xylitol® are also good sugar substitutes (see p 15).

   Beyond this, eat what makes you feel the best. Everyone is different, but foods that are high protein and low carbohydrate are most likely to help you feel the best.

2. **Sleep**. Can and do you sleep at least 8 hours a night? If you do, great! Deep sleep is the way your body heals the causes of pain. **Eight to nine hours of quality sleep a night is critical for pain to heal!** If you are not sleeping at least 8 to 9 hours a night, make the time. If you still can't get 8 hours sleep at night, here's what to do. Begin with natural remedies (unless you prefer to start with prescriptions because your insurance covers them). For natural sleep support, add remedies in the following order as needed:

   A. Use the Revitalizing Sleep Formula, 1 to 4 capsules either at bedtime or 30 to 90 minutes before bedtime if you have trouble falling asleep (see p 19).
   B. Take 5-HTP, 200 to 400 mg at bedtime (takes 6 to 12 weeks to work). Only take 200 mg if you are on anti-depressants (see p 19, 326).
   C. Add calcium, 500 to 600 mg at bedtime.
   D. Take Melatonin, ½ to 1 mg at bedtime.

If the natural therapies are not strong enough to get yo
plus hours at night, add the prescription sleep medicatio
They can be added in the following order as needed to g
8 hours a night without waking or hangover. See Appendix B: Pain Treatment Protocol for treatment directions. If you have phases where your sleep quality worsens, adjust the treatments as needed to get at least 8 hours sleep a night. Here's the order:

A. Ambien®
B. Klonopin®
C. Flexeril®
D. Soma®
E. Neurontin®
F. Zanaflex®
G. Gabatril®
H. Sonata®
I. Elavil® (or related Rx)
J. Desyrel®
K. See Appendix B: Pain Treatment Protocol for more options

3. Hormonal Support:

A. You may have suboptimal thyroid function or need thyroid support if you have: chronic fatigue, heavy periods, constipation, easy weight gain, cold intolerance, dry skin, thin hair, or a body temperature that tends to be on the low side of normal. If so, even if your blood tests are normal, ask your doctor to prescribe a low dose of thyroid hormone.
B. You may have suboptimal adrenal function or need more adrenal support if you have recurrent infections, "crashing" during stress, hypoglycemia (irritability when hungry), low blood pressure or dizziness upon first standing and/or an elevated Sedimentation Rate blood test. If so, consider Adrenal Stress End, 1 to 2 in the morning and perhaps 1 at lunch, and/or take Cortef®, 5to 20 mg per day.
C. If female, you may have suboptimal ovarian function and need more natural estrogen (not the dangerous kinds discussed in the media). If you have worsening of pain before your period or decreased vaginal lubrication, you may need more natural estrogen.
D. If your "free testosterone" blood test is in the lowest quarter of the normal range, consider treatment with natural testosterone. This applies to both males and females.

4. Treat the infections that can drive the pain.

If you have any of these:

A. Chronic sinusitis and nasal congestion
B. Spastic colon, gas, bloating, constipation, and/or diarrhea
C. A history of frequent antibiotic use
D. Recurrent or ongoing skin, nail, or vaginal fungal infections
E. Itchy ears or anus, recurrent aphthous ulcers (painful ulcers in the mouth where the lips meet your gums that last 5 to 10 days), sugar cravings, **and/or**
F. The presence of widespread achiness without inflammation (i.e. fibromyalgia/chronic fatigue syndrome)

Then:

Treat for yeast:

A. Use Acidophilus Pearls (see p 48), 2 pearls, twice a day for 5 months
B. Take Phytostan, 2 tablets twice a day and/or Citricidal®, 100 mg tablets, 2 times a day for 5 months
C. Avoid sweets (except for chocolate) and antibiotics
D. Take Nystatin®, 2, twice a day for 5 months and Diflucan®, 200 mg a day for 6 to 12 weeks
E. If symptoms recur months to years later, simply repeat the above for 6 weeks.

Other infections:

If you have bowel symptoms, check for parasites (at GSML labs, see p 322). Treat **any** parasites that are present.

If you have recurrent temperatures over 98.6 F; if you have lung congestion; if your pain or other chronic symptoms improved (even briefly) while you were taking antibiotics for something else; or if you have inflammatory arthritis, consider a 6 to 24 month treatment course of the antibiotics Cipro®, doxycycline, or Zithromax®.

If you have chronic nasal congestion or sinusitis, treat for yeast and use the prescription sinusitis nose spray from Cape Apothecary and the "silver" nose spray (see p 321).

Now go to the sections that apply to you.

## Section 2 Neuropathic Pain

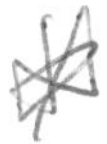

1. Neuropathies are characterized by pain that is burning, shooting (often to distant areas), or stabbing. It also has an "electric" quality about it. "Tingling or numbness" (paresthesias) and increased sensitivity, with normal touch being painful (allodynia), are also commonly seen.
2. Neuropathic pain can come from malfunction of nerves or the brain (e.g. diabetes, low thyroid, etc.), infections (e.g. shingles), pinched nerves, nutritional deficiencies (e.g. vitamins B6 and B12), injury (e.g. stroke, tumors, spinal cord injury, and multiple sclerosis), and medication/treatment side effects.
3. Do blood testing to check for diabetes, low thyroid, or vitamin B12 deficiency.
4. Nutritional support is critical! This can be done simply by taking the Energy Revitalization System vitamin powder/B complex plus lipoic acid, 300 mg, 3 times a day.

### *Types and Causes of Neuropathic Pain*

1. **Diabetic Nerve Pain**. Be sure to take the vitamin powder and B complex capsule because vitamins B6 and B12, as well inositol, can be very important for nutritional support. Take lipoic acid, 300 mg, 3 times a day. Then follow the directions below for nerve pain as needed.
2. Did the pain follow an attack of shingles/herpes zoster (a linear painful rash on one side of your body)?

   **If yes**, consider Postherpetic Neuralgia and treat with Lidoderm® patches and a gel containing a combination of Neurontin® and Ketamine®. If pain persists, take Neurontin® and Elavil® orally with the other medications below as needed.
3. **Nerve Compression**. This is often a muscular problem with the tight muscles pinching the nerves. See Chapter 9 for the treatment of muscle tightness. If the pain is from disc disease, Intravenous Colchicine, 1 mg once or twice weekly for a total of 6 to 8 doses will usually eliminate this pain.
4. Does your pain manifest as horribly severe pain in one hand or foot (often following trauma to that extremity or the associated hip/shoulder) so that you make sure no one touches it?

   **If yes**, consider Reflex Sympathetic Dystrophy (CRPS). Treat this with Neurontin® (at least 2400 mg daily), Elavil® (25 mg at bedtime), topical gels containing high levels of Ketamine®, and Lidoderm® patches. For refractory cases consider Intravenous Ketamine®.

5. Is the pain excruciating, consisting of attacks of pain in the lips, gums, cheek, or jaw, usually lasting no more than a few seconds or minutes? Do the painful attacks also recur frequently throughout the day and night for several weeks at a time (usually occurring in the middle-aged and elderly)?

   **If yes**, consider Trigeminal Neuralgia (tic douloureux). Begin treatment with Tegretol®, 100 mg a day (taken with food), and increasing slowly up to 200 mg 4 times a day as needed. This eliminates the pain in 75 percent of patients. Nutritional therapies can also be helpful and I recommend beginning with the vitamin powder and lipoic acid, 300 mg 3 times a day. Several studies have shown that giving niacin (nicotinic acid 100 to 200 mg IV daily for several days) and vitamin B1 intravenously can also help. The other treatments listed below can also be helpful. If these treatments fail, surgical options are available.

## *General Principles for Treating Neuropathies/Nerve Pain*

Many medications can be helpful for nerve pain. Allow them each 2 to 6 weeks to start working. If pain is severe, you may want to begin with Ultram® or narcotics immediately, as well as topical treatments, which will let you be more comfortable while waiting for these other therapies to work. For small areas, begin with the Lidocaine® patch (Lidoderm®). Up to 4 patches can be used at a time, and they can be left on for 12 to 18 hours a day (leave the patch off for at least 6 hours daily). You can add topical gels or use them instead of the patch. Consider putting the patch over the gels. It can take 2 weeks for these to work. For large areas, or if topical/local treatments are not effective, use the oral medications below. They can be tried in the order listed. Appendix B: Pain Treatment Protocol gives directions for using each medication. It may take 2 to 6 weeks to see the effect of a given treatment.

If pain is severe, you can try 2 medications at a time so that you can get relief more quickly. This is especially true if you're combining a topical and an oral medication. It may take a higher dose of medicine to eliminate nerve pain than for other types of pain. Side effects are less likely if you start with a lower dose and work your way up as is comfortable. If the first treatment for any given family (number) is helpful but poorly tolerated, try the next one in the same group. If the medication does not help significantly, skip down to the next numbered treatment (i.e. if medications for level 1A help but have too many side effects, try level 1B. If 1A simply does not help, go to treatment group 2).

## Treatment Order for Neuropathies

Begin with the vitamin powder and lipoic acid, 300 mg, 3 times a day. For localized areas add the Lidoderm® patch and pain gels (effects seen in 2 weeks). Begin all these simultaneously as well as:

1A. Neurontin®—may take 2400 to 3600 mg daily for nerve pain
1B. Gabatril®—average effective dose for nerve pain is 16 mg a day

2. Tricyclic anti-depressants, 10 to 50 mg at bedtime
2A. Elavil®
2B. Tofranil®
2C. Nortriptyline®
2D. Doxepin®

3A. Effexor®, 75 mg 3 times a day
3B. Paxil®, 20 to 80 mg per day

4. Ultram®, 50 mg, 1 to 2 tablets up to 4 times a day. Four tablets a day works very well. Above this dose sometimes causes nausea. It can start to work immediately.
5. Topamax® (Topiramate®), 200 to 300 mg a day. Side effects are less if you start with a low dose and work up.
6. Lamictal® (Lamotrigine®), 300 to 400 mg a day. Lower doses are less likely to be effective.
7. Zanaflex®, although more likely to be helpful for muscle pain at a dose of 4 to 8 mg daily, it can help nerve pain in doses of approximately 24 mg a day.
8. Keppra®, 1000 to 1500 mg, 2 times a day
9. Trileptal® (oxcarbazepine), usually requires approximately 150 to 300 mg twice daily
10. Dilantin®, 100 mg, 3 to 4 times day
11. Narcotics
12. Benadryl®, 25+ mg, 3 to 4 times a day

As you can see, there are many treatments that can eliminate nerve pain.

## Section 3 Fibromyalgia and Myofascial Pain Syndrome

See Section 1 The Basics.

1. Fibromyalgia and myofascial (muscle) pain syndrome are associated with shortened, tight muscles. In fibromyalgia, the pain is widespread, with pain being present in both the upper and lower and left and right portions of the body. It is also usually associated with fatigue and insomnia. Myofascial/muscle pain is more likely to be localized in one or two areas. In these situations, pain often comes from a structural problem (i.e. an uneven leg length or repetitive stress injuries). Pushing deeply on the area reproduces the pain.

2. To release the muscles and eliminate pain, four key areas need to be treated. These are sleep, hormonal support, nutritional support, and the treatment of underlying infections. For localized pain, structural or other triggers should also be looked for and eliminated. If you do this, you have a 91 percent chance of improving (see the study at www.vitality101.com).

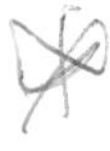

3. For nutritional support take the vitamin powder long-term. Add NAC, 500 to 650 mg, coenzyme Q10 (use the Vitaline® form) 200 mg, and acetyl l-carnitine 1000 mg a day for 3 to 4 months if you have fibromyalgia.

4. For sleep, take the Revitalizing Sleep Formula combined with medications, as needed, to get at least eight hours of sleep a night. Excellent medications for sleep include Ambien®, Klonopin®, Trazodone®, Soma®, Zanaflex®, doxepin, and Elavil®.

5. Most patients with fibromyalgia benefit from a trial of thyroid hormone. If you have low blood pressure, irritability that goes away with eating, crash with stress, or have an elevated sedimentation rate blood test, I recommend adrenal support with Adrenal Stress End and Cortef®.

6. Treat the underlying infections—especially yeast. If you have bowel symptoms or nasal congestion/sinusitis, yeast overgrowth is especially likely (although controversial). Treat yeast by avoiding sugar (except for chocolate), taking Acidophilus Pearls, Phytostan®, and Citricidal®. You can also take nystatin and Diflucan®. If you have a recurrent low-grade fever or lung congestion, consider the antibiotics doxycycline or Cipro®. If you have bowel symptoms, perform a stool test for parasites at the Great Smokey Mountain Labs.

7. For symptomatic relief while waiting for the underlying problems to be eliminated, a number of medications can be helpful. These do

**not** include Tylenol® (which can deplete a critical nutrient called glutathione) or NSAIDs (like Motrin®), which are only effective approximately 10 percent of the time. Instead, Celebrex® is much more likely to be helpful, even though it has similar mechanisms of action. Other medications that are very helpful include Ultram®, Skelaxin®, Neurontin®, Baclofen®, Zanaflex®, Permax®, and a not yet released medication called Pregabalin®.

## Section 4 Arthritis

1. Do not presume that joint pain is arthritis. Joint pain can also come from the muscles, tendons, and ligaments around the joint. This is so even if x-rays are abnormal.
2. The most common type of arthritis is osteoarthritis, known as "wear and tear arthritis." The joints mainly affected by osteoarthritis are the finger, knee, and hip joints. There may be joint deformities, but there should not be inflammation.
3. If inflammation is present, consider rheumatoid or infectious arthritis. In these situations, in addition to standard treatments, I recommend adding the antibiotic doxycycline, 100 mg twice daily, and an anti-inflammatory diet low in meat and high in fish oil. It is a good idea to take fish oil (1 to 2 Tbsp daily) as well. Many other nutrients are also critical, so be sure to take the vitamin powder.
4. If you have psoriasis or "pitting" in the fingernails, which looks like someone stuck a needle tip into several places in the nails (even without the skin changes/rash), your arthritis may be from the psoriasis.
5. If you have an elevated uric acid blood test and sudden pain and swelling in the joints (especially the big toe), consider gout. The NSAID medications plus colchicine can work well for the acute phase. Allopurinol® can be used to prevent further attacks. Your doctor is likely to be familiar with the treatment for gout.
6. I recommend you begin with a natural treatment program, which will decrease inflammation and help to repair the joints. This treatment has four main components:

   A. Repair. The joint cartilage can be repaired using a combination of glucosamine sulfate (most important, 500 mg 3 times a day for at least 6 weeks), MSM (3 to 6 grams a day), and Condroitin® (less important). It is also critical that you get the other nutrients present in the vitamin powder to promote wound healing. The powder naturally increases your SAMe levels. Increasing these levels has been shown to help arthritis. After 6 weeks, this combination decreases pain.

B. Use other anti-inflammatories to prevent damage and decrease or eliminate pain. I recommend a combination of several natural remedies, many of which can be found in combination. The mix I like the most combines boswellia, willow bark, and cherry (all present in the End Pain formula). It takes 6 weeks to see the full effect. Begin with 2 capsules 3 times a day for 2 to 6 weeks until your pain is controlled. You can then lower the dose.

C. Restore function with stretching, exercise, weight loss, and heat. Exercise at least twenty minutes a day. Swimming, walking, and yoga are good choices. Use a heating pad or moist heat for up to 20 minutes at a time to give relief.

D. Rule out and treat infections and food allergies that can aggravate arthritis. Most blood tests (except the ones from Elisa Act Technologies) are not reliable. NAET (see www.NAET.com) is a wonderful way to test for and eliminate food sensitivities. A related technique called JMT (see www.jmt-jafmeltechnique.com) is also an excellent way to treat rheumatoid and osteoarthritis naturally using energy medicine.

7. For symptomatic relief, prescription therapies, including NSAIDs such as Motrin®, COX 2 inhibitors like Celebrex®, Tylenol®, Lidoderm® patches and Ultram® can all be helpful.

## Section 5 Inflammatory Pain

1. Inflammation is a common cause of pain and many other medical problems that we experience in Western society. For example, anything that ends in the letters "itis" means that the problem is inflammatory. This includes things like arthritis, tendonitis, bursitis, spondylitis, appendicitis, etc.

2. Many inflammatory problems cause a secondary fibromyalgia, which may be causing most of the symptoms. If you have widespread pain, fatigue, and insomnia, look for and treat the associated fibromyalgia.

3. Much of our increased tendency to inflammation occurs because of the high amounts of animal fats relative to fish and vegetable oils in our diets. Increasing fish, nuts and seeds, berries, free range chicken and grass fed meats, spices and herbs, and green leafy vegetables (not potatoes and grains) can be a helpful start if you want to decrease inflammation.

4. For acute injury, remember the old standbys. These have the initials R.I.C.E., which stand for Rest, Ice, Compression, and Elevation.
5. In addition to dietary changes, natural remedies can be helpful in settling down inflammation. These include antioxidants, which are abundantly present in the vitamin powder. In addition, fish oil can be helpful. Begin with 1 to 2 Tbsp daily. You can then lower the dose to 1 tsp a day after 2 to 6 months as the inflammation settles. Many herbals such as willow bark, boswellia, and tart cherry are also excellent. These three herbals are all present in the End Pain formula – see Appendix C).
6. Anti-inflammatories like Motrin® and Celebrex® can be helpful but are more likely to cause side effects and long-term problems. Natural therapies are safer and more likely to help heal the body over time, while also decreasing pain.

## Section 6 Osteoporosis and Bone Pain/Fractures

1. Taking calcium plays only a modest role in improving bone strength. Take 1000 to 1500 mg per day (with evening meals or at bedtime, and not within 6 hours of taking thyroid hormone).
2. Also take the vitamin powder, which contains magnesium, boron, folic acid, copper, manganese, zinc, and vitamins B6, B12, D, and C, all of which are important in treating osteoporosis.
3. Take strontium, 680 mg per day as well. This nutrient can markedly increase bone density by 4 to 7 percent a year safely and inexpensively. It can also help osteoarthritis. Take it on an empty stomach in the morning at a different time than the calcium.
4. DHEA, testosterone, and estrogen replacement (use the safer, natural forms—the problems reported on in the media are predominantly with synthetic forms) can also help.
5. Fosamax® (Rx), 70 mg once a week can also help.

## Section 7 Cancer Pain

1. It is unacceptable for cancer patients to be in pain, and the treatments discussed in this book can also be helpful in eliminating cancer pain. Most pain is coming from tissue/nerve invasion or muscle spasm. Treat these pains as discussed elsewhere in the book (see Chapter 22 on prescription therapies).

2. It takes much less medication to prevent pain than to make it go away once it occurs. Because of this, if you have chronic pain, take the medication before you expect the pain to hit (or at first sign of it coming back) instead of waiting for it to be severe. You'll need less pain medicine and have fewer side effects.
3. I recommend that any patient with a significant cancer order a search of medical studies done on their specific type and stage of cancer from Health Resources (Call Jan Guthrie at 800-949-0090 for more information). I have seen "incurable cancers" go away when the patient combines the best of standard and complementary therapies.
4. For uncontrollable nausea, use ABHR cream (applied to an area of soft skin, such as the wrist). This prescription cream can be made by compounding pharmacists, who can also guide you in its proper use. It contains lorazepam, Benadryl®, Haldol®, and metoclopramide.
5. Treatments that improve bone density (see osteoporosis above) may decrease bone pain as well.

## Section 8 Headaches

1. Tension Headaches cause moderate pain on both sides of and across the forehead, tend to both start and fade away gradually, and are the result of muscle tightness in the sterno-cleidomastoid muscles of the neck. If the pain is coming from the suboccipital muscles at the base of the skull, the pain is often behind the eyes and/or on top of the head.
2. Because tension headaches are muscular, the same treatments discussed in Chapter 9 that cause your muscles to relax will often eliminate the recurrence of these headaches. Paying attention to structural factors can also help.
3. Many medications can be used to prevent chronic tension headaches. These include anti-depressants such as Remeron®, 15 to 30 mg, or Elavil®, 10 to 50 mg at bedtime.
4. To treat the acute pain of headaches, begin with herbal remedies such as the End Pain formula, which contains willow bark, boswellia, and cherry. This can be helpful for acute attacks, but it takes 2 to 6 weeks to **fully** kick in. A physical therapy technique called stretch and spray, which approximately 10 percent of physical therapists are familiar with, is also an excellent and pain-free way to

release your muscles and eliminate a tension headache. In addition, there are the old standbys of Tylenol® and Motrin®/Advil®. Other medications that can be quite helpful include Midrin® and Ultram®. I would begin with the natural therapies first, however, as I think these are both more effective and safer.

## *Migraine Headaches*

1. These headaches can be very severe and usually last for several days. Migraines are often preceded by an "aura," which may consist of visual disturbances such as flashing lights. And the headaches are often associated with nausea, sweats, dizziness, and light and sound sensitivity.
2. In the U. S., medications in the Imitrex® family still remain the first choice for the treatment of acute migraines. A combination of indomethacin (a "super-aspirin"), prochlorperazine (for nausea and to enhance absorption), and caffeine in suppository form is commonly used in Italy (it can be made up by compounding pharmacies). Midrin®, which is a mix of three medications, can also be effective. Take two capsules immediately followed by 1 capsule every hour until the headache is relieved (to a maximum of 5 capsules within a 12 hour period).
3. A fascinating study can guide you on when to use Imitrex® family medications vs. when to go with other therapies. Seventy-five percent of migraine patients get painful sensitivity to normal touch (e.g. from eyeglasses) around their eyes. Studies showed that when participants used Imitrex before the tenderness/pain around the eyes began, it knocked out the migraine 93 percent of the time. If the pain/tenderness around the eyes had already set in, Imitrex only eliminated the migraine 13 percent of the time, although it still helped the throbbing. In other words, if you are one of the lucky ones who does not get pain around the eyes, the Imitrex can knock out your migraine at any time. If you are one of those who do get pain/tenderness around the eyes, it is a race against the clock to take the Imitrex before the pain starts. This means take the Imitrex early in the attack (the first 5 to 20 minutes) before the skin hypersensitivity gets established. For example, use it at the earliest warning signs, like painful scalp or discomfort from your wearing glasses or earrings or from shaving. If pain has already fully set in before you take the Imitrex, consider using one of the other treatments.

4. Anti-nausea medications can also be helpful. Phenergan® or Compazine® suppositories can be helpful. Another excellent anti-nausea alternative is ABHR cream, which is applied to an area of soft skin, such as the wrist. This prescription cream can be made by compounding pharmacists, who can also guide you in its proper use. It contains lorazepam, Benadryl®, Haldol®, and metoclopramide.
5. Butterbur is an herb that can both prevent and eliminate migraines. Take 50 mg 3 times a day for 1 month and then 1 50 mg dose twice a day to prevent migraines. You can take 100 mg every 3 hours to eliminate an acute migraine. In the hospital emergency room or doctor's office, intravenous magnesium can very effectively and quickly eliminate an acute migraine.
6. For patients with severe migraines who often need to go to the hospital emergency room, and if the above treatments are not adequate, it is helpful to have a "rescue medication" that can be used at home. ACTIQ (fentanyl lollipops) can be used at home and are as effective as intravenous morphine. The average dose needed is 800 mcg (see page 126).

## *Migraine Prevention*

1. Natural therapies can prevent many, if not most, migraines. I would begin by taking the Energy Revitalization System vitamin powder plus 300 mg of Vitamin B2 in the morning, plus 200 mg of magnesium at night. If the cost is not prohibitive, add butterbur, 75 mg 2 times day (you can use 100 mg once a day but it is not as effective). Natural approaches can help eliminate even frequent and horribly severe migraine problems, but remember that it usually takes 2 to 3 months to see the effect. So give them time to work.
2. Avoiding hidden food allergies can reduce or eliminate migraines in as many as 85 percent of patients. The most common reactive foods are: wheat in 78 percent of patients; oranges in 65 percent; eggs in 45 percent; tea and coffee in 40 percent each; chocolate and milk in 37 percent each; beef in 35 percent; and corn, cane sugar, and yeast in 33 percent each. Clinical experience also suggests that the artificial sweetener aspartame (NutraSweet®) can trigger migraines and other headaches, although this is controversial. You may find that instead of avoiding foods that trigger your migraines for the rest of your life, you can eliminate the sensitivities/allergies using a powerfully effective acupressure technique called NAET (see www.NAET.com).

3. If the migraines are predominately around your periods or associated with taking estrogen, see page 129.
4. Prescription therapies for prevention can reduce the number of headache days per month by an average of 50 percent. These include Neurontin®, beta-blockers (Inderal®—avoid this if you have asthma or fatigue), calcium channel blockers, Depakote®, Topamax®, Elavil®, and Doxepin®.

## *Other Headaches*

1. Sinusitis is another common cause of headaches. It is usually associated with pain and tenderness over the sinuses, by the cheeks, or above the eyes. Nasal congestion, often with yellow/green nasal mucus, is also common. Interestingly, we have found that most cases of chronic sinusitis are caused by fungal overgrowth in your body, especially your bowels, which can then cause gas, bloating, diarrhea, or constipation. Chronic sinusitis routinely resolves when we treat it with Diflucan® and the other yeast/anti-fungal therapies. It is also helpful to use a special prescription nose spray that contains anti-bacterials and anti-fungals. Your doctor can order it by calling Cape Apothecary at 410-757-3522. Use 1 to 2 sprays in each nostril twice a day. Silver spray taken with it can also be effective. (see page 321)
2. Caffeine withdrawal headaches are common in people who drink a lot of coffee. It is especially common in the morning before people get their coffee "fix" and often occurs approximately 18 hours after the last cup of coffee. Weaning off excess caffeine is the solution.
3. Cluster headaches occur as a repeating series of headaches that can each last 30 to 90 minutes and are very severe. They cause excruciating, piercing pain on one side of the head (often centered around one eye) and are much more common in men. Many medications can help. These include anti-seizure medications like Valproic Acid, 500 to 1000 mg a day, or Topamax®, 50 to 100 mg a day. These often start to work in 1 to 2 weeks.
4. Trigeminal Neuralgia is characterized by excruciating attacks of stabbing, shooting pain in the lips, gums, cheek, or chin that last for a few seconds to minutes. It occurs almost exclusively in the middle-aged and elderly. It often responds well to treatment with the medications Tegretol® and/or Neurontin®.
5. Temporo Mandibular (Jaw) Joint Dysfunction (TMJ/TMD) is a common cause of facial pain and headaches. Although classically

considered to come from the jaw joint (the area just in front of your ears), in many cases the pain is actually coming from tightness of the Masseter muscles. Following the principles discussed above for myofascial/muscle pain (and information in Chapter 13) will often make this pain go away.

## Section 9 Back Pain

1. By eliminating the tissue swelling using intravenous colchicine, disc pain can be eliminated approximately 70 percent of the time without surgery. Sciatica, or back pain in which the pain goes down the leg, is often a form of disc disease.
2. Sleep on a medium firm mattress instead of a firm mattress.
3. Add glucosamine sulfate, 1500 mg a day and Chondroitin® sulfate, 2500 mg per day. Give it a 6 to 12 week trial.
4. Lamictal® and/or Lidoderm® patches can also be helpful in reducing back pain.
5. Most other back pain, unless it is coming from your chest or abdominal organs (which is rare and usually can be found by your internist) is muscular, arthritic, or from ligaments. Using the treatments in Chapters 9 and 10 on myofascial pain and arthritis, and also taking care of any underlying structural/ergonomic problems, can routinely eliminate this pain. In addition, chiropractic (see Chapter 21), Prolotherapy (see Chapter 23) and mind-body approaches developed by Dr. Sarno (see Chapter 24) can also be helpful, as can many forms of body work.

## Section 10 Indigestion and Digestive Enzymes

1. Indigestion is usually not caused by excess stomach acid. Due to poor digestion or stomach infections, any stomach acid can hurt. Although it helps you feel better in the short-term, turning off stomach acid long-term can markedly worsen digestion and overall health. Food processing (used to prolong grocery store shelf life) destroys the digestive enzymes present in food. This contributes dramatically to indigestion. Coffee, alcohol, and aspirin/Motrin® products can also cause indigestion and ulcers.

2. To get off of acid blocker medications comfortably do the ing for 4 to 8 weeks:

   A. Use plant-based digestive enzymes (e.g. Complete Gest by Enzymatic Therapy). Taking 2 capsules with each meal will help you digest your food properly. In addition, drink warm liquids with meals, because cold liquids inactivate your digestive enzymes. If the enzymes are irritating to the stomach, switch to a brand called GS Similase until your stomach feels better.
   B. Take mastic gum (any brand), 1000 mg twice a day for 2 months, then as needed.
   C. Take DGL Licorice, 380 mg (not the sugar-free type) from Enzymatic Therapy or Rhizinate from PhytoPharmica. Chew 2 tablets 20 minutes before meals.
   D. Take Heartburn Free. After your stomach is feeling better, take 1 capsule every other day for 20 days. It may initially aggravate reflux, but 10 capsules can give long term-relief by eliminating the stomach infection.
   E. In 4 to 8 weeks, when your stomach is better, you can wean off the antacids (with your doctor's OK).

## Section 11 Spastic Colon

1. The most effective way to eliminate spastic colon is to treat the underlying cause, which is usually infection. In my experience most patients' spastic colon resolves when underlying bowel infections are treated. What is most important is to treat the Candida/fungal overgrowth in the gut (see Chapter 16 for recommended treatment). In addition, many patients have parasitic infections. Unfortunately, many, if not most, labs are clueless about how to do a proper stool parasite exam and will miss the vast majority of these infections. Because of this, I would do the parasitology testing by mail at the Great Smokey Mountain Labs or the Parasitology Center (see Appendic C: Resources). In addition, I recommend a stool test for Clostridium Difficile. This is a toxin-producing bacteria and testing for it can be done at any laboratory.

2. For symptomatic relief while treating the underlying problems, consider taking peppermint oil. This must be in an enteric-coated capsule, or it could be quite irritating. Take 1 to 2 capsules 3 times a day between meals (**not with food**) for spastic colon.

3. Prescription medications that can be helpful include antispasmodics such as Hyoscyamine®, and Valium® family medications

such as Librax®. These can be used on an "as needed" basis. If constipation is a predominant symptom, adding fiber and water plus the magnesium contained in the vitamin powder can be helpful. If these are not adequate, you can take the prescription Miralax®. In addition, you can add Zelnorm®, 6 mg twice a day for both constipation and pain.

## Section 12 Non Cardiac Chest Pain

1. Once your doctor has ruled out heart or lung problems as a source of your chest pain, it most often turns out to be muscle/cartilage pain (Costochondritis) or indigestion/acid reflux.

2. Costochondritis pain tends to be aggravated by movement, deep breathing, or position change. It tends to be sharp, nagging, aching, or pressure-like, and it is usually well-localized, although the pain may radiate. It is usually along the sides of the sternum (the chest bone in the center of the chest), 2 inches below the left nipple, or in the Pectoral muscles in the upper chest. Reproducing the chest pain by pushing on the area suggests that the pain is coming from the muscles or ligaments of the chest wall. Hot compresses and relaxing the muscles with your mind can be helpful, as can the rest of the treatments for muscle pain. For severe cases, Lidocaine® patches can be helpful, as well as the pain creams recommended earlier for muscle pain.

3. If the pain is in your solar plexus and mid-chest and relieved by taking a few ounces of Maalox® or Mylanta® or other antacids, or is affected by eating, it is likely indigestion. See Chapter 15 for information on treating indigestion.

4. The most worrisome causes of chest pain, are, of course, angina and heart attacks. These pains are usually associated with tightness and pain that radiates down the left arm, shortness of breath, and sweats, and is made worse with walking or exercise. Everyone is different, however, and sometimes these pains can be atypical. It is always best be on the safe side and have a family doctor check out the source of the pain to be sure it is not coming from something dangerous.

## Section 13 Pelvic Pain

1. For menstrual pain, begin with over-the-counter Advil® or Aleve®. For severe menstrual cramps, the prescription Bextra®, 20 mg twice a day can be even more effective.

2. Interstitial Cystitis(IC) is a bladder problem characterized by **severe** urinary urgency, frequency, burning, and pain. Once bacterial infections have been ruled out, I prescribe Elavil®, 25 mg at bedtime plus Neurontin®, 300 to 900 mg at bedtime and perhaps during the day as well. If these are ineffective after 6 weeks, a trial of Sinequan® and the other anti-seizure medications is worthwhile. The medication pyridium, which numbs the bladder (and turns the urine and sweat light orange) and Urispaz®, an anti-spasmodic, can be helpful as well. I also treat the patient for presumptive Candida with oral Diflucan® for 3 months.

3. It is important to avoid certain foods that aggravate symptoms and to recognize that any vitamins, especially the B vitamins and any nutrients that are acidic (including the vitamin powder), can dramatically irritate the bladder in some patients with IC.

4. Conversely, some practitioners have found that patients with interstitial cystitis often have chronic alkaline urine. This can be aggravated by excessive coffee and cola intake. pH strip paper can be obtained cheaply at most pharmacies and one can test multiple urine samples at home to see if the pH is regularly over 7.0. Also take the enzyme product URT (enzyme product No. 24), 4 capsules 5 times a day between meals. During flares, add the enzyme product called "Kidney," 2 capsules every 20 minutes as needed. In 2 to 4 weeks the symptoms may subside and the products can then be taken as needed (products are available by phoning 410-573-5389).

5. If the above products do not work, try Elmiron®, a 100 mg capsule 3 times a day with water at least 1 hour before, or 2 hours after, eating. In addition, consider adding MSM (Methyl Sulfonyl Methane) at a dose of 6 to 18 grams a day, L-Arginine®, 500 mg 3 times day, and the herbal "saw palmetto," 160 mg twice a day. These may all take 3 months to work.

6. Vulvodynia is defined as chronic vulvar itching, burning, and/or pain that is significantly uncomfortable. In this condition, vulvar/vaginal pain can either occur only during intercourse, or be constantly present. I put almost all women with pelvic pain on tricyclics

such as Elavil® or nortriptyline combined with Neurontin®. In my experience, vulvodynia seems to occur as 3 main types:

A. Neuropathic—this pain appears to be caused by nerve irritation and is sharp, burning, and/or shooting (like nerve pain). In this case, apply the treatment principles in Chapter 8 on neuropathic pain. Begin with tricyclic anti-depressants (nortriptyline, desipramine, imipramine, doxepin, or Elavil®) at 25 to 150 mg each night and/or Neurontin®, 100 mg to 3600 mg daily, and proceed from there.
B. Inflammatory—this pain type is associated with local inflammation/irritation. In this situation, I would avoid topical creams. I routinely give at least a 3 month trial of oral Diflucan®, 200 mg a day.
C. Muscle pain—if the pain is deep seated and not triggered by touching the outer vagina, it may be coming from spasm of the deep pelvic muscles. In this situation, the pain may occur or be accentuated during the deep thrusting of intercourse. For this pain, the general principles for treating muscle pain apply.

7. Prostate pain—this pain is fairly common in men. When no infection is found, it is called prostadynia. I suspect that prostadynia often occurs because of subtle infections, and it usually improves when I treat these. Interestingly, the bioflavonoid vitamin Quercetin, 500 mg twice a day, decreases prostate symptoms in both prostadynia and prostatitis.

8. Endometriosis—if you have pelvic and/or abdominal pain that is much worse around your periods (and not simply muscle cramps), consider endometriosis. See the book *Endometriosis* by Mary Lou Ballweg and the Endometriosis Association for more information.

## Section 14 Wrist, Hand, Shoulder, Leg, and Foot Pains

1. Carpal tunnel syndrome is characterized by pain, numbness, and tingling that occurs in one or both hands. It often wakes people from their sleep, leaving them feeling like they have to "shake their hands out" to make the pain and symptoms go away. In almost all of my patients, their carpal tunnel syndromes have resolved by using vitamin B6 (250 mg daily), Armour Thyroid hormone (see Appendix B: Pain Treatment Protocol for information on how to adjust the dose) and a "cock up" wrist splint at night for 6 weeks.

2. Thumb tendonitis is characterized by pain along the side of the hand going from the thumb joint towards the wrist. The pain gels/creams can work very well for this. Give them several weeks to work.

3. If you get a shoulder injury or pain, be sure to maintain range of motion to prevent frozen shoulder.

4. Nighttime leg cramps—Take magnesium, 150 to 250 mg, and calcium, 500 to 1000 mg, at bedtime and increase the potassium in your diet (e.g. bananas, V8®, or tomato juice). Stretch your calf muscles before you go to sleep. This can be done by pulling your toes towards you when you're sitting on your bed. Wearing socks at night can also help, since cold feet will sometimes be a trigger. Quinine can be helpful for nighttime leg cramps as well.

## Section 15 Natural Therapies

1. Natural remedies can be very powerful tools. Unfortunately, most medical doctors have a strong bias against natural remedies due to a lack of awareness of the scientific data.

2. Many natural therapies can be very helpful for pain. My three favorite pain relieving herbals are willow bark, boswellia, and tart cherry. All three can be found in combination in the End Pain formula by Integrative Therapeutics. Begin with 2 tablets 2 to 3 times a day, as needed, until maximum benefit is achieved (approximately 4 to 6 weeks) and then you can use the lowest effective dose.

3. Take the vitamin powder, which has many nutrients that help pain, and add sleep herbals if needed for 8 hours sleep a night (see Section 1 The Basics above). The sleep herbals in the Revitalizing Sleep Formula decrease pain as well.

4. If you have arthritis, or back pain from arthritis of the spine bones (vertebrae), take Glucosamine Sulfate (500 mg 3 times a day—takes 6 weeks to work), and consider MSM (3 grams a day for 2 to 5 months).

5. If you have nerve pain, take lipoic acid, 200 to 300 mg, 3 times a day (takes weeks to months to help).

6. Joint Gel® by NF Formulas is an over-the-counter, natural pain reliever that is applied directly on the skin. Joint Gel contains many different natural products that provide relief from aches and pains. It can be used for pain of backaches, muscle sprains, and strains.

Massage Joint Gel into your skin over the painful area until it is absorbed. You can use Joint Gel every day as needed, up to 3 to 4 times daily.

7. Digestive enzymes can actually digest away inflammation. Ultrazyme and MegaZyme can be helpful in aiding **digestion of your food** when taken **with** meals. I recommend that you take them **on an empty stomach**, however, because enzymes are most effective at reducing pain and inflammation when you take them between meals. For acute pain, enzymes can be taken for a few days as needed. For chronic pain, begin by taking either of the above regularly (2 to 3 tablets, 3 times a day) between meals for 6 to 12 weeks to see how much it helps, or until the pain and inflammation are gone. Then you can take the enzymes as needed.

8. A major problem in chronic pain is that the areas that hurt often have decreased blood flow. This is one reason why using the intravenous "Myers Cocktails" nutritional therapies can be so effective. A less expensive way to get the blood vessels to open wide is to take a B vitamin called niacin (**not** niacinamide, which does not cause flushing). Take 100 to 500 mg of niacin 3 to 4 times a day as needed to cause a "flushing" feeling, which will occur within approximately 10 to 20 minutes. This can significantly help pain and is inexpensive. Try to keep the dose at 1000 mg a day or less, if this is enough to cause flushing, because higher doses can sometimes (but rarely) cause liver inflammation or unmask diabetes. The flushing may be intense. Do not worry—it is not dangerous and it can help your muscles to heal while decreasing pain. It also lowers cholesterol levels at doses at or over 1000 mg per day.

9. Treat food allergies and sensitivities. As discussed earlier, the best approach I have found for the elimination of food and other sensitivities/allergies is a technique called NAET (see www.NAET.com).

10. Homeopathics can be helpful (see discussion in Chapter 20).

11. Consider home remedies like "Purple Pectin for Pain" (especially arthritis): Purchase Certo® in the canning section of your local grocery. It is the thickening agent used to make jams and jellies. Certo contains pectin, a natural ingredient found in the cell walls of plants. Use 1 to 3 Tbsp of Certo in 8 ounces of grape juice 1 to 2 times daily. If it's going to help, you'll likely know in 7 to 14 days. You can lower the dose as you feel better.

12. Consider hypnosis and/or magnets. Acupuncture and structural therapies such as chiropractic, osteopathy, and numerous types of body work can also be powerfully effective.

## Section 16 Prescription Therapies

1. The use of topical delivery systems for pain medications is a major leap forward in pain management. It allows high doses of multiple medications to get right to your area of pain—usually with no side effects!
2. Begin by going after the perpetuating factors (i.e. nutritional, hormonal, sleep deficiencies, and underlying infections discussed above in Section 1 The Basics), followed by adding in natural remedies. Then use the prescription pain creams. The oral followed by IV medications below can (and should) be added if needed because it is unhealthy to be in pain. On the other hand, it is also reasonable to begin immediately with prescription pain medications like Ultram®, and sometimes even narcotics, for immediate pain relief while you're waiting for the other treatments to take effect.
3. Give the creams at least 1 to 2 weeks to work, and be willing to continue adjusting the mix until you find what works. This is a list of just some of the medications that can be added to the creams: Ketoprofen®, piroxicam, diclofenac, or ibuprofen (these four are NSAID anti-inflammatories); Neurontin®, clonidine, amitriptyline, Cyclobenzaprine®, Baclofen®, Ketamine®, Lidocaine®, guaifenesin, capsaicin, cortisone, and/or Sarapin®.
4. Because your physician may not be familiar with compounded pain creams, the pharmacist at Cape Apothecary (phone 410-757-3522) can help guide your doctor and can mail you the cream if prescribed.
5. The chapters in which we discussed the different kinds of pain (e.g. neuropathic, muscular, arthritic, etc.) and the summary sections on these chapters (see above) give the order in which to try the medications for pain. If you are not clear on the source/type of your pain, there are many orders, or sequences, in which to try the medications. One order I recommend is listed below. When there are several medications on the same line, if the first medication helped but was not tolerated because of side effects, go to the next medication on the same line. If it did not help significantly, go to the next line. If you get partial benefit from a medication, continue it and

add the next medication, as needed, to get pain free.
Here is the order:

A. Lidocaine® patches or gels for localized area of pain
B. Tylenol®
C. Motrin®, Voltaren®, or Daypro® (your insurance company prefers that these be tried before Celebrex® because of cost)
D. Celebrex®
E. Skelaxin® (for muscle pain/achiness
F. Ultram®
G. Neurontin®, Gabitril®, and/or Pregabalin®
H. Flexeril® (for muscle pain/achiness)
I. Elavil®, Doxepin®, Desipramine® (norpramin), or nortriptyline (Pamelor®)
J. Zanaflex®
K. Effexor
L. Baclofen® (for muscle pain/achiness)
M. Klonopin® (for muscle pain/achiness)
N. Topamax
O. Lamictal®
P. Keppra®
Q. Narcotics®
R. Benadryl®

Appendix B: Pain Treatment Protocol gives the directions on how to use each of these medications. Other medications are also discussed in Appendix B.

6. For refractory pain consider IV nutrients (see Appendix F: Myers Cocktails), IV Lidocaine®, Ketamine®, or Prolotherapy.

## Section 17 Prolotherapy

1. Prolotherapy is a series of injections of a natural solution (something as simple as a sugar or salt solution, cod liver oil (known as sodium morrhuate), or herbal extract) into the area where the ligaments have either been weakened or damaged through injury or strain. This stimulates proliferation of **normal** tissue, which helps the body to repair painful areas.

2. Its effectiveness for pain is wide-ranging and includes pain associated with the back, the neck, all joints throughout the body, arthritis, migraine headaches, fibromyalgia, sciatica, herniated discs, and Temporo Mandibular Joint Dysfunction (TMJ).

3. Chronic musculoskeletal pain is often due to weakness of ligaments and tendons. The injection is given at the point where the ligament or tendon connects to the bone. Many points may require injection. The injection causes the body to heal itself through the process of controlled inflammation and production of growth factors.

## Section 18 Sexual Dysfunction, Depression, Mind-Body Aspects of Pain

1. Sexual dysfunction and loss of libido is common in chronic pain. Pain can cause a low testosterone level, as can treatment with codeine/narcotics. Check a free testosterone level and take natural testosterone supplements if the level is in the lowest 25$^{th}$ percentile of the normal range. For men, use Androgel®, 25 to 50 mg, 1 to 2 times a day rubbed onto your skin. For women, 2 to 6 mg a day of natural testosterone is usually adequate and can help pain, as well as loss of libido. Keep the free testosterone blood test in the upper 30$^{th}$ percentile of the normal range (lower if you get acne).

2. Depression is also common in chronic pain, and it is important to be able to talk about your feelings with your doctor and family. Usually, depression can be reversed naturally by taking the vitamin powder, taking fish oil (1 Tbsp daily), getting exercise (if able), taking the herb St. John's Wort (1000 to 2000 mg a day of a standardized product), taking 5-HTP (200 to 400 mg a day (use the lower dose if on anti-depressants), and natural hormones including Armour Thyroid and testosterone as needed. If depression persists, use anti-depressants, which can also decrease pain. The mineral Rubidium, 500 mg daily with food, can help even resistant depression. It takes 1 month to work and is available from compounding pharmacies without a prescription.

3. Anti-depressants can also cause sexual dysfunction. The herb ginkgo biloba, 120 mg twice a day can often reverse this after 6 weeks.

4. Work by Dr. John Sarno, M.D., has shown that emotional stress can also contribute to pain. He found that the mind often decreases the blood flow to areas of the body because of repressed anger/rage and/or an attempt to distract us from uncomfortable emotions by causing pain. To overcome this, learn to "feel" and express your feelings. In addition, when you feel pain, tell your mind that you will repeatedly use the pain as a signal to look for and feel those uncomfortable emotions for 10 to 15 minutes—then do so. The pain will often leave within 6 weeks.

5. Read my book *Three Steps to Happiness: Healing through Joy!* It will help you get from where you are to feeling great in 144 pages.
6. By treating the things that your pain is pointing out, the pain signal decreases and often stops. In addition, the filtering system of your mind now knows that it is okay to ignore any residual pain signal.

## Section 19 Eliminating the Weight Gain

1. The average weight gain in fibromyalgia/chronic pain is 32 pounds.
2. Several factors contribute to the weight gain. These include inadequate thyroid and adrenal function, poor sleep, yeast overgrowth, and sometimes decreased ability to exercise because of the pain.
3. Treating these problems can result in marked weight loss. See Section 1 The Basics, for details on how to do this. ■

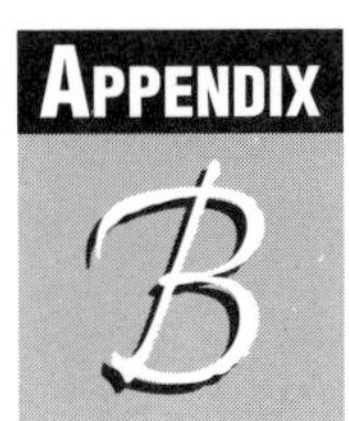

# Pain Treatment Protocol

*(Supplies can be ordered by phoning 800-333-5287 or online at www.endfatigue.com)*

Below is a form that lists the more common treatments that can be helpful with pain and associated problems. It will give you and your doctor treatment options and directions on how to use the recommended treatments. If you would like a more comprehensive and frequently updated form with over 280 treatment options, see my website at www.endfatigue.com.

I recommend you use this form as a record of your treatments and have it with you for your doctor visits. Occasionally you may see "___" for your doctor to fill in a dose. Here are some points on how to use the form most effectively:

- Write the date started in front of a treatment.
- Draw a line through the number in front of any treatment you stop and note the reason stopped and the date. Although it can take 6 weeks to see a treatment's benefits, most medications' side effects will usually occur within the first few days of starting a treatment.

Also, note these important points about the treatments listed on the form:

- Do not take any treatments that you are allergic to or that have caused prohibitive side effects.
- Do not get pregnant during treatment or drive if sedated. It is normal for a woman's periods to be irregular during the first 3 to 4 months of treatment.
- If a recommended (i.e. checked-off by your health practitioner) treatment has a double asterisk ** by its number, it is a **most important** treatment. If it has a single *, it is an **important** treatment, and no * means the treatment is **helpful** but not critical. If you choose to simplify your program, you can begin treatment with the

double asterisk items followed by the single asterisk items, and then the no asterisk items.

- Except for treatments #1 through 14, which can all be started in the first 1 to 3 days, add in 1 new treatment each 1 to 3 days. If a side effect occurs, stop the treatments begun in the previous week for a few days and see if it goes away. If the side effect is acute or worrisome, call your family doctor (or go to the hospital emergency room) immediately.
- On average, it takes 3 months to start resolving the underlying causes of your pain. You can begin to slowly taper off most treatments when you feel well for 6 months. Stop treatments one at a time and do so gradually (e.g. one pill every 1 to 2 weeks) so you can see if you still need a specific treatment. If needed, however, most of these treatments can be used for a lifetime (usually **not** necessary).
- Prescription items have an "Rx" after their names. Some prescriptions can be obtained at a much lower cost from Consumers Discount Drug Company (phone 323-461-3606). For example, 90 Sporanox tablets (100mg) generally cost $820.00 at a local food chain pharmacy as compared to $600.00 at Consumers Discount Drug. Another good source to see what you should be paying for generic prescription drugs is www.costco.com (click on pharmacy).
- I have listed natural/over-the-counter alternatives for most prescription therapies that can be substituted for and/or added to the prescription items. I often recommend products made by Enzymatic Therapies or Integrative Therapeutics as these have proven potency and purity. I do not accept money from any company whose products I recommend. I direct that all royalties for products I make be donated to charity.

## Nutritional Treatments

___ 1.** **Energy Revitalization System** (for powerful, overall nutritional support)—take ½ to 1 scoop of the powder a day (as feels best) blended with milk, juice, water, or yogurt with 1 capsule of the included Daily Energy B-Complex (also available separately). If uncomfortable gas or diarrhea occurs, mix the powder with milk and/or start with a lower dose and work your way up to the dose that feels best, or divide the daily dose into smaller doses and take twice a day. These products are available on line at www.endfatigue.com and at most health food stores. One scoop contains over 35 tablets

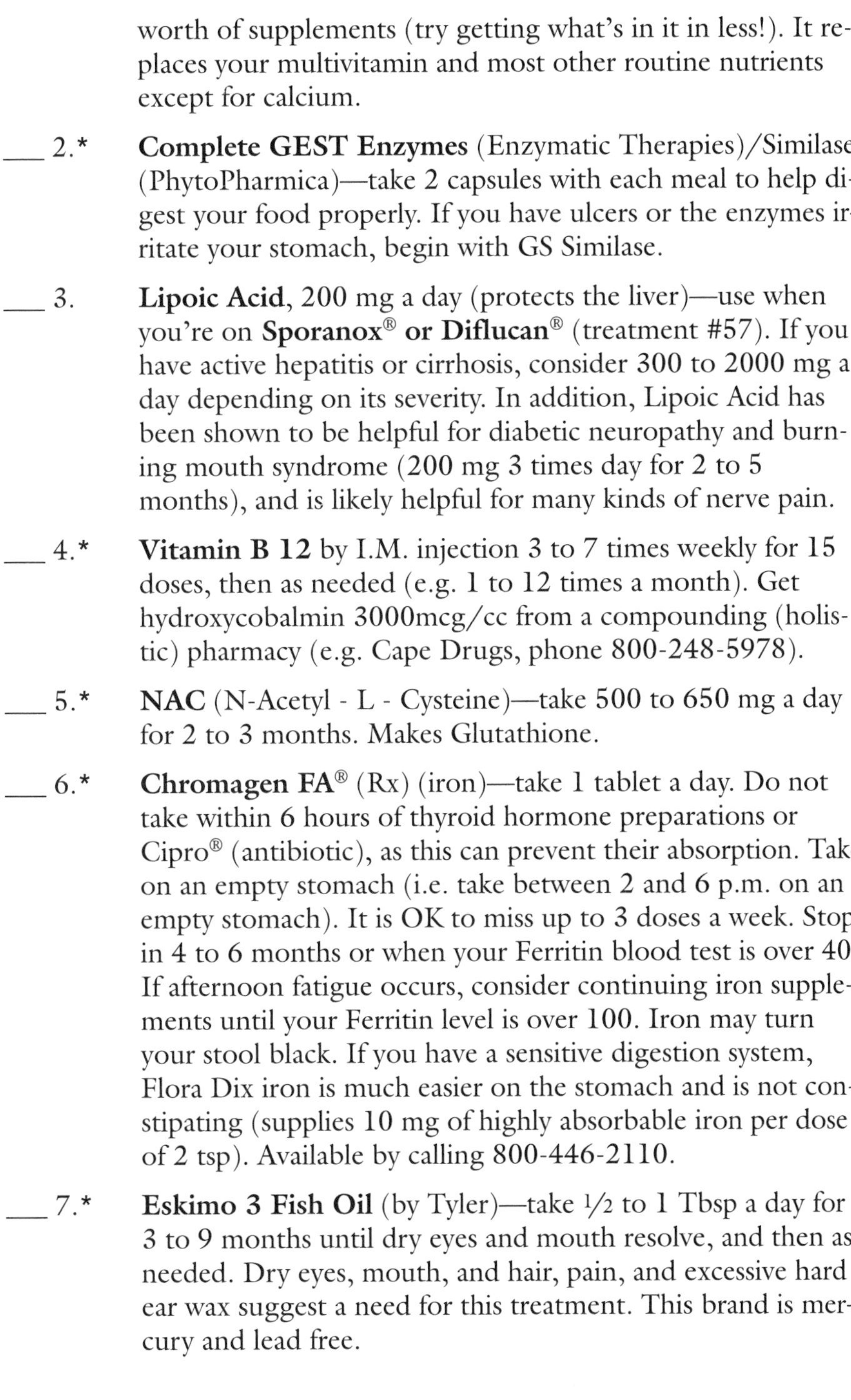

worth of supplements (try getting what's in it in less!). It replaces your multivitamin and most other routine nutrients except for calcium.

___ 2.* **Complete GEST Enzymes** (Enzymatic Therapies)/Similase (PhytoPharmica)—take 2 capsules with each meal to help digest your food properly. If you have ulcers or the enzymes irritate your stomach, begin with GS Similase.

___ 3. **Lipoic Acid**, 200 mg a day (protects the liver)—use when you're on **Sporanox® or Diflucan®** (treatment #57). If you have active hepatitis or cirrhosis, consider 300 to 2000 mg a day depending on its severity. In addition, Lipoic Acid has been shown to be helpful for diabetic neuropathy and burning mouth syndrome (200 mg 3 times day for 2 to 5 months), and is likely helpful for many kinds of nerve pain.

___ 4.* **Vitamin B 12** by I.M. injection 3 to 7 times weekly for 15 doses, then as needed (e.g. 1 to 12 times a month). Get hydroxycobalmin 3000mcg/cc from a compounding (holistic) pharmacy (e.g. Cape Drugs, phone 800-248-5978).

___ 5.* **NAC** (N-Acetyl - L - Cysteine)—take 500 to 650 mg a day for 2 to 3 months. Makes Glutathione.

___ 6.* **Chromagen FA®** (Rx) (iron)—take 1 tablet a day. Do not take within 6 hours of thyroid hormone preparations or Cipro® (antibiotic), as this can prevent their absorption. Take on an empty stomach (i.e. take between 2 and 6 p.m. on an empty stomach). It is OK to miss up to 3 doses a week. Stop in 4 to 6 months or when your Ferritin blood test is over 40. If afternoon fatigue occurs, consider continuing iron supplements until your Ferritin level is over 100. Iron may turn your stool black. If you have a sensitive digestion system, Flora Dix iron is much easier on the stomach and is not constipating (supplies 10 mg of highly absorbable iron per dose of 2 tsp). Available by calling 800-446-2110.

___ 7.* **Eskimo 3 Fish Oil** (by Tyler)—take ½ to 1 Tbsp a day for 3 to 9 months until dry eyes and mouth resolve, and then as needed. Dry eyes, mouth, and hair, pain, and excessive hard ear wax suggest a need for this treatment. This brand is mercury and lead free.

## Anxiety—Natural Treatments

___ 8. **Inositol** (helps depression, anxiety, bipolar and other psychological stress states)—take 3 to 6 tsp a day. Use just like sugar. Takes 3 to 6 weeks to work. You can purchase inositol as bulk powder.

___ 9. **Thiamine** (Vitamin B1), 500 mg—take 1 to 3 times day. Can help anxiety within 1 to 4 weeks.

## Mitochondrial Energy Treatments

Use these treatments for 4 to 9 months, then as needed.

___ 10.* **Acetyl-L-Carnitine**, 500 mg—take 1 capsule once or twice a day for 3 months. Then 250 to 500 mg/day, or stop it. Although important in CFS/FMS, it is even more important to take this if you also have Mitral Valve Prolapse, MS, and/or elevated blood triglycerides. This also helps with weight loss.

___ 11. **Coenzyme Q10**, 200 mg—take once a day. Especially important if taking cholesterol lowering prescriptions (e.g. Mevacor®), which **can cause** severe muscle pain. (I do not recommend they be used in pain patients.) Take with vitamin E or a meal that has fat or oil supplements or in an oil-based form to improve absorption. I strongly recommend the Vitaline® brand.

___ 12. **Magnesium/Potassium Aspartate**—take two 500 mg capsules 2 times a day. Use a "fully reacted" brand for 3 to 4 months.

___ 13. **NADH** (Enada brand)—use 10 mg sublingual tablets. Dissolve 1 tablet under the tongue (or swallow two 5 mg tablets) each morning. Take on an empty stomach first thing in the morning (leave by your bedside in the bottle or in foil wrap with a glass of water) at least ½ hour before eating; It takes 2 months to see results.

___ 14. **Magnesium Glycinate**, 75mg/Malic Acid 300 mg (Fibrocare)—take 2 tablets 3 times a day for 8 months, then 2 tablets a day (less if diarrhea is a problem). Start with 1 to 2 tablets a day and slowly work up as able without getting uncomfortable diarrhea. You can take up to 10 a day for constipation. Taking the tablets with food may lessen diarrhea. If pain or fatigue recurs on lowering the dose, increase it. Taken at bedtime, it helps with sleep.

## **Sleeping Aids

You can try these in the order listed or as you prefer based on your history. **Adjust the dose as needed to get 8 to 9 hours of solid sleep without waking or hangover**. No going to the bathroom if you wake up during the night unless you still have to go 5 minutes after waking. Mixing low doses of several treatments is more likely to help you sleep without a hangover than a high dose of a single medication. Do not drive if you have next day sedation (adjust your treatment to avoid this). If you're not sleeping 8 to 9 hours a night without waking, let your physician know so your medications can be adjusted.

Ambien®, Klonopin®, Xanax® and Soma® are considered potentially addictive, but in the dose and form that I use, this is rarely a problem. If you have next day sedation, try taking the medications (except for Sonata and Ambien) a few hours before bedtime. The anti-depressants (e.g. Prozac®/Paxil®) can improve sleep after 6 weeks. Taking calcium and magnesium at bedtime can help sleep. **In addition, you can try the other natural and/or nonprescription products in combination first to see if they give you 8 hours of sleep a night. Add them in this order: treatment #16, 19, 20, 29, 21**.

___ 15.** **Ambien**® (Rx) (zolpidem), 10 mg—take ½ to 1 ½ at bedtime. If you tend to wake during the night, leave an extra ½ to 1 tablet at your bedside and you can take it as needed to help you sleep through the night.

___ 16.** **Revitalizing Sleep Formula** (by Enzymatic Therapies and PhytoPharmica), contains Valerian 200 mg, Passion Flower 90 mg, L-Theanine 50 mg, Hops 30 mg, Jamaican Dogwood 12 mg and Wild Lettuce 28 mg. Take 2 to 4 capsules each night 30 to 90 minutes before bedtime. The formula can also be used during the day for anxiety. If Valerian energizes you (occurs in 5 to 10 percent of people), use the other components. Do not take more than 8 capsules a day.

___ 17. **Desyrel**® (Rx) (trazodone), 50 mg—take ½ to 6 at bedtime. Although sedating, it can be used (50 to 250 mg at a time) for anxiety. Do not take over 450 mg a day (or 150 mg a day if on other anti-depressants).

___ 18.* **Klonopin**® (Rx) (clonazepam), ½ mg—begin slowly and work your way up as sedation allows. Take ½ tablet at bedtime and increase up to 6 tablets at bedtime as needed. Can be **very** effective for sleep, pain, and restless leg syndrome.

Klonopin may be addictive. Taking 1/4 to 1/2 tablet in the morning (not more) can actually decrease brain fog in some patients.

___ 19.* **5 HTP** (5 Hydroxytryptophan), 200 to 400 mg at night—naturally stimulates serotonin. Don't take over 250 mg a day if you are on antidepressants such as Prozac®, Paxil®, Zoloft®, Desyrel®, or Celexa®. Can help with pain and weight loss at 300 mg a day for at least 3 months. Or you can take Tryptophan, 500 mg caps—1 to 6 capsules at bedtime. Available at www.Vitaganza.com ($65 for 180 capsules).

___ 20. **Calcium,** 500 to 600 mg, and **Magnesium**, 100 to 200 mg at bedtime helps sleep.

___ 21. **Doxylamine®** or **Benadryl®** (antihistamines), 25 mg at night. May also help pain.

___ 22.* **Neurontin**(Rx) 300 mg (see treatment #140A)—take 1 to 3 capsules at bedtime. Also helps pain and restless leg syndrome.

___ 23.* **Zanaflex®**(Rx) (see treatment #150A), 4 mg—take 1/2 to 2 at bedtime for sleep (higher doses for pain). Stop if it causes nightmares.

___ 24. **Sonata®** (Rx), 10 mg—take 1 to 2 capsules during the night if you wake after 3 a.m. or if you only have trouble falling (vs. staying) asleep. Its sedation only lasts 3 to 4 hours.

___ 25.* **Soma®** (Rx) (carisprodol)—take 1/2 to 1 at bedtime. This is very good if pain is severe. May be addictive.

___ 26.* **Flexeril®** (Rx) (cyclobenzaprine), 10 mg—take 1/2 to 2 at bedtime. A muscle relaxant; can cause dry mouth.

___ 27.* **Doxepin®** (Rx) (Sinequan, a powerful antihistamine), 5 to 10mg—take 1 to 3 capsules at bedtime or Doxepin liquid, 10mg/cc. If you need a lower dose, start with 1 to 3 drops at night. Some people get the greatest benefit with the least next-day sedation with a dose of less than 5 mg a night.

___ 28. **Elavil®** (Rx) (amitriptyline), 10 mg—take 1/2 to 5 tablets at bedtime. May cause weight gain or dry mouth. Good for nerve pain and vulvadynia.

___ 29. **Melatonin®**, 1/2 to 1 mg at bedtime. If you feel wide awake at bedtime, try 5mg 3 to 5 hours before bedtime. Don't use a higher dose unless you find it more effective (.5 mg is usually as effective as 5 mg, and may be safer).

___ 30.* **Gabitril**®(Rx), 2 mg twice a day (see treatment #140B)—increase by a maximum 4 mg daily each week to a maximum of 24 mg a day (optimal effect is seen at an average dose of 16 mg/day). Even 5 mg at bedtime can markedly improve deep sleep and can sometimes decrease next-day sedation. The main side effects are sedation, dizziness, and gastric upset.

___ 31. **Xanax**® (Rx) (alprazolam), ½ mg—take ½ to 4 tablets at bedtime. This is short-acting and gives a good 3 to 5 hours sleep with less hangover in the morning. May be addictive.

___ 32. **Seroquel**® (Rx), 25mg—take 1 to 3 at bedtime (an anti-schizophrenic medication).

## Hormonal Treatments

### *Thyroid Supplementation*

Several studies show that thyroid therapies can be very helpful in treatment of fibromyalgia/pain, even if your blood tests are normal.

Thyroid treatment is very controversial, even though it's usually very safe. All treatments (even aspirin) can cause problems in some people though. The main risks of thyroid treatment are:

1. Triggering caffeine-like anxiety or palpitations. If this happens, cut back the dose and increase by ½ to 1 tablet each 6 to 8 weeks or more (as is comfortable). Sometimes taking vitamin B1 (thiamine) 500 mg 1 to 3 times a day will also help after about one week. If you have severe, persistent racing heart, call your family doctor and/or go to a hospital emergency room.

2. Like exercise (i.e. climbing steps), if one is on the edge of having a heart attack or severe "racing heart" (atrial fibrillation), thyroid hormone can trigger these occurrences. However, research suggests that thyroid hormone treatments may actually decrease the risk of heart disease. If you have chest pain, go to the hospital emergency room and/or call your family doctor. It will likely be chest muscle pain (not dangerous) but better safe than sorry. To put it in perspective, I've **never** seen this happen in my years of treating thousands of patients with thyroid hormone. Increasing your thyroid hormone dose to levels **above** the **upper** limit of the normal range may accelerate osteoporosis, which is already common in pain. Because of this, you need to check your thyroid (Free T4, **not** TSH) blood levels after 4 to 8 weeks on your optimum dose of thyroid hormone. I find treatments with thyroid hormone **safer** than aspirin and Motrin®. If you have risk factors or angina, do an exercise

stress test to make sure your heart is healthy before beginning thyroid hormone treatment. Risk factors for angina include: diabetes, elevated cholesterol, hypertension, smoking, personal or family history of angina, gout, and age over 50 years old.

There are several forms of thyroid hormone, and one type often will work when another does not. Do not take thyroid within 6 hours of iron or 2 to 4 hours of calcium supplements or you will not absorb the thyroid. It can take 3 to 24 months to see the thyroid hormone treatment's **full** benefit.

___ 33. **Levoxyl®** or **Synthroid®** (Rx) (L-Thyroxine), 50mcg (100 mcg=.1mg)—see the paragraph below and thyroid hormone treatment information above.

___ 34.** **Armour Thyroid** (Rx), 30 mg (½ grain = 30 mg)—this is a natural thyroid glandular. If treatment #37 (Cortef®) is prescribed, begin the Cortef and/or adrenal support 1 to 7 days before starting the thyroid treatment. See paragraph below and thyroid hormone treatment information above. For both of these treatments (#33-34), take ½ tablet each **morning** on an empty stomach for 1 week and then 1 tablet each morning. Increase by ½ to 1 tablet each 1 to 6 weeks (until you're taking 3 tablets or a dose that feels best). Check a repeat Free T4 blood level when you're on 3 tablets a day (or your optimum dose) for 4 weeks. If okay, you can continue to raise the dose by ½ to 1 tablet each morning each 6 to 9 weeks to a maximum of 5 a day and then recheck the Free T4 level 4 weeks later. Adjust to the dose that feels the best (lower the dose if you are shaky or if your resting pulse is regularly over 88/minute). Although it may take as many as 10 tablets a day to see the optimal effect, **do not exceed 5 tablets** a day without discussing it with your doctor. When on your optimum dose, you can often get a single tablet at that strength. If your energy wanes too early in the day, you can also take part of your thyroid dose between 11 a.m. and 3 p.m. Some people find that taking part of their thyroid hormone treatment dose at night feels better. You can divide your thyroid dose through the day to see what feels best.

**And/Or**

___ 35. **Iodine** (**Iodoral®** tablets from Optimox)—take ½ to 1 a day for 2 to 4 months if you have daytime body temperatures under 98.3 degrees, breast cysts or tenderness, **or** ovarian cysts.

These tablets contain 12.5 mg iodine (iodine 5 mg and iodide 7.5 mg). May flare Hashimoto's thyroiditis and rarely may suppress thyroid function with long term use.

___ 36.* **Cytomel®**, pure active T3 (Rx), 5 and 25 mcg tablets—in fibromyalgia, resistance to normal thyroid doses may occur and patients often need very high levels of T3 Thyroid to improve. For example, Dr. John Lowe's research group feels that the average dose needed in fibromyalgia is 75 to 125 mcg each morning—**much** higher than your body's normal production. Because you are often going above normal levels with T3, the risks/side effects noted above increase. Because of this, if you have risk factors, it is important to consider an exercise stress test to make sure your heart is healthy (i.e. no underlying angina) before beginning this protocol. Also, consider a Dexa Scan (for osteoporosis) before treatment and then each 6 to 18 months while on the treatment. There may be initial bone loss the first year (see osteoporosis treatments), then increased bone density. In my experience this treatment has been quite safe and, in some FMS patients, dramatically effective. Begin with 5 mcg each morning and continue to increase by 5 mcg each 3 days until you feel well, or you're at 75 mcg a day, whichever comes first, and then increase by 5 mcg a day each 1 to 6 weeks until:

1. You reach 125 mcg each morning (or 60 mcg if you're over 50 years old unless approved by your physician).
2. You feel healthy.
3. You get shakiness, worsening **significant** palpitations (occasional "flip flops" are common), anxiety, racing heart, sweating, or other uncomfortable side effects. If this happens, lower the dose to where side effects resolve for 2 to 4 weeks and then try raising it again until you experience significant improvement **without** uncomfortable side effects.

Blood tests for thyroid hormone or TSH are not reliable or useful on this regimen. If you feel no better even on the maximum dose, taper off. Decrease by 5 mcg each 3 days until you reach 15 mcg a day. Take 15 mcg a day for 3 weeks and then drop to 5 mcg a day for 3 weeks, then stop. After being on the treatment for 3 to 6 months, some patients can lower the T3 dose or stop it. Feel free to try lowering the dose. If you feel better initially and then worse (beginning more than 4 weeks after starting a new dose), you probably need to lower the dose. If you lose too much weight, try to eat more (discuss this with your physician) and lower the dose.

## *Adrenal Hormones, Glandulars and Support*

These treatments help your body deal with stress and maintain blood pressure.

___ 37.** **Cortef®** (Rx), 5 mg tablets—take 1/2 to 2 1/2 tablets at breakfast, 1/2 to 1 1/2 tablets at lunch and 0 to 1/2 tablets at 4 p.m. Use the lowest dose that feels the best. Most patients find that 1 to 1 1/2 tablets in the morning and 1/2 to 1 tablet at noon is optimal. Take it with food if it causes an acid stomach. Do not take over 4 tablets a day without discussing the risks with your physician. Take Calcium if on Cortef. If taken too late in the day, Cortef can keep you up at night. You can double the dose for up to 1 to 3 weeks (to a maximum 7 tablets a day) during periods of severe stress (e.g. infections—see or call your doctor for an infection and let him or her know that you're raising the dose). If routinely taking over 4 tablets a day (at your doctor's direction), wear a "Med-Alert Bracelet" that says "on chronic Cortisol treatment." After 9 to 18 months, you can start to wean off Cortef (decrease by 1/2 tablet a day each 2 weeks), if you feel OK (or no worse) without it.

**Or Treatment #38 and/or #39**

___ 38.** **Adrenal Stress End** (from Enzymatic Therapies or PhytoPharmica)—take 1 to 2 capsules each morning (or 1 to 2 in the morning and 1 at noon). Take less or take with food if you experience upset stomach.

___ 39. **Isocort®** (Adrenal Glandular)—may contain approximately 2 1/2 mg Cortisol (Cortef) per pellet (see treatment #37 above for directions). You can order Isocort by phoning 800 743-2256.

___ 40.* **DHEA** _____mg—take each morning or twice daily. Lower the dose if acne or darkening of facial hair occurs. Some experts recommend that the entire dose be taken in the morning. Keep your DHEA-Sulphate levels between 140 to 180 mcg/dL for females and 300 to 500mcg/dL for males. If you have breast cancer, do not use without your physician's OK.

## *Other Hormones*

___ 41.* **Natural Estrogen** (Rx)—take **Estrace®** (estradiol) 1 mg, 1 to 2 times a day, **or** put a **Climara®** .05 to .1 mg patch on each Sunday, **or** take **Biestrogen,** 2 ½ mg 1 to 2 times a day. If you have not had a hysterectomy, you **must** be on progesterone with the estrogen to prevent uterine cancer. If you are on the patch and it seems to stop working the last 1 to 2 days of the week, you can change the patch every 5 days.

Use the estrogen ____ every day; ____ day 1 through 25 of your cycle (day 1 of your period is day 1 of your cycle). It is normal for your periods to be irregular for 3 to 4 months. If your symptoms (including migraines and anxiety) worsen for the week you are off the estrogen, you can add a Climara .025 mg patch for that week. If symptoms worsen a few hours before you take the estrogen by mouth, divide up the dose through the day (e.g. ½ tablet, 4 times a day as compared to 2 tablets each morning). If you order your estrogen/progesterone capsules from Cape Apothecary (phone 800-248-5978 or 410-757-3522), they will be glad to work with you in adjusting the dose.

**Or**

___ 42.* **Biest®** 2.5mg, plus **Progesterone** 50 mg, plus **Testosterone** 2 mg all in 1 capsule—take one capsule 1 to 2 times day. If you order your estrogen/progesterone capsules from Cape Apothecary (phone 800-248-5978 or 410-757-3522), they will be glad to work with you in adjusting the dose.

**Or**

___ 43. **Ortho-novum** 1/35 (Rx)—begin the Sunday after your next period. Its effectiveness as birth control begins after you've been on it the first week. If you miss taking a pill, add alternate contraception that cycle. Its effectiveness as birth control is decreased while on Doxycycline® or Amoxicillin®/ Augmentin family antibiotics. If you feel poorly the week off the pill, you can take it every day until you get your period (or for 5 months, whichever comes first). Then stop the pill for 5 to 7 days, and then repeat this cycle.

___ 44.* **Natural Progesterone** (Rx) (**Prometrium®**, available in most pharmacies)—take 100 mg daily if over 48 years old **or** 200 mg a day for the $16^{th}$ to $25^{th}$ day of your cycle if under 48 years old. Take it at night.

___ 45.* **Testosterone** (Rx)—females take 2 mg tablets or cream, 1 to 2 times a day(less if acne or darkening of facial hair occurs). Make 4 mg/gm of cream. Rub the cream into an area of thin skin on the abdomen or inner thigh. The cream is available by prescription from Cape Apothecary (phone 410-757-3522).

___ 46.* **Testosterone** (Rx)—males take 25 to 50 mg (order 100mg/gm of cream) 2 to 3 times a day (less if acne occurs). Rub the cream into an area of thin skin on the abdomen, or inner thigh. The cream is available by prescription from Cape Apothecary (phone 410-757-3522) and can be mailed to you.

**Or**

____**Androgel**(Rx)____25 mg or____50 mg—apply gel 1 to 2 times a day. Consider also checking estrogen and DHT levels when you check your testosterone blood levels. If the DHT level elevates too high, it can cause hair loss, which can be prevented by Proscar® (Rx) or Saw Palmetto, 160 mg 2 times day. If estrogen levels elevate too high, this can be blocked by Arimidex® (Rx), 1 mg a day. If you are taking thyroid tablets, be aware that adding testosterone can increase your thyroid blood levels. If you become moody, anxious, or experience racing heart, check blood levels for your thyroid and consider lowering the dose.

## Anti-Viral Agents

(See the article "Treating Respiratory Infections Without Antibiotics.")

___ 47. **Colloidal Silver**—Use Argentyn 23, available online from my web site at www.endfatigue.com, or purchase wholesale at www.natural-immunogenics.com. For acute infections or aggressive treatment take 2 Tbsp by mouth in the morning, 1 Tbsp before lunch, and 1 Tbsp 20 minutes before dinner. Silver should be taken on an empty stomach (at least 10 minutes before eating or drinking). If you get a "die-off" reaction (flaring of symptoms) as the infection dies, lower the dose to 1 tsp a day and increase more slowly. Use the higher dose (a 240 oz. bottle is enough for an 8 day course of treatment) for 8 to 12 weeks for chronic viral infections. Taking 1 tsp a day is a good maintenance dose (a 240 oz. bottle lasts 48 days) after the infection resolves.

___ 48. **Monolaurin®**, 300 mg capsules—take 9 capsules once a day on an empty stomach for 1 week, followed by 6 capsules once a day for 20 days. Take Lysine, 1500 mg, twice a day while on Monolaurin.

## Anti-Yeast Treatments

For a non-prescription approach, use treatments #49, 51, 52, 53, and 54.

___ 49.** **Avoid Sweets**. This includes sucrose, glucose, fructose, corn syrup, or any other sugars until the doctor says that it is okay to include them in your diet again. Avoid fruit **juices**, which are naturally loaded with sugar. Having 1 to 2 fruits a day (whole fruit as opposed to juice) is okay. Stevia (treatment #50) is a great sugar substitute. Inositol (treatment #8- helps relieve anxiety and depression) and Xylitol (helps osteoporosis) are also excellent and healthy sugar substitutes that look and taste like just like sugar.

___ 50. **Stevia** is a wonderful herbal sweetener. Use all you want. A great tasting brand is from Body Ecology, available by phoning 800-478-3842.

___ 51.** **Acidophilus Milk Bacteria** (use the Pearls form by Enzymatic Therapy/ Phyto Pharmica)—take 2 twice a day for 5 months. Then consider 1 a day to help maintain a healthy bowel. Do **not** take within 6 hours of taking an antibiotic (e.g. take it midday, if you take the antibiotic morning and night). The Enzymatic Therapy/PhytoPharmica Acidophilus or Probiotic Pearls form contains approximately 2.8 billion units per pearl, even though the box says only 1 billion. I use only this brand, because in many other brands the bacteria are not viable.

___ 52. **Primal Defense Tablets**—take 2-4 tablets 2-3 times day for 3 to 5 months along with acidophilus pearls.

___ 53.* **Phytostan®** (NF Formulations/ITI), an excellent natural antifungal mix—take 2 twice a day for 3 to 5 months.

___ 54. **Citricidal®**, 100 mg—1-2 tablets twice a day.

___ 55. **Mycelex® Oral Lozenges** (Rx), for Thrush and/or "in the mouth" sores—suck on 1 lozenge 5 times a day for 1 to 4 days (as needed). After sucking on it awhile (e.g. 10 minutes), put a piece of the lozenge up against the sore(s) until you are tired of it being there.

___ 56.* **Nystatin®** (Rx), 500,000 units—take 2 tablets 2 to 4 times a day. Begin with 1 a day and increase by 1 tablet a day until you are up to the total recommended dose. Your symptoms may initially flare as the yeast dies. If this occurs, stop it and take Actos® (Rx) 45 mg a day for 10 days. On the 7th day of taking Actos, resume the Nystatin and raise the dose more slowly or stop for a while, if die off is still severe. The Nystatin is usually taken for 5 to 8 months. If nausea occurs, take 2 twice a day and/or switch to the Nystatin powder in capsules or mixed in water (available from Kronos Pharmacy, phone 800-723-7455) in 1 million unit capsules. These are much cheaper and better tolerated but need to be refrigerated. Repeat Nystatin for 4 to 6 weeks anytime you take an antibiotic or have recurrent bowel symptoms.

___ 57.** **Diflucan®** (Rx)(fluconazole), 200 mg a day for 6 weeks. **Important**: begin taking the Diflucan 4 weeks after starting the Nystatin. See the paragraph below.

**Or**

___ ** **Sporanox®** (Rx) (itraconazole), 100 mg, take 2 each day (simultaneously) with food. Begin taking the Diflucan or Sporanox 4 weeks after beginning the Nystatin. If symptoms have improved and then worsen when you stop the antifungal medications, refill the prescription for another 6 weeks. (**Note:** A six-week supply costs over $500, but generic Diflucan is now available for only $42!) If your symptoms flared when you began the Nystatin, begin with ¼ to ½ the above dose for the 1st week. Do not take cholesterol lowering agents related to Mevacor® while on Diflucan or Sporanox, or antacids (e.g. Tagamet®) while on Sporanox. Also, taking Betaine HCL (stomach acid to help digestion, available at most health food stores) at the same time as the Sporanox, can dramatically increase Sporanox's absorption and effectiveness. Lipoic Acid(#3) may decrease the risk of liver inflammation from the Diflucan or Sporanox. If you need to stay on these medications more than 3 months, check liver blood tests (ALT, AST) every 3 months. If you feel well and symptoms (especially bowel symptoms) recur over time, consider re-treating yourself with Acidophilus Pearls, 2 twice a day; Nystatin; and Sporanox (or Diflucan) for 6 weeks, as needed.

### *Immune Stimulants*

___ 58.** **Thymic Protein** (AKA Proboost and Bio Pro A)—**Very Powerful**. Dissolve the contents of 1 packet **under your tongue**—any that is swallowed is destroyed! Take it three times a day for 12 weeks, then 1 a day for 6 weeks. Also take it 3 times a day at first sign of any infection until the infection resolves (cost is approximately $1.80 a packet). Available from my office (phone 800-333-5287) or online at www.Vitality101.com. Works in the first 24 hours for acute infections but takes 2 to 3 months to work for chronic infections.

___ 59.* **Colloidal Silver** (available online at www.natural-immunogenics.com or phone 888-328-8840). See treatment #47 for dosage instructions.

## *Treatments for Parasites, Bowel, and Other Infections

If your stool test shows parasites, recheck the stool test 3 to 4 weeks after finishing the treatment below. See the Comprehensive Treatment Protocol online at www.Vitality101.com for information on how to treat specific parasites or antibiotic sensitive infections.

___ 60.* **Vermox®** (Rx), 100 mg—chew 1 twice a day for 3 days. 1 week later chew 1 twice a day for 1 day. Good as an "empiric" therapy if you suspect parasites but cannot isolate them.

___ 61* **Neomycin®** (Rx)—take 500 mg 3 times a day for 10 days. Used for small bowel bacterial overgrowth.

___ 62.* **Multi-pure Water Filter**—most other filters, except reverse osmosis, are ineffective (available from Bren Jacobson, phone 410-224-4877 or order online at purewatermd.tripod.com, do not type in www before the web address). Decreases the risk of re-infection.

### *Chronic and Acute Sinusitis*

___ 63.* **Sinusitis Nose Spray** (Rx)—available from Cape Apothecary (phone 800-248-5978). Contains Sporanox, Xylitol, Bactroban, Beclamethasone and Nystatin. Use 1 to 2 sprays in each nostril twice a day for 6 to 12 weeks. If it irritates the nose, dilute it with saline. Use with silver spray below.

___ 64.* **Nasal Silver Spray**—use 5 to 10 sprays in each nostril 3 times a day for 7 to 14 days until the sinusitis resolves (available online at www.endfatigue.com, or order wholesale from Immunogenics at www.natural–immunogenics.com).

___ 65. **Nasal Irrigation** (Rx)—use 1 liter of normal saline with 100 mg Amphotericin B and a second liter with 80 mg gentamycin. Use 1 ounce of each in each nostril as a nasal rinse twice a day as needed(from compounding pharmacies).

### *Kills Many Infections*

___ 66. **Colloidal Silver**—See treatment #27.

### *E.Coli Bladder Infections*

___ 67. **D-Mannose**—take 1 tsp (2 grams) stirred in water every 2 to 3 hours while awake for 2 to 5 days for acute bladder infections (may use up to 1 to 2 times a day long term if needed for chronic infections) caused by E.Coli (this causes approximately 90 percent of bladder infections). If not much better in 24 hours, get a urine culture and consider an antibiotic. Continue taking it for 2 to 3 days after the last symptom resolves. Taking it 1 hour before and immediately after intercourse can also prevent bladder infections. D-Mannose is available from BioTech (phone 800-345-1199), from my office or www.endfatigue.com.

### *Chronic Lyme*

___ 68. **Una D'gato TOA Free Cats Claw Drops** (Allergy Research)—use 5 drops 3 times a day for 12 months for Lyme disease. If symptoms flare, start with a low dose and work up as comfortable.

## Other Treatments

### *Food and Other Sensitivities*

___ 69.** **NAET**—wonderful for elimination of sensitivities/allergies (see www.naet.com for more information). In Annapolis, phone Laurie Teitelbaum at 410-266-6958.

___ 70. **Food Allergy Elimination Diet**—instruction sheet is available online at www.endfatigue.com. Click on the "useful articles" link.

## IV Nutritional Support

___ 71.** **Myers Cocktail** IV nutritional therapies (very helpful). In Annapolis, phone Rhonda Kidd at 443-994-0126 or Kim Weiss at 410-280-1655.

## * Detoxification

There are several simple things that you can do that can be very helpful:

___ 72. **Sweating** can remove toxins, especially if you shower immediately after, and can be very helpful for health. "Far infrared" saunas taken for one half hour 3 to 7 times a week can help detoxification.

___ 73. **Detox Baths**—some of you may be more comfortable with hot baths. This is one recipe that was given to me by a wonderful practitioner (Anette Mnabhi, DO in Montgomery, IL).

Recipe for Detox Bath
(helps with general muscle aches and pains)
Epsom Salts—2 cups
Baking Soda—1 cup
Hydrogen Peroxide—1/3 cup

Fill tub with hot water and add above ingredients. Soak for 20 to 30 minutes. You will sweat in the tub and lose toxins, which causes you to lose some water as well. It is important to drink plenty of water while you soak. You can make fresh lemon juice and mix with water and drink, or drink plain water, but it is essential to drink while you take the bath. If you have a tendency to get light headed easily, be cautious when getting out of the tub, or have someone nearby the first time you take a detox bath. Take a lukewarm to cool shower after getting out of the tub to rinse off the salts, or you may itch. Rest for 30 minutes after the bath.

___ 74. Two excellent products can be used intermittently to eliminate toxins. These are___**Whole Body Cleanse** and___**Metal Magnet** by Enzymatic Therapy. Simply follow the labeled instructions.

### *Energy Boosters*

___ 75. **Dexedrine®** (Rx) (dextroamphetamine), 5 mg—take 1 to 2 tablets in the morning; plus ½ to 1 ½ tablets at noon; or take Concerta®, 18 mg, 1 to 2 each morning and/or_____Provigil® (Rx), 200 mg, ½ to 1 tablet in the morning and at noon, as needed for energy. Dexedrine is an amphetamine family stimulant similar to Ritalin® and may be addictive. Take less if you have caffeine-like shakiness. Most patients use 1 to 3 tablets of Dexedrine in the morning and ½ to 2 at noon. If appetite suppression and/or weight loss is a problem, you can add Periactin® (Rx), 4 mg (antihistamine and anti-serotonin) up to 5 tablets a day.

### *Anti-depressants*

These help pain even if you are not depressed.

___ 76. Hypericum (St. John's Wort)—take 300 to 625 mg 3 times a day (takes 6 weeks to see the anti-depressant effect). Use one standardized to at least .3 percent hypericum. Can take 2/3 of the total daily dose at night to help sleep. Can take up to 2000 mg Hypericum a day if not on other anti-depressants (otherwise limit to 1000 mg a day).

___ 77. **Effexor®** (Rx) (venlafaxine)—take 37 ½ mg_____tablets_____times a day.

___ 78. **Prozac®** (Rx) (fluoxetine)—take 20 mg_____capsule(s) each morning. Begin with 10 mg a day the first week if the full dose makes you hyper.

___ 79. **Celexa®** (Rx)—take 20mg____tablet(s) a day **OR** treatment #109.

___ 80. **Zoloft®** (Rx) (Sertraline)—take 50 mg_____tablet(s) each morning or evening.

___ 81. **Paxil®** (Rx) (paroxetine)—take 20 mg_____tablet(s) each morning.

___ 82. **Wellbutrin®** (Rx) (bupropion)—take_____mg_____times a day. Not sedating.

___ 83. **Meridia®**(Rx) (Sibutramine)—take 10 or 15 mg each morning. Causes weight-loss.

___ 84. **Cymbalta®**(Rx) 60 mg one-two times a day—helps pain and causes weight loss.

## Sexual Dysfunction

Make sure your testosterone levels are optimal.

___ 85. Anti-depressant induced sexual dysfunction can be treated with___**Ginkgo Biloba** 120 mg twice daily____**Dexedrine®(see #75)** 25 mg each morning, ____**Symmetral®**(Rx) 100 mg twice daily, or switching to Wellbutrin (see treatment # 82).

___ 86. **Viagra®**(Rx), 100 mg—for erectile dysfunction, take 1/4 to 1 tablet 1 hour before intercourse on an empty stomach. **Do not use with nitroglycerin or underlying heart disease**.

___ 87. **Cialis®**(Rx), 20 mg—for erectile dysfunction, take 1/2 to 1 tablet 15 minutes before intercourse. **Do not use with nitroglycerin or underlying heart disease**.

## Spastic Colon—IBS

Treat the yeast and parasites and the IBS will usually go away. For symptomatic relief:

___ 88. **Peppermint Oil** (Enteric/stomach coated) .2cc capsules—take 1 to 2 capsules 3 times a day between meals, **not** with food, for spastic colon. You can use **Peppermint Plus** from Enzymatic Therapies or **Mentharil** from PhytoPharmica.

___ 89. **Simethicone** (Mylicon), 40 to 80 mg—**chew** 1 tablet 3 times a day as needed for abdominal gas pains.

___ 90. **Iberogast** (digestive system herbal)—take 20 drops 3 times a day in warm water with meals. Very helpful for indigestion (takes 4 to 8 weeks to work). Available from Phyto Pharmica.

## Osteoporosis

In addition to weight bearing and estrogen replacement, DHEA and testosterone replacement can also be beneficial in the treatment of osteoporosis. In addition to calcium, numerous nutrients (e.g. magnesium, boron, etc) are critical for building bone strength. Except for calcium, strontium, and vitamin K, most of these are contained in the Energy Revitalization System (see treatment #1), which contains over 50 nutrients. Take this plus calcium and:

___ 91. **Strontium®**, 680 mg/day—take on an empty stomach and at a different time of day than the calcium because calcium can block strontium's absorption. Early data also suggests that strontium may be helpful in the treatment of osteoarthritis. Available at www.EndFatigue.com.

___ 92. **Fosamax®**(Rx), 70 mg—take once a week on an empty stomach with a full glass of water. It is best to take it immediately upon waking and then stay upright for 30 minutes so gravity helps get it past the stomach quickly (because it can irritate the stomach). For those on the 35 mg a week prevention dose, be aware that the 35 and 70 mg tablets cost exactly the same amount. You can save half the cost by getting a 70 mg tablet and breaking it in half!

___ 93. **Xylitol**—use this powder instead of sugar (increases bone density and tastes and looks like sugar).

### *Constipation*

You can adjust these treatments as needed to have one soft bowel movement a day. Increasing your water, fiber (e.g. 1 bowl of whole grain cereal in the morning) and magnesium intake is also helpful.

___ 94. **Miralax® Laxative** (Rx)—take 1 heaping Tbsp once a day in 8 oz of water (comes in 14 oz and 26 oz bottles).

___ 95. **Prunes** and/or **Prune Juice**.

___ 96. **Zelnorm®**(Rx), 6 mg—take twice a day for spastic colon associated with constipation.

___ 97. **Sorbitol®** 70 percent—take 1 to 3 tsp 3 times a day as needed.

## Migraine Therapy

### *Prevention*

For migraine prevention, Magnesium (see treatment #1 plus take an extra 200 mg at bedtime) is very important. I recommend adding vitamin B2 and butterbur (or feverfew if the butterbur is too expensive). It can take 3 months to see the effect of these preventive measures! If your migraines are predominately around your period or associated with taking estrogen, they can often be eliminated by adjusting estrogen dosing. Many medications, which are elsewhere on this form, can also be helpful for the prevention of migraines when taken regularly. These include Neurontin®, Topamax®, Elavil®, and Doxepin®. Inderal® XL can also be helpful but may aggravate fatigue, asthma, or depression. Food allergies should also be addressed.

___ 98.** **Food Allergies** are also very important to consider in the production of migraines. To tell if foods are playing a role, it is helpful to do a food elimination diet. Although a very limited diet is needed for 5 days (eat only pears and lamb, and drink only bottled spring or distilled water), this kind of strict elimination diet for 5 days will make it easier to tell if true food allergies are present and triggering your migraines when you reintroduce the withheld foods into your diet. In one study, by avoiding the ten most common food triggers, there was a dramatic reduction in the number of headaches per month, with 85 percent of participants becoming headache free. The most common reactive foods in participants were: wheat in 78 percent of patients; oranges in 65 percent; eggs in 45 percent; tea and coffee in 40 percent each; chocolate and milk in 37 percent each; beef in 35 percent; and corn, cane sugar, and yeast in 33 percent each. If you have severe and frequent migraines, it is worth exploring food allergies. You may find that instead of avoiding these foods for the rest of your life, you can eliminate the sensitivities/allergies using an acupressure technique called NAET (see www.NAET.com).

___ 99.* **Vitamin B2** (riboflavin)—take 400mg each morning to prevent migraines.

___ 100.* **Petadolex** (butterbur)—take 50mg 3 times a day for 1 month and then twice a day to prevent migraines. Can take 2 every 3 hours up to 6 capsules for acute migraines. Use Enzymatic Therapy or ITI brands because others often have impurities and do not contain the amount of butterbur the label claims. Petadolex can be highly effective in headache treatment.

___ 101. **Feverfew**—take 250mg 1 to 3 times a day to prevent migraines.

___ 102. **Zonegran**®, 100 mg. See #159

## *For Acute Migraines*

___ 103.* **Petadolex (butterbur),** 50mg—take 2 capsules every 3 hours up to 6 capsules for acute migraines.

___ 104.* **Imitrex®**—for the treatment of acute migraines, medications in the Imitrex family still remain the first choice. Imitrex comes in 25, 50, and 100 mg tablets, and up to 100 mg may be taken at a time. The 50-100 mg dose is a reasonable dose to start with. If pain persists at 2 hours, you can take another dose of up to 100 mg. In addition, Imitrex is also available by nasal spray. I recommend using a dose of up to 20 mg initially, followed by 1 more spray of up to 20 mg 2 hours later, if needed. Another alternative is a 6 mg subcutaneous injection, which can also be repeated 1 hour later, if needed. I recommend trying these different forms to see what works best for your migraines. You may also want to try a newer medication cousin, called **Amerge®**(Rx). Use 2.5 mg initially. This dose may be repeated 4 hours later, if needed.

___ 105. **Axert®**(Rx) (Almotriptan)—use 6.5 or 12.5 mg. Can repeat the dose after 2 hours. This medication is a cousin to Imitrex but is less expensive.

___ 106. **Magnesium,** 1 to 2 grams IV administered over a time period of 15 to 30 minutes will usually knock out acute migraine attacks.

___ 107. **Midrin®**(Rx) —take 2 capsules immediately followed by 1 capsule every hour until the headache is relieved (to a maximum of 5 capsules within a 12 hour period). It can also be helpful for tension headaches in a dose of 2 capsules 4 times a day as needed.

___ 108. **Metoclopramide®**(Rx) 10 mg, plus **Lysine Acetylsalicylate®** (compounded) 1620 mg, or **Aspirin** 900 to 1200 mg, (chewed). Metoclopramide returns the absorption of aspirin to normal during migraine attacks and also combats nausea and vomiting. In two placebo-controlled studies, this combination (using lysine acetylsalicylate) was more effective than 100 mg of Imitrex by mouth and was better tolerated.

**Or**

___ 109. **Indomethacin®**(Rx) (a "super-aspirin"), **Prochlorperazine®** (Rx) (for nausea), and **Caffeine** in suppository form (also compounded)—eliminates an acute migraine in 49 percent of patients.

___ 110. **ACTIQ** (Rx) (Fentanyl® lollipops), 200 to 1600 mcg—this powerful narcotic should be used only for breakthrough pain that is not relieved by other medications (i.e. used instead of going to the hospital emergency room—see information in Chapter 13: Headaches for use).

___ 111. **Phenergan® Rectal Suppositories** (for nausea), 25 mg—take 1 every 4 hours as needed for nausea (up to 5 a day).

___ 112. **Diamox®** (Rx) (a diuretic), 125-500 mg—taking Diamox once or twice daily may decrease severe pressure headaches. Carbonated beverages will taste funny while you're on this medication.

## Pain Treatments

Anti-depressants often help pain. Natural treatments can be substituted for or added to prescription pain medications. If side effects occur, they often can be avoided by starting medications at a low dose and raising the dose every 3 to 7 days as your body gets used to the medication. It may take 2 to 6 weeks for a treatment to start working.

### *Natural Pain Therapies*

___ 113. **Rolfing**, **Trager**, **Myofascial Release**, **Chiropractic**, **Body Work and Manipulation Modalities**, and/or **Acupuncture**. In Annapolis Maryland, Bren Jacobson (phone 410-224-4877), does superb Rolfing.

___ 114. **End Pain Formula**—contains Willow Bark, Boswellia, and Cherry. Take 2 tablets 3 times day. It takes 2 to 6 weeks to see the full effect. At that time, you can often lower the dose to 1 tablet 3 times day or as needed.

___ 115. **NAET**—treat food and other sensitivities and pain often resolves. See www.NAET.com and the book, *Say Goodbye to Pain*. Other related techniques such as **JMT** (see www.JMT-jaffemeltechnique.com) can be very helpful for rheumatoid and osteoarthritis problems.

___ 116. **Niacin** (not niacinamide or "flush free" niacin)—take 100 to 500 mg (100 mg is usually enough to cause the desired flush) of niacin 3 to 4 times a day on an empty stomach as needed to cause a "flushing" feeling, which occurs within approximately 10 to 20 minutes. This can significantly help pain by flushing nutrients into and toxins out of painful areas. Try to keep the dose at 1000 mg a day or less if this is enough to cause flushing, because higher doses can cause liver inflammation (rarely) or unmask diabetes. This treatment also helps to lower cholesterol and decrease brain fog.

___ 117. **NF Joint Gel**—for best results, massage Joint Gel into your skin until absorbed. You can use Joint Gel up to 3 to 4 times daily.

___ 118. **Lipoic Acid**, 200-300 mg—use 3 times a day for neuropathic pain. Benefit usually begins to be seen by 2 to 3 months. It has been shown to be helpful for diabetic neuropathy and burning mouth syndrome (200 mg 3 times day for 5 months).

___ 119. **Glucosamine <u>Sulfate</u>**, 500 mg—use 3 times a day (for arthritis). Takes 6 weeks to see if it will help. When the maximum benefit is seen, you can decrease to the lowest dose that maintains the desired effect.

___ 120. **MSM**—use 1.5-3 grams a day for arthritis.

___ 121. **Fish Oil** (see treatment # 7 for recommendations)—can markedly decrease inflammation and pain. Dry eyes and mouth suggest you need fish oil.

___ 122.* **Megazyme** (from Enzymatic Therapies) or **Biozyme** (from PhytoPharmica)—works like a super Wobenzyme. Take 2 to 4 capsules 3 times a day between meals. May dissolve clots in the blood vessels. Can be helpful for pain and other symptoms (takes days to weeks to work). Especially helpful for inflammatory pain.

___ 123 **Purple Pectin for Pain** (especially arthritis)—purchase Certo® in the canning section of your local grocery. It is the thickening agent used to make jams and jellies. Certo contains pectin, a natural ingredient found in plants. Take 1 to 3 Tbsp of Certo in 8 oz of grape juice 1 to 2 times a day (1 to 2 Tbsp a day is enough for most people, but you can try more). If it's going to help, you'll likely know in 7 to 14 days. As the pain disappears, the dose can be reduced to 1 tsp in grape juice once or twice a day as needed. Many people have found this simple, safe and cheap treatment to be very effective!

___ 124. **Heel Lift**____inches for____foot—for uneven hip heights.

___ 125. **John Sarno, M.D.'s Approach for Localized Pain**—the mind can decrease blood flow to muscles to distract us from uncomfortable emotional feelings. When you feel pain, tell your mind you will use the pain as a signal to look for and feel uncomfortable feelings for 10 to 15 minutes, then do so. The pain will often leave within 6 weeks. Also read my book *Three Steps to Happiness—Healing through Joy!* available in my office because this will help you to let go of feelings that may be buried and causing pain.

___ 126. **Rhus Tox** (homeopathic treatment)—dissolve under the tongue as directed on the bottle. Use as needed for muscle pain.

___ 127. **Magnets**—start with spot magnets, insoles, and seat. If they help in 2 months, consider a mattress pad. Available from Bren Jacobsen (phone 410-224-4877) or Amy Podd (phone 410-757-7295).

___ 128. **Copper/Magnet Bracelet**—use nail polish remover to remove any coating on the inside of the bracelet so the copper is in direct contact with your skin.

___ 129 **Quercetin** (for prostate pain)—taking 500 mg twice a day decreases symptoms in both prostadynia and prostatitis.

___ 130. **Flexyx**—can be very effective as a brainwave biofeedback system. See www.flexyx.com for more information.

___ 131. **Cetyl Myristoleate**, 385 mg capsules—take 3 capsules 2 times a day for 10 days. You can raise the dose to a maximum of 17 gm a day. For pain, benefits often persist after the 10 days of treatment.

## *Pharmacologic Pain Treatments*

If you are not clear about the source/type of your pain, there are many sequences in which to try the medications. One order in which to try them is listed below. It can take 2 to 6 weeks to see the full effect of the medication. When there are several medications with the same number (e.g. treatment #139 A, 139B, 139C), if the first medication helped but was not tolerated because of side effects, go to the next medication of the same number. If it simply did not help significantly, go to the next number. If you get partial benefit from a medication, continue it and add the next medication, as needed, to get pain free. I recommend the following order to try pain medications: #136, 135, 133, 134,

137,139,142,141,140A, 147A, 150A, 148A, 143, 151, 155, 157, 154, narcotics.

___ 133. **Tylenol®** (acetaminophen)—for many people, this can be a safe and effective pain medication. Simply be aware that chronic use at too high of a dose can cause liver and sometimes kidney problems. Do not take over 4000 mg a day, and for chronic use it is best to stay under 2000 to 3000 mg daily. If you are taking over 1500 mg of acetaminophen a day on a regular basis, get an extra 500 to 650 mg of NAC from your health food store (or online at www.Vitality101.com) and take it each day along with the vitamin powder. Otherwise, you will deplete a key antioxidant, which is why Tylenol can damage the liver.

___ 134.* **Ultram®** (Rx) (Tramadol), 50mg—take 1 to 2 tablets up to 4 times a day, as needed, for pain. Side effects are less with 4 or fewer tablets a day. May cause nausea/vomiting. **Caution:** Ultram may very rarely cause seizures or raise serotonin too high when combined with anti-depressants.

## *Topical treatments*

___ 135.* **Arizona Pain Formula Cream** (Rx)—rub a pea-sized amount onto painful areas 3 times a day as needed. (Available from Cape Apothecary, phone 410-757-3522, ask for Tom.) You can use this on 3 or 4 "silver dollar" sized areas at a time.

___ 136.* **Lidocaine® Patches** (Lidoderm) (Rx)—can be cut into pieces to put over different areas. Leave the patch on for 12 to 18 hours, and then take it off for the rest of the day. It can help localized pain (i.e. right under the patch). Up to 4 patches can be used at one time each day. It can take 2 to 3 weeks to see if it works.

## *NSAIDs*

Aspirin family medications can cause stomach bleeding. Take with an antacid or food if it upsets your stomach. If gastritis persists, stop the medicine or lower the dose. If you have a black stool (and are not taking iron tablets or Pepto Bismol®), this may represent a life threatening stomach bleed (the stool will often have a very foul smell). If this occurs, go to the hospital emergency room immediately.

___ 137. **Daypro®** (Rx), 600 mg—take 2 each morning as needed.

___ 138. **Voltaren®** (Rx) 50-75 mg 2 times a day as needed.

## *COX-2 Inhibitors*

___ 139A. ***Celebrex®** (Rx) (Celecoxib), 100 to 200 mg—take 1 to 2 times a day for pain. Do not take if you're allergic to sulfa or aspirin (e.g. hives). Do not use over 200 mg a day while on Sporanox® or Diflucan®. The End Pain formula (treatment #114) is a natural form, and it is safer.

___ 139B. **Bextra®** (Rx) (Valdecoxib)—take 10 to 20 mg once a day. Take twice a day for menstrual pain.

## *GABA Agonists*

___ 140A. ***Neurontin®** (Rx) (Gabapentin)—take____mg____times a day (to a maximum of 3600 mg a day). Cut back and increase by 100 mg a day each 4 to 5 days if it causes any uncomfortable or unusual neurologic symptoms or excessive sedation. Begin with 100 to 300 mg at night. Slowly increase to 300 to 900 mg 3 times a day, as is comfortable. In some, pain relief is immediate with a low dose. In others, it can take a minimum of 2400 mg a day. You can increase to 3600 mg a day.

___ 140B. **Gabitril®** (Rx) —take 2 to 4 mg twice a day and increase by a maximum 4 mg daily. Then increase each 3 to 7 days to a maximum of 24 mg a day. Helps both pain and deep sleep. The main side effects are sedation, dizziness, and gastric upset.

___ 140C. **Pregabalin®** (Rx) is helpful for pain, increasing deep sleep, and relieving restless leg syndrome. The main side effects are dizziness and drowsiness, which tend to decrease over time. Unfortunately, it also has another side effect of causing weight gain, ranging between 2 to 5 pounds per month (less with lower doses).

## *Muscle Relaxants*

___ 141. **Flexeril®** (Rx) (cyclobenzaprine), 10 mg—take ½ to 2 at bedtime. This muscle relaxant can cause dry mouth.

___ 142.* **Skelaxin®** (Rx) (metaxolone), 800 mg—take 1 tablet 4 times a day as needed for pain. This is usually not sedating.

___ 143. **Baclofen®** (Rx), 10 to 30 mg—take 1 to 3 times a day (sedating).

___ 144. **Norflex® Tablets** (Rx)—take 1 tablet twice a day.

___ 145. **Dantrium®** (Rx), 25 mg—for muscle spasm take 1 a day for 1 week. Then take one 3 times a day for 1 week, then 2 tablets 3 times a day for 1 week, then 100 mg 3 times a day. Adjust to the lowest dose that feels the best. Stop or lower dose if severe diarrhea occurs. Check liver blood tests at 6, 12, and 24 weeks and then each 1 to 6 months to make sure there is no liver inflammation.

___ 146. **Robaxin®** (Rx) (methocarbimol), 750 mg—take 1 to 2 capsules 3 to 4 times a day, as needed, for pain (sedating).

## *Anti-depressants*

Do not presume that your pain specialist thinks that you have a psychological problem if you're offered an anti-depressant. Tricyclic anti-depressants (e.g. Elavil®/amitriptyline, Doxepin®, etc.) can be dramatically beneficial (even at very low doses) for neuropathic pain. They also improve sleep problems caused by pain. SSRI anti-depressants such as Prozac®, Effexor®, and Celexa® can also be highly effective for pain. These medications raise serotonin, which lowers levels of a major pain messenger (substance P).

## *Tricyclics*

___ 147A. **Elavil®** (Rx) (amitriptyline), 10 mg—take ½ to 5 tablets at bedtime. May cause weight gain or dry mouth. Good for relieving nerve pain and vulvadynia.

___ 147B.***Desipramine®** (Rx) (norpramin)—25 to 150 mg at bedtime or____nortriptyline (Rx) (Pamelor®)—10 to 25 mg at bedtime causes less sedation and fewer side effects than Elavil®, and may be as effective. If sedation is still a problem, consider switching to Doxepin, 10 to 40 mg at bedtime.

___ 147C. ***Doxepin**® (Rx) (Sinequan), 5 to 10 mg—take 5 to 80 mg at bedtime or use Doxepin liquid 10 mg/cc. If a lower dose is needed you can start with 1 to 3 drops at night. A powerful antihistamine. Some people get the greatest benefit with the least next-day sedation with a dose of less than 5 mg a night.

## *SSRIs*

___ 148A. **Effexor**® (Rx) (venlafaxine), 37 1/2 mg—take_____tablets_____times a day.

___ 148B. **Prozac**® (Rx) (fluoxetine), 20 mg—take_____capsule(s) each morning. Begin with 10 mg a day the first week if the full dose makes you hyper.

___ 148C. **Celexa**® (Rx), 20mg—take____tablet(s) a day.

___ 149. **Cymbalta**® (Rx) (duloxetine) 60 mg one-two times a day—a norepinephrine and serotonin reuptake inhibitor. It has fewer side effects and does not cause weight gain. It has been shown to be very helpful in treating FMS pain.

## *Alpha 2 Adrenergic Agonists*

___ 150A. ***Zanaflex**® (Rx) (tizanidine), 4 mg—take with food, 1/2 to 2 tablets 1 to 2 times a day as needed for spasm and/or pain (sedating). Begin with 2 to 4 mg at night. If side effects occur, raise the dose more slowly. Stop if it causes nightmares.

___ 150B. **Catapres® TTS 1 Patch** (Rx)—wear 1 to 3 at a time and change patch weekly. Related to Zanaflex® but cheaper and lowers blood pressure more. Helps pain and raises growth hormone.

## *NMDA Receptor Antagonists*

___ 151.* **Klonopin**® (Rx) (clonazepam), 1/2 mg—begin slowly and work your way up as sedation allows. Begin with 1/2 tablet at bedtime increasing to 1 to 2 mg 3 times a day as needed. Can be very effective for sleep, pain and anxiety (it is in the Valium® family). Klonopin may be addictive. Taking 1/4 to 1/2 tablet in the morning (not more) can actually decrease brain fog in some pain patients.

___ 152. **Dextromethorphan**® (Rx) (DM), 25 mg—take 2 times a day. If on narcotics, (e.g., Codeine/Vicodin®) makes the narcotic more effective and less likely to lose effectiveness. Available from Cape Drugs, phone 800-248-5978.

___ 153. **Amantadine®**(Rx) 100 mg—taking 1 to 3 tablets each morning may help nerve pain and this also is an anti-viral. The most common side effects include visual blurring, dizziness, and nausea.

## *Other Medications*

___ 154. **Keppra®** (Rx) is a new anti-seizure medication that we are just starting to explore and which has been effective when other treatments have not helped. The recommended dose is 250 to 1500 mg twice daily. Can help "burning pain."

___ 155. **Topamax®** (Rx) (topiramate)—begin with 25 to 50 mg daily, and increase by 25 to 50 mg a week until you get the desired effect. This medication is usually given twice a day at a total daily dose of 50 to 100 mg/day for migraines and 200 to 300 mg a day for nerve pain, although lower doses can be effective. This is a medication that I have seen work wonderfully in patients who failed numerous other treatments and it sometimes starts working within a few days. If you get side effects, decrease the dose and perhaps later increase it more slowly until you get the desired effect. The most common side effects are diarrhea, loss of appetite, sedation, and nausea. The nausea will often go away after one has been on the Topamax for 3 months. Along with pain relief, it also has the benefit of causing weight loss. Besides sedation, its most worrisome (albeit unusual) side effect is that it can make your body very acidic, to the point where it is dangerous. Because of this, I recommend checking a blood bicarbonate level every so often (especially if you start developing symptoms such as fatigue) to make sure that the level is over 17.

___ 156. **Benadryl®**—taking 25 or more mg 3 to 4 times daily can often markedly decrease pain (worth trying).

___ 157. **Lamictal®** (Rx) (Lamotrigine), 25mg—take 1 at bedtime for 1 week. Can then increase to one 3 times a day for 1 week. You can go as high as 100 mg 4 times a day. Although rare, it can cause a rash that, if you stay on the medication, can be fatal. Although the vast majority of rashes would not be this dangerous type, to be on the safe side, **STOP LAMICTAL AT FIRST SIGN OF ANY RASH!**

___ 158. **Trileptal®** (Rx)—take 150 mg twice a day. Can go as high as 600 mg 2 times a day.

___ 159. **Zonegran®** (Rx) 100 mg—an anti-seizure medication. Begin with 100 mg a day for 2 weeks and then increase to 2 tablets a day. The maximum dose is 400 mg daily, although most of the benefit occurs at the first 200 mg. Because there have been rare occurrences of a life threatening rash (most rashes caused by the medication are not, however), **stop the medication immediately if you get a rash**.

___ 160. **Permex®** (Rx) (Pramipexole), 1/4 mg—begin with 1 a night and increase by 1 tablet weekly as needed to a maximum of 6 mg. In one study, taking Permex resulted in a 50 percent reduction in pain after 2 months at an average dose of 1.5 mg at bedtime. If stomach pain occurs, Nexium® or similar medications are used during the first month. If restless leg syndrome worsens, Klonopin® is also added at bedtime. Both side effects generally go away as the dose is increased.

___ 161. **Humibid®** (Rx) (guaifenisin), 600 mg—
take_____tablets_____times a day.
No aspirin or herbals can be taken while on Guaifenisin.
GuaiLife, a shorter acting form, may be more effective.
See www.fludan.com for more information.

___ 162. **Risperdal®**(Rx) (Risperidone)—take 1/4 mg to 1 1/2 mg a day (not more). Begin with 1/4 mg and increase by 1/4 mg each 6 weeks. Going above the optimal dose will cancel out the effect. Takes 2 weeks to work. Blocks serotonin (not dopamine) at this low dose. Helps pain, anxiety and sleep.

## *Acetylcholine Raisers*

___ 163. **Aricept®** (Rx) (Donepezil)—take 5 mg in the a.m. (or 2 1/2 mg a.m. and noon) to a maximum of 20 mg a day. This central acetylcholinesterase inhibitor decreases both pain and opiate-induced fatigue by 50 percent in cancer patients. Effects begin within 1 week.

## *Cannabinoids*

___ 164. **Marinol®**(Rx), 5 mg capsules—take 1 to 2 twice a day. As this is a THC extract, it may cause sedation and increased appetite.

## For Opiate Side Effects

___ 165. Constipation is common as an opiate side effect. (See constipation section, treatments #94 – 97.) In addition, opiates can lower testosterone and this should be checked for and treated if loss of libido occurs. They can also cause B2 vitamin deficiencies, so be sure to take the B-complex (see treatment #1). Provigil® (treatment #75) or Aricept® (treatment #163) can also decrease opiate induced fatigue.

## IV Treatments

___ 166. **Lidocaine®** (IV) (Rx)—use 100-500 mg (60-100 mg 1st dose) IV each 3 to 20 days as needed. Give 75 mg IV over a 10 to 15 minute time period, followed by up to 120 mg per hour (total dose 200 to 500 mg). Take with IV Myers Cocktail (see Appendix F). For the first dose, give 60 mg over a ½ hour time period first, and only continue if blood pressure is stable.

## For Interstitial Cystitis

___ 167. **Elmiron®**(Rx), 100 mg 3 times a day. It may take 3 months to work. Take with water at least 1 hour before or 2 hours after eating.

___ 168. **MSM** (Methyl Sulfonyl Methane)—using a dose of 6 to 18 g a day can mimic the effect of DMSO and may be helpful.

___ 169. **Alkaline Urine**—some practitioners have found that patients with interstitial cystitis often have chronic very alkaline urine. This can be aggravated by excessive coffee and cola intake. pH strip paper can be obtained cheaply at most pharmacies and one can test multiple urine samples at home to see if the pH is regularly over 7.0. Also take the enzyme product **URT** (enzyme product No. 24) 4 capsules 5 times a day between meals. During flares, add the enzyme product called **KDY** (kidney) 2 capsules every 20 minutes, as needed. In 2 to 4 hours, the symptoms may subside and the products can then be taken just as needed. (Products are available from my office by phoning 410-573-5389.)

___ 170. **L-arginine**, 500 mg—take 3 times a day for 3 months.

___ 171. **Saw Palmetto**—take 160 mg twice a day for 6 weeks.

## Heartburn, Indigestion or Reflux

For detailed information on how to get off acid blockers naturally, see the article on my web site at www.endfatigue.com (click the "useful articles" button on the left sidebar). Using chronic acid blockers (e.g. Prilosec®) is a poor long-term solution for these problems, because it worsens digestion and your defense against bowel infections. Use the treatment(s) checked off below. After 1 month you can stop your prescription acid blocker and switch to Tagamet® (cimetidine, available over-the-counter), up to 400 mg 3 times a day, as needed. Then taper off the Tagamet as able. Use treatment #2 (Complete Gest Digestive Enzymes) as well and sip warm liquids with meals instead of cold water (digestive enzymes work poorly at cold temperatures). Taking a minute to relax before eating and chewing your food will also help digestion. Coffee (including decaf), colas, aspirin, and/or alcohol can markedly worsen indigestion and increase reflux.

___ 172. **Mastic Gum**, 500 mg—take 2 capsules twice a day for 2 months. Then take as needed.

___ 173. **Heartburn Free** (Enzymatic Therapies)—take 1 every other day for 20 days (may initially aggravate reflux).

___ 174. **DGL Licorice/Rhizinate**, 380 mg (not the sugar-free one)—chew 2 tablets 20 minutes before meals. Available from Enzymatic Therapies/PhytoPharmica.

___ 175. **Saventaro Cat's Claw**—take 1 twice a day (see treatment #66). ■

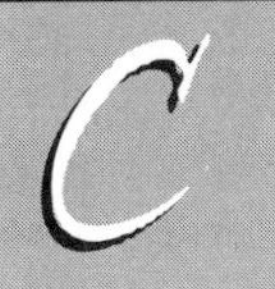

# Resources

## 1. Finding a Physician
## 2. Supplies and Services
## 3. Tools and Products That Help You Get Well

## Finding a Physician

### *Physicians Specializing in Pain and Fibromyalgia:*

1. The sophisticated computerized educational program on my website can analyze your medical history (and laboratory test results, if available) to determine the most important underlying metabolic problems in your case. It will create a treatment protocol tailored to your case that you can institute on your own and will assist and support your doctor in giving you the best possible care. The long form can also create a complete medical record of your case. To do this program go to www.endfatigue.com This web site also has a referral list of practitioners that have done my workshop(s).

2. For physicians specializing in pain (who may or may not be familiar with these metabolic therapies) go to the American Academy of Pain Management web site. This is an outstanding medical society of pain specialists! Go to: www.aapainmanage.org and click on "Patients"

3. I see patients from all over the world in consultation at my office at the following address:

   Jacob Teitelbaum, M.D.<br>
   466 Forelands Road<br>
   Annapolis, MD 21401<br>
   Phone: 410-266-6958<br>
   Fax: 410-266-6104

### *Other Physician Organizations:*

Physicians who can treat the underlying nutritional, sleep, and hormonal deficiencies, as well as the infections that drive your pain (i.e. metabolic therapies) are holistic/comprehensive physicians. They are often familiar with effective pain and fibromyalgia therapies. The following are two of many organizations of physicians who take a comprehensive/holistic approach to medicine:

American College for the Advancement of Medicine
P.O. Box 3427
Laguna Hills, CA 92654
http://www.apma.net

American Holistic Medical Association (AHMA)
4101 Lake Boone Trail, Suite 201
Raleigh, NC 27607
Phone: 919–787–5146
Provides speakers through its Speakers Bureau.

### *Psychological Counseling by Phone:*

Bren Jacobson is an excellent Rolfer, who has spent decades working with people in pain. He is also a minister and does brilliant personal pastoral counseling in person or by phone. He can be reached by phone at 410-224-4877.

### *Physicians Trained in Prolotherapy:*

To find physicians that have been trained in Prolotherapy, please refer to http://www.aaomed.org/ (American Association of Orthopedic Medicine) and http://www.getprolo.com/.

## Supplies and Services

### *To Purchase Natural Products and Prescription Pain Creams:*

Most of the nonprescription supplements I recommend are readily available in most health food stores, and most are also available on my website at www.vitality101.com. You may notice that I often recommend products by Enzymatic Therapy (which sells to health food stores) and Integrative Therapeutics (which sells predominately to practitioners). This is because in my 28 years of practice I have found them to be an incredibly reliable source for natural products. One never has to worry about the purity or potency of their products. I was amazed to find that they both voluntarily registered with the FDA as pharmaceutical companies (even though they only make natural products). Because of this, their products are subject to an incredibly high level of testing. This is almost unheard of in the natural food industry, yet both of these companies did this so you could be sure that what you are getting is the best quality supplement possible. (Now you can see why I do not take money from any company whose products I recommend. I am very opinionated and picky!)

## *To Find the Supplements You Need:*

Online, go to www.Vitality101.com or call 410-573-5389 (my web site and office number).

**Note from Dr. Teitelbaum:** *Most of the products recommended in this book are available through my office and the Vitamin Shop section of my website. The website also contains a sophisticated computer program that will tailor a treatment protocol to your case (we actually hold the patent for a computerized physician—making this was necessary to make effective treatment available for everyone).*

**A word about products bearing my name:** *I developed these products to meet the needs of my patients and others suffering from pain, fibromyalgia, and chronic fatigue. I know that when I see a "Dr. Smith's Formula," I worry that Dr. Smith "sold out." Because of this, I direct any company making my formulas to donate all of my royalties to charity. I also never accept any money from anyone whose products or services I recommend.*

www.enzy.com (to find stores near you that carry these products)

## *For Health Practitioners (to make wholesale purchases):*

1. Integrative Therapeutics carries many of the natural products discussed in this book.
   Phone: 800-931-1709
2. Klabin Marketing makes ProBoost, the best immune stimulant on the market.
   Phone: 800-933-9440
3. Stevia is available from Body Ecology.
   Phone: 1-800-4Stevia

4. For homeopathics, I recommend HEEL. They are the makers of Traumeel Cream
5. Colloidal Silver-Argentyn 23 is available from Natural Immunogenics.
   Phone: 888-328-8840

**For stool culture and sensitivity tests** (does an excellent job with stool testing for ova and parasites, yeast, and bacterial infections), I recommend:

Great Smokies Diagnostic Laboratory (GSML)
63 Zillicoa Street
Asheville, NC 28801
Phone: 800–522–4762
Fax: 828–252–9303
www.gsdl.com

Or

Parasitology Center, Inc.
903 South Rural Road, Suite 101-318
Tempe, AZ 85281
Phone: 480–777–1078 (call Urokeep at 602–545–9236 to get the stool test kit)
Fax: 480-777-1223

## *For Water Filters That Actually Work Well:*

Pure Water
Bren Jacobson
103 Second Street
Annapolis, MD 21401
Phone: 410–224–4877
Web: purewatermd.tripod.com (do not type in www before the web address)
Consultant on health and environmental concerns, especially water, and distributor of Multi-Pure water filters.

### *Compounding Pharmacies:*

To find a compounding pharmacy near you call the Pharmaceutical Compounding Association at 800-221-8768 or the International Academy of Compounding Pharmacies at 800-927-4227 (www.iacprx.org)

My favorite compounding pharmacy (and they ship anywhere in the world) is:

Cape Apothecary
1384 Cape St. Claire Road
Annapolis, MD 21401
Ph. 800–248–5978 or 410–757–3522 or 410–974–1788
Fax: 410–626–7226
www.rxstat.com/capedrug

Cape Apothecary is a holistic compounding pharmacy that fulfills mail orders. Among other products, they can supply pain gels and creams, the sinusitis nose spray, natural testosterone cream, pure dextromethorphan (DM), sustained-release T3 (thyroid hormone), high-dose injectable vitamin B12, natural biestrogen, testosterone, and natural progesterone. Tom the pharmacist lectures at Johns Hopkins and will work with you to adjust pain cream and hormonal formulations to provide the optimum dosage and combination of medications for your case. Cape Apothecary can also supply ingredients for Myers Cocktails.

## Tools and Products That Help You Get Well

### *Energy Revitalization System Vitamin Powder with B-complex*

I developed this product so that my patients could easily get the nutritional support they need without taking handfuls of tablets. As noted above, 100 percent of my royalties go to charity, and the product is available in most health food stores (or at www.Vitality101.com). One good tasting drink and one capsule replaces over 35 tablets of supplements a day. The "Energy Revitalization System" contains over 50 nutrients (almost all in optimal forms and amounts), and can supply outstanding nutritional support for almost everyone. It contains almost all the key nutrients that you need to get from your diet except iron (which is toxic to take unless you are iron deficient), calcium (which blocks thyroid hormone absorption, and should be taken at nighttime), and essential fatty acids (oil and water don't mix). Many people find that simply taking this product for optimal nutritional support can help them feel much better while decreasing and sometimes eliminating their pain. It can replace your multi-vitamin and almost all of the nutritional supplements that most people take.

Some people will develop diarrhea from magnesium-containing products. Most people, however, find that it simply makes them wonderfully regular. If diarrhea or stomach upset is a problem, one can cut the dose of the powder in half or take it with milk, and this will usually take care of the problem. In addition, any supplement containing B vitamins can turn your urine bright yellow. This is normal.

### Energy Revitalization System Vitamin Powder with B-complex Ingredients

Powders can be adjusted (e.g. taking 1/4 to 1/2 scoop 1 to 2 times day in sensitive patients)

This system provides improvement in energy, endurance, and vitality. Often less pain is seen after 2 to 8 weeks. Below are 30 of the over 50 nutrients it contains:

- <u>Vitamin A</u> (7000 IU)—Critical for mucosal immunity and zinc function.
- <u>Vitamin C</u> (750 mg/day)—Critical for immune, **adrenal** and **antioxidant** function.
- <u>Hesperidin</u> (bioflavonoid), (500 mg/day)—blood vessel integrity, immune function, protects against pollutants, decreases prostate pain.
- <u>Vitamin E</u> (100 IU)—**Antioxidant**, blood thinning.
- <u>Vitamin D</u> (600 IU /day)—**bone** strength, **cognitive**, visual, immune function, and can decreases pain.
- <u>Minerals:</u>
    - <u>Boron</u> (2-mg)—**bone** strength. May decrease arthritis. Essential to human health and behavior.
    - <u>Iodine</u> (150 mcg)—**thyroid** function, **temperature** control.
    - <u>Magnesium</u> (200 mg/day as glycinate)—presume deficiency! Most critical nutrient in > 300 reactions and it's **critical for pain management**, Muscle relaxation, **mood, energy**, etc.
    - <u>Zinc</u> (15 mg/day)—deficient in FMS, critical to **immune function, wound healing**.
    - <u>Selenium</u> (200 mcg/day)—**antioxidant, immune** function.
    - <u>Copper</u> (1/2 mg)—may be high or low, for SOD function, superoxide dismutase is one of the body's natural free-radical scavengers that reduce pain and inflammation.
    - <u>Chromium</u> (200 mg)—helps insulin function , **hypoglycemia, weight loss.**
    - <u>Molybdenum</u> (250 mg)—**allergies, sensitivities** (e.g. sulfites).

- Amino Acids:
  - o Serine (500 mg )—antioxidant, immunity, energy.
  - o Lysine (550 mg)—helps make **L-Carnitine**, which is used by the body to transport long chain fatty acids to the mitochondria in your cells, where they are burned for energy. L-Carnitine deficiencies can also appear as mental confusion or cloudiness, angina, and weight gain. Can be antiviral.
  - o Taurine (500 mg)—helps make **energy**.
  - o Tyrosine (500+ mg/day)—**dopamine, norepinephrine, which can decrease pain and increase energy**.

- N-Acetyl-Cysteine (NAC 650 mg initially; 250 to 650 mg maintenance), + Glutamic acid (1000 mg) + Glycine (500 to 1000 mg). These three make **glutathione**, a **critical antioxidant** that maintains antioxidants and vitamins C and E in their reduced (active) forms; plays a role in the **detoxification** of many xenobiotics (foreign compounds); helps **immune** response.

- Malic acid (900 mg/day)—**energy and may decrease muscle pain**.

- B-vitamins—RDA's inadequate, critical for **energy, immunity, nerve/brain** function, treating in preventing nerve pain, etc.
  - ○ B1 (thiamine- 75 mg)—**cognitive** and **muscle**/heart function.
  - ○ B2 (riboflavin-75 mg)—**energy**; helps **migraines**.
  - ○ Niacin (50 mg)—**energy.**
  - ○ B6 (pyridoxine 85 mg)—**energy**, **cognition**, nerve (CTS), swelling, energy etc.
  - ○ Choline (100 mg) methyl group donor, nerve impulses, fat metabolism.
  - ○ Folic acid (800 mcg)—**immunity**, birth defects, etc.
  - ○ Pantothenic acid (50 mg)—**adrenal** function, **energy**.
  - ○ Vitamin B12 (500 mcg) is low or absent in brain in CFS despite normal labs. Critical nutrient-nerve function and pain, cognition, **no** scavenger, blood cells,
  - ○ Biotin (200 mcg)—cofactor for enzyme reactions, healthy skin and nails.
  - ○ Inositol (750 mg)—**anxiety**, mental health, **nerve function and pain**.

## *Fatigued to Fantastic!® Revitalizing Sleep Formula*

This formula helps you get to sleep faster and maintain a healthy sleep cycle through the night so you wake up energized and with less pain. Lack of sleep at night can lead to daytime sleepiness and pain, and negatively impact your daily activities. These herbs also decrease pain directly by acting as muscle relaxants, and they also decrease stress/and anxiety.

Key ingredients in each capsule include:

- Valerian (200 mg)
- Passionflower (90 mg)
- L-Theanine (50 mg)
- Hops (30 mg)
- Wild lettuce (18 mg)
- Jamaica Dogwood (12 mg)

For optimum results, use 1 to 4 capsules taken ½ to 1 ½ hours before bedtime.

## *End Pain Formula*

This natural formula contains:

- Willow bark (40 mg Salicin)
- Boswellia (300 mg)
- Tart Cherry (333 mg)

These are wonderful ingredients for relief of inflammation and pain. For chronic pain, it can take 2 to 6 weeks to see the full effect. Begin with 2 capsules, 3 times a day. After 6 weeks, you can often lower the dose to 1 capsule 3 times day or take it as needed.

## *Fish Oils*

Fish oil deficiencies can contribute to pain and many other problems. I have seen people come off of chronic morphine by taking fish oil. I strongly recommend using the "Eskimo 3" brand because it does not contain mercury, lead, or other toxins. Most other fish oils do contain these toxic elements. It is also not rancid and nasty tasting, and is less likely to come back up and "repeat on you" like most other fish oils. Do you really want every cat in the neighborhood looking up at you when you burp and wondering, "What's that fishy smell?" The usual dose is ½ to 2 Tbsp daily for 3-9 months. Dry eyes, dry mouth, and inflammation are indicators of inadequate fish oil in the body. Health food stores only carry the "Eskimo 3" capsules. The liquid, which is the form I recommend (cheaper and easier than a handful of capsules), is available from health practitioners, pharmacies, and from www.Vitality101.com.

## *Sugar Substitutes*

Here are some points to consider about sugar substitutes:

- Russell Stover® has a whole line of sugar free chocolates that are outstanding.
- There are many healthy sugar substitutes. Stevia is excellent, healthy, and easy to use. The best tasting Stevias I've found are from Body Ecology (phone: 1-800-4-stevia or online at www.vitality101.com) and Stevita (in many shops).
- Inositol (helps anxiety and nerve pain) and xylitol (decreases osteoporosis) look and taste just like sugar. Outside of occasionally causing loose stools, these are healthy and you can use all you want.
- Saccharin® (comes in the pink packets) is also OK.
- I suspect Splenda® will also turn out to be OK.
- I do not recommend aspartame (NutraSweet®).
- Some sugar substitutes can cause diarrhea.

## *Enzymes for Pain Relief and Inflammation*

My favorite enzyme supplements for pain and inflammation are MegaZyme by Enzymatic Therapy and Ultrazyme by Integrative Therapeutics. Ultrazyme and MegaZyme are very helpful in aiding **digestion of your food** when taken **with** meals (but I would rather you use CompleteGest for this). I recommend that you **take them on an empty stomach**, however, because enzymes are most effective at reducing pain and inflammation when you take them between meals so they get absorbed into your body, instead of being used for digestion. For acute pain, enzymes can be taken for a few days as needed. For chronic pain, begin by taking either MegaZyme or Ultrazyme regularly (2 to 3 tablets 3 times a day) between meals for 6 to 12 weeks to see how much it helps or until the pain and inflammation are gone. Then you can take the enzymes as needed. ■

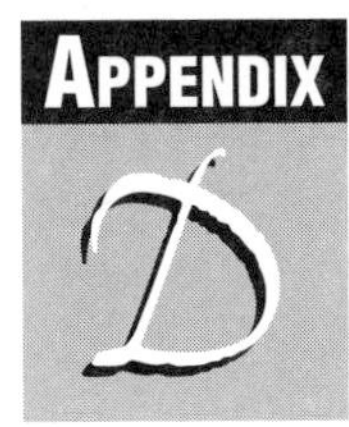

# 1. Study Abstract: Effective Treatment of Chronic Fatigue Syndrome and Fibromyalgia

# 2. Editorial: "Effective Treatment of Fibromyalgia and Myofascial Pain Syndrome: A Clinician's Perspective," by Hal Blatman, M.D., *Journal of the American Academy of Pain Management*

## Study Abstract

Effective Treatment of Chronic Fatigue Syndrome and Fibromyalgia—A Randomized, Double-Blind, Placebo-Controlled, Intent to Treat Study, *Journal of Chronic Fatigue Syndrome* Vol. 8, No. 2, 2001, p.3-28.

Jacob E. Teitelbaum, MD*[1]; Barbara Bird, M.T.,C.L.S.*; Robert M. Greenfield, MD[1]; Alan Weiss, MD[1]; Larry Muenz, PhD[2]; Laurie Gould, BS*[3] [*Annapolis Research Center for Effective FMS/CFIDS Therapies, 466 Forelands Rd., Annapolis, MD 21401; 1) Anne Arundel Medical Center, Annapolis, MD; 2) Gaithersburg, MD; 3) USDA, Beltsville, MD] *No outside funding*

Background: Hypothalamic dysfunction has been suggested in Fibromyalgia (FMS) and Chronic Fatigue Syndrome (CFS). This dysfunction may result in disordered sleep, subclinical hormonal deficiencies, and immunologic changes. Our previously published open trial showed that patients usually improve by using a protocol which treats all the above processes simultaneously. The current study examines this protocol using a randomized, double-blind design with an intent-to-treat analysis.

Methods: Seventy-two FMS patients (thirty-eight active: thirty-four placebo; sixty-nine also met CFS criteria) received all active or all placebo therapies as a unified intervention. Patients were treated, as indicated by symptoms and/or lab testing, for: (1) subclinical thyroid, gonadal, and/or adrenal insufficiency, (2) disordered sleep, (3) suspected NMH, (4) opportunistic infections, and (5) suspected nutritional deficiencies.

Results: At the final visit, sixteen active patients were "much better," fourteen "better," two "same," zero "worse," and one "much worse" versus three, nine, eleven, six, and four, respectively, in the placebo group ($p < .0001$, Cochran-Mantel-Haenszel trend test). Significant improvement in the FMS Impact Questionnaire (FIQ) scores (decreasing from 54.8 to 33.2 versus 51.4 to 47.7) and Analog scores (improving from 176.1 to 310.3 versus 177.1 to 211.9) (both with $p < .0001$ by random effects regression), and Tender Point Index (TPI) (31.7 to 15.5 versus 35.0 to 32.3, $p < .0001$ by baseline adjusted linear model) were seen. Long-term follow-up (mean 1.9 years) of the active group showed continuing and increasing improvement over time, despite patients being able to wean off most treatments.

Conclusions: Significantly greater benefits were seen in the active group than in the placebo group for all primary outcomes. Using an integrated treatment approach, effective treatment is now available for FMS/CFS.

The full text of this and a previous study can be viewed online at www.vitality101.com.

## Editorial: *Journal of the American Academy of Pain Management*

April 2002
by Hal Blatman, M.D.

### Effective Treatment of Fibromyalgia and Myofascial Pain Syndrome: A Clinician's Perspective

In 1983 Drs. Janet Travell and David Simons published the first volume of their work *Myofascial Pain and Dysfunction, The Trigger Point Manual.* Their textbooks have become the foundation of education for treating myofascial pain syndrome (MPS). Although much of the text focused on anatomical and structural aspects of MPS, chapter 4 was dedicated to a discussion of the numerous metabolic perpetuating factors that contribute to the disorder. These factors are thought to contribute to causation as well as preventing recovery. Chapter 4 offers 294 references that support the importance of metabolic perpetuating factors.[1]

During the last several years, public awareness of Fibromyalgia has greatly increased. Practitioners have noted that much of the pain of FMS is related to myofascial trigger points, and that MPS plays a critical role in the disorder. Many physicians have postulated that FMS represents a generalized MPS that is perpetuated by the metabolic factors. Clinical experience and the scientific literature suggest that many of these perpetuating factors need to be treated despite laboratory blood testing falling within the normal range.

With this in mind, it was very exciting to read the recent randomized, double-blind, placebo-controlled study by Teitelbaum et al.,[2] which, years later, finally validates the work of Drs. Travell and Simons. Titled "Effective Treatment of Chronic Fatigue Syndrome and Fibromyalgia - a Randomized Double-blind Placebo-controlled Study," the study found that treating Fibromyalgia patients for the perpetuating factors below resulted in a dramatic improvement vs. placebo ($P<0.0001$):

1. Hormonal deficiencies. Dr. Teitelbaum postulated that hypothalamic dysfunction is a key process in the etiology of Fibromyalgia. Patients with lab tests for thyroid, adrenal and ovarian/testicular function that fell in the normal range were still treated if their clinical picture suggested a hormonal deficiency.

2. Opportunistic infections. As a number of infections can perpetuate MPS, and since FMS is associated with immune dysfunction and opportunistic infections, possible parasitic and fungal infections were treated.

3. Sleep disorders. Lack of adequate deep sleep has been shown to be a factor in chronic pain disorders and FMS. Dr. Teitelbaum treated this very aggressively.

4. Nutritional inadequacies. Nutritional deficiencies were suspected to contribute to chronic, pathologic muscle shortening despite lab testing sometimes being in the normal range. In this study, nutritional needs were aggressively considered and treated.

In the history of medicine, people with undiagnosed and unrecognized diseases such as rheumatoid arthritis, polio and Lyme's disease were often considered to be hypochondriacs until diagnostic tests were developed. Tests are now in development that will likely be specific for the diagnosis of FMS. In the interim, this study by Dr. Teitelbaum et al. confirms what years of clinical success have shown -that the treatment approach described in chapter 4 of The Trigger Point Manual is effective, that subclinical abnormalities are important and that the comprehensive and aggressive metabolic approach to treatment in Teitelbaum's study is highly successful and makes FMS a very treatable disorder. The study by Dr. Teitelbaum et al. and years of clinical experience makes this approach an excellent and powerfully effective part of the standard of practice for treatment of people who suffer from FMS and MPS— both of which are common and devastating syndromes. It is very exciting that this research helps to usher in a new, more effective era in medical care by treating the patient and not only the laboratory tests! ■

1. Travell J, Simons DG, Simons L: Perpetuating Factors. Chapter 4. In: *Myofascial Pain and Dysfunction: The Trigger Point Manual.* Ed.2. Williams and Wilkins, Baltimore MD, 1999.
2. Teitelbaum JE, Bird B, Greenfield RM ,Weiss A., Muenz L, Gould L. Effective Treatment of CFS and Fibromyalgia—A Randomized, Double-blind, Placebo-controlled, Intent to Treat Study. *The Journal of Chronic Fatigue Syndrome.* Volume 8(2), 2001,p. 3 –28.

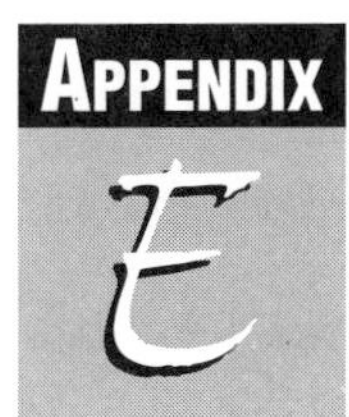

# Why Physicians Do Not Focus on Pain Medicine

by Jacob Teitelbaum, M.D.

Clearly, if pain management is to be adequate, it is necessary for medical schools to do a better job training physicians and/or to recognize that it may be necessary for non M.D.s to be given the legal rights to prescribe, so that they may appropriately take a lead in this role.

With pain being such a common problem, one would wonder why more physicians don't specialize in its treatment. As is often the case in medicine, it boils down to dollars and cents.

Insurance companies pay very poorly for a doctor's time unless they are doing a procedure. For example, if a doctor is performing surgery, a heart catheterization, or even setting a broken bone, he or she will be paid handsomely. If, on the other hand, the doctor is predominantly spending time listening, data-gathering, or conducting an examination so that he or she can make a proper diagnosis, the insurance company will often pay less than the physician's overhead! Basically, the insurance companies pay for the average eight-minute doctor visit. If a doctor spends more than eight minutes on your case, without performing other procedures or tests, the doctor is likely going to lose money. Doctors can afford to do this once in awhile, but they will go bankrupt if they do it on a regular basis.

To give you an idea of the severity of the problem, Ohio has only 335 physicians who designate themselves as pain specialists, with 74 percent of these being anesthesiologists, who often, though not always, are more interested in doing procedures that tend to be invasive. It is estimated that 2.3 million people in Ohio have chronic pain. This means that there is one pain specialists for every 6,865 people suffering with chronic pain. Treating chronic pain is fairly time intensive, and seeing 20 patients a day is a very full day. If the chronic pain patient is only seen every three months, doing the math shows that we need 25 times more pain specialists that we currently have.[1]

The evaluation of pain is a complex and time-consuming process. For reasons that escape me, insurance companies by and large will also not pay for time spent doing simple yet highly effective pain management procedures such as trigger point injections or stretch and spray.

In fact, insurance companies are shooting both themselves and you in the foot by this approach. By not paying adequately for safe and effective procedures, more and more patients are forced into surgery, medications, or nerve blocks, which are often far more expensive, riskier, and less effective than other pain reduction treatments. If your physician spends the necessary time to take a proper history, do a proper examination, and learn and use trigger point injections and/or the stretch and spray procedure, it is unlikely that your doctor will be able to stay in business if he or she accepts what your insurance company considers payment in full.

In addition to being poorly reimbursed by insurance companies (unless they perform procedures, testing, or surgery), pain specialists are often faced with patients who require narcotics for severe and chronic pain. Because of the current political climate, pain specialists often are threatened with loss of their medical license, and sometimes are even arrested for the very appropriate prescribing of these medications. After over a decade of training, would you be willing to lose your license, be driven into bankruptcy, and even be thrown in jail? This is the risk pain specialists face every time they prescribe a narcotic medication—no matter how appropriate it is to give it. Although there are a few doctors who unscrupulously maintain narcotic "pill mills," even pain specialists who are simply providing excellent patient care are being arrested and treated like drug kingpins in the government's "war against drugs." This causes major problems for pain doctors, pharmacists, and suffering patients. In a front-page article in the *Washington Post*, Attorney General John Ashcroft was quoted as saying that arrests of pain specialists who prescribe Oxycontin show "our commitment to bring to justice all those who traffic in this very dangerous drug." The doctor is presumed guilty until proven innocent, and is often judged by people who are hostile to the use of narcotics in chronic pain patients. In the same article, Russell Portenoy, a pain specialist at Beth Israel Medical Center in New York, who is considered one of the fathers of modern pain management, notes that "15 years of progress in treating patients in chronic pain could really be wiped away if these prosecutions continue...treating people in pain isn't easy and there aren't black-and-white answers...but what's happening now is that the medical ambiguity is being turned into allegations of criminal behavior. We have to draw a line in the sand here, or else the treatment will be lost, and millions of patients will suffer." In the same article, Rebecca Patchin, a pain specialist who is a board member of the AMA, notes that an estimated 50 million Americans live with chronic pain. She says that almost half of all Americans will seek care for persistent pain sometime during their lives, but that many will not receive the treatment they need. She notes that "Doctors hear what's happening to other physicians... and that makes them very reluctant to prescribe opiates that patients might well need.[2]

Unfortunately, it will not be doctors who get these misguided laws changed. Doctors attempting to get the laws changed can make themselves targets for those who would take away their medical licenses. The change will come when patients make it clear to their senators and representatives (and the president) that they demand the right to proper care without being treated like drug addicts. Otherwise, government officials will continue to live by the adage, "all pain is tolerable as long as it is somebody else's!" We live in a democracy; be heard, be clear, and make your vote count! The article in the *Washington Post* mentions a group called the "Pain Relief Network" (see www.PainReliefNetwork.org) that is fighting for your right to be pain-free.

The good news is that the large majority of patients with pain can become pain-free without narcotics using the principles in this book. Although I recommend that you make your voice heard, I would direct most of your energy into getting your life back. You can do this now, without waiting for the government to act!

More good news is that things are already starting to change. Doctors are interested in learning more about pain management, and many are aware of their own ignorance in this area. For example, a survey of 247 physicians from various specialties showed that 96 percent were dissatisfied with the training they received in medical school about opiates, and 84 percent were dissatisfied with such training during residencies and fellowships. For patients with persistent pain, 82 percent of providers were uncomfortable prescribing opiates for more than 3 months; 42 percent said they were not prescribing opiates properly, and 34 percent weren't sure whether they were properly prescribing them. Nearly all (94 percent) said that further courses in opioid management would help them in their practices.[3]

## The Relationship Between Prescription and Natural Medicine

Standard allopathic medicine, which focuses predominantly on prescriptions and surgery, offers powerful new techniques that fall outside of what's found in nature. Because they are tailored to specifically suppress certain reactions in the body, they can at times be more powerful than natural medicines. Experience shows, however, that they are also far more likely to be toxic. As the pharmaceutical industry is driven largely by financial motivations (this is not necessarily a bad thing—it's simply how our capitalist system is structured), the ability of a prescription to make money is usually the predominant driving force for its creation. Sadly, this financial influence has resulted in "modern" medicine being more closed minded than scientific. Although physicians are well-meaning, they sometimes attempt to make sure that anyone who is of a different religion than "scientism," is legally prevented from practicing. They also ignore any scientific data that does not fit their belief system!

### *Can We Rely on the Results of Scientific Studies?*

I wish we could. Unfortunately, both clinical experience and research has shown that "troubling financial links between pharmaceutical firms and academic scientists are pervasive and may impact research process." In recent study published in the *Journal of the American Medical Association*, researchers led by Yale's Cary Gross found that industry funding makes it 3.6 times more likely that a study result will be favorable to the sponsor! What makes this interesting is that many doctors and academics would not dream of publishing or relying on a study that is not placebo-controlled, because this increases the chance of a positive outcome by 30 percent. On the other hand, that fact that a drug company paying for a study increases the chance of a positive outcome by 360 percent, does not seem to affect whether they will rely on or publish that study. The Yale study also showed that one quarter of medical researchers have financial ties to companies whose products they're studying, and approximately two thirds of research schools have financial ties these companies as well.

A drug company paying for a study can affect results in a number of ways. As a physician, I have often seen study designs that markedly favor the sponsor's drug. For example, a study would use the proper dose of the sponsor's drug, but too low a dose of the competitor's drugs. In addition, if the study did not give a favorable outcome, the company would not allow the data to be published. Adding to the bias is the fact that research journals are less likely to publish studies showing a negative outcome because this is considered boring or less important. The exception to this, however, is that the journals are happy to publish studies that reflect negatively on natural remedies, no matter how poorly the study was done. Yet they are often unwilling to publish studies that show a positive effect from natural therapies.

The Center for Science in the Public Interest notes, "there is a lot of idealism about how science is isolated and objective. Unfortunately, that's not the case. Money can absolutely influence scientists." In addition, despite the heavy biases of studies that are paid for by the drug companies, the FDA still uses that data in assessing whether drug will be approved. As drug companies funded nearly 60 percent of medical research in United States (spending over $30 billion last year), in addition to spending an enormous amount on television and other advertising, they have enormous clout with both the medical and media establishments. Basically, upsetting them by saying anything bad about them and their products can be a very expensive mistake. A medical journal editor tries very hard to maintain objectivity. But, when given a choice between publishing a study that will result in the journal getting hundreds of thousands of dollars of advertising versus losing this money, the editor may be biased toward publishing the study—people are human.[4] This is one reason for my policy of not taking money from any company whose products I recommend (or for that matter, from any company period).

### *Why Is There a Conflict Between the Two Systems?*

Medicine is evolving. When I was in medical school in the early 1970s, the focus of treatment was on how to poison one body system to bring about balance in another. For example, Prozac® poisons the system that brings serotonin back into the cell, thus raising serotonin levels outside of the cell. This can work well to raise serotonin and treat depression, but poisoning one system to bring balance often throws other systems out of balance. For example, Prozac causes sexual dysfunction and other side effects in upwards of one-third of people who use it. Nonetheless, in a society based on economics and quick fixes, the use of prescription medications such as Prozac moved forward quickly, and squeezed out other branches of the healing arts. This had certain benefits, but often these benefits came at great cost to you, the patient.

It is worth looking at how things came to be the way they are. This gives us both understanding and the ability to choose where we want to go. In the 1800s, there was little research and regulation in the healing arts. The healers and wise women in the tribe would learn what worked from experience and pass on the information to their apprentices in a tribal chain that dated back thousands of years. As world wars and the expansion of Western civilization began to destroy long-standing social structures on the planet, much of this ancient information and experience was lost. Natural medicine declined. In areas where there were not enough well-trained healers/herbalists, accountability was also lost, and we began to see the rise of the "snake oil salesmen."

It was in this context that science began to come to the forefront. People longed for something more valid, from groups in which there was accountability. Scientists provided this, using techniques that allowed ideas to be tested, reproduced, and validated. Because of the natural competition among scientists, their ideas had to make it through much skepticism before being accepted. Testing and validation began to take hold in the healing arts.

As in any system that generates a large amount of money and power, however, financial influences began to have their say. In the early 1900s, research focused on both biophysics (i.e. treatments that affected the body's energy systems) and biochemistry. Politics being what it is, the biochemists gained the upper hand, and research and treatment using biophysics was marginalized and suppressed. Seeing which way the political winds of change were blowing, many of the greatest names in modern medicine switched from biophysics to biochemistry. Medical schools were established (which initially focused on using natural therapies). Standardized curriculums and tests were developed, and it became possible to develop reliable conditions for licensing doctors. To counteract "snake oil salesman," who were preying on the public, state governments developed licensing requirements for the practice of the healing arts, bringing more credibility, power, and respect to the field. Medicine was therefore able to attract those people who were compassionate healers. The fields of allopathic medicine and biochemistry blossomed.

As our understanding of chemistry evolved, it began to change the face of our country. We went from almost no foreign chemicals in our environment, to tens of thousands of new chemicals that our bodies had to detoxify. These chemicals are added to our food, water supply, building materials, clothing, and not surprisingly, to our medications. In addition, where a natural substance could not be patented, new chemicals could be. As a patent prevents competition, more money can be made from a patented chemical (e.g. for indigestion, patentable acid blockers can cost over $2 a pill, where non patentable calcium carbonate may cost a nickel). People realized that there was a lot of money to be made in medicine and in patentable medications. This money was used to influence legislation and people's perceptions in an attempt to eliminate the competition.

Language was added to legislation to consolidate allopathic medicine's power. As the FDA was (appropriately) developed to protect public safety in the face of creating thousands of new chemical medications, language was added saying that a manufacturer could not claim that something was effective for treating an illness unless it went through the FDA approval process. As this process costs $400 to $800 million per treatment, only things that are patentable (i.e. not natural) can recoup these enormous costs. Vitamin B6 used for carpal tunnel syndrome is an excellent example. Treating carpal tunnel syndrome with 250 mg of Vitamin B6 daily for six weeks costs about $9 per patient. Vitamin B6 manufacturers would therefore find it impossible to recoup the cost of getting FDA approval for this treatment, and cannot advertise the vitamin for the treatment of carpal tunnel syndrome. Because of this, most patients instead spend between $2,000 and $4,000 to have surgery. This situation is the same for hundreds of other non patentable, effective, inexpensive, and relatively safe treatments. The FDA has even been fighting to make it illegal for stores that sell supplements to hand out copies of well-conducted scientific studies showing the effects of the supplements!

In one legislative stroke, it became illegal for the manufacturer of natural medicines/products to advertise or even to give you information about how these natural products can help you get well, regardless of how good the scientific data supporting the claim was. Legislation was also pushed through saying that anyone who was not an M.D. or an osteopathic physician could not diagnose or treat you. In addition, it was illegal for manufacturers of natural products to give the patient the research studies and information needed to make an informed decision. At the same time, we were (mistakenly) taught in medical school that nutritional and natural therapies had no scientific basis and were only use by "quacks." We were told that only "old-fashioned" (i.e. uneducated and stupid) doctors would use these treatments. Thus, despite large amounts of scientific data supporting natural medicine, you'll find that your doctor will usually not know about this data, may be hostile to it, and will sometimes even refuse to look at the studies. Modern medicine went from using the wonderful tool of science to becoming the "religion" of Scientism.

Fortunately, as always, life moves forward seeking balance and growth. Although it had its strengths, people also began to recognize allopathic medicine's weaknesses. Research continued on natural and energy (e.g. acupuncture) therapies despite lack of funding and acceptance by mainstream journals. Many practitioners, seeing how effective natural therapies were, explored this expanding body of research. As medicine was hostile to and turned a blind eye to this research, those who were M.D.s (like myself) were often introduced to this information by our patients.

I came out of medical school with the impression that if an important treatment existed for an illness, I would know about it. If someone claimed he or she could effectively treat a non treatable disease, that person was a quack. If such a treatment existed, I would surely have been taught about it.

I was wrong.

When I first started my practice, patients would ask me if I knew about certain herbal or nutritional treatments for illnesses. For example, one patient asked me if I had ever heard about using coenzyme Q10 for congestive heart failure. "That's nonsense," I answered. "If coenzyme Q10 helped congestive heart failure, don't you think I would have been taught to use that instead of doing heart transplants?" I said that I would look into it, however.

Joyce Miller, the Anne Arundel Medical Center librarian, has always been happy to obtain studies for me (and she has obtained many thousands over the years). When she did a literature search on coenzyme Q10, she found a number of studies showing it could be very beneficial in treating congestive heart failure. I thought that was curious. Over the next few months, this scenario was played out again and again. I decided to keep notes on these rare "pearls" in a thirty-page spiral notebook. My notes are now over a thousand pages long.

The area of natural medicine has been growing tremendously in the last few decades and is now able to help give you your life back! As an example, combining natural and prescription therapies has allowed us to research and develop highly effective treatments for people with chronic fatigue syndrome and fibromyalgia. These syndromes are characterized by exhaustion, widespread pain, brain fog, and insomnia—crippling over 6 million Americans. Most doctors tell patients that nothing can be done and they simply have to live with the illness. Natural practitioners, however, know that this is not the case. "Gold standard" placebo-controlled research demonstrates that over 91 percent of patients can now get marked improvement using an Integrative Medicine approach (the full text of the studies can be seen at www.vitality101.com). In fact, natural medicine is now able to markedly improve the treatment of most illnesses!

Please recognize that because most physicians were trained in university hospitals, over ninety-five percent of the clinical training that your M.D. received was in treating severe, life-threatening illnesses. I was taught more about how to tell whether fluid coming from the patient's nose was from a skull fracture than I was taught about how to treat a common cold! It was somehow presumed that if we could save your life in acute life-threatening emergencies, we would also magically know how to treat common non-emergency problems. As most of you with pain, fatigue, hormonal, or other day-to-day problems have learned, this is sadly not the case.

The good news is that as more and more doctors familiarize themselves with the scientific literature, many are becoming more open minded to therapies that can help you. They are trying to do the best they can, and progress is occurring. Comprehensive Medicine, which combines the best of natural and prescription therapies, is well on its way to becoming the medicine of the future! ■

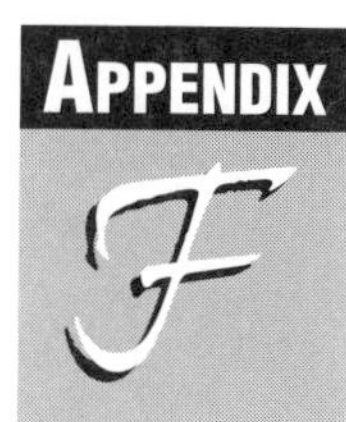

# Myers Cocktail

**The following are instructions for making up and administering the slow IV Myers Push (MP).**

| Supplies Needed | Amount |
|---|---|
| **1.** Bacteriostatic water | 7 cc |
| **2.** Ascorbic acid (500 mg/ml), preservative-free | 1 to 10 cc |
| **3.** Magnesium sulfate ($MgSO_4$), 50 percent (0.5g/ml) | 2 to 4 cc |
| **4.** Pyridoxine (100mg/ml), preservative free | 1 cc |
| **5.** Hydroxycobalamin (3,000 mcg/ml) | 1 cc (give IM) |
| **6.** B-Complex 100 | 0.5 to 1 cc |
| **7.** Dexpanthenol (250 mg/ml) | 0.5 cc |
| **8.** Glutathione, 200 mg per cc (optional) | 2–5 cc *(Push in separately. Do not mix in the same syringe with other nutrients)* |
| **9.** 20-cc or 25-cc syringes | |
| **10.** 18 gauge, 1 to 1 1/2-inch needles | |
| **11.** 25 gauge, 3/4-inch butterfly sets | |
| **12.** Calcium gluconate, 10 percent, preservative-free (optional) | 4 to 10 cc |

ms 1 through 3 and 6 through 12 can be ordered (among other ces) from Harvard Drug Company (Phone: 800-783-7103). Item 4 n be obtained from compounding pharmacies, including Pathways and Wellness and Health Pharmaceuticals. Item 5 can be purchased from G.Y. and N. Most of the above items are also available from McGuff (Phone: 800-854-7220) or Cape Apothecary (Phone: 800–248–5978 or 410–757–3522 or 410–974–1788).

To make the Myers Push (MP), draw up each ingredient using a separate syringe/needle and squirt it into the mouth of a 20-cc to 25-cc syringe. Attach the 25-gauge butterfly to the large syringe, pushing fluid through the butterfly tubing until the entire tubing and needle are filled. Now the mixture is ready for venipuncture and a slow IV push. The glutathione should be kept in the initial syringe (not mixed with other nutrients) and pushed in over 1 to 10 minutes (1 cc every one to two minutes).

The dose of $MgSO_4$ typically begins at 2 cc. If the patient feels comfortable, without dizziness, nausea, or hypotension (warmth in the neck, face, chest, abdomen, groin, and/or extremities is normal, and is a sign of physiological action of the magnesium as a vasodilator), I usually increase the $MgSO_4$ to 4cc and give it over 10 to 40 minutes. Alternately, all these nutrients can be added in an IV bag and allowed to drip in over 30 to 60 minutes.

The desired result is to inject at a rate at which the patient feels comfortable warmth without **excessive** flushing or feeling ill—that is, dizziness, nausea, and headache- symptoms that are rare.

Prior to the injection, it is important for the patient to be instructed to give frequent feedback about any developing warm feeling early on, so that the injection may be slowed down, or even temporarily stopped, before excessive, uncomfortable flushing occurs. Likewise, feedback by the patient needs to be given when the warm feeling has mostly subsided so that the injection may be resumed at a reduced rate. Eventually, the infusion will find the "happy medium" rate of injection, which maintains the "comfortable warmth" (see above).

Also, prior to the first few MP injections, explain that a taste of B vitamins usually appears during the infusion, often early in the push.

The physician needs to consider one major option, which has become routine in many quarters—the possible addition of calcium gluconate, 10 percent injectable. Some of the major reasons for deciding to include calcium are:

- If the patient feels consistently unwell for any reason after the MP (weakness, fatigue, sleepiness, palpitations—all rare and mild, if present).
- If the patient has a history, or laboratory evidence, of calcium deficit.
- If the physician's clinical judgment dictates it for any reason.

The dose of calcium gluconate 10 percent injectable varies from 4 cc to 10 cc, depending on the clinician's judgment. The key is to maintain balance without diluting the magnesium's positive effects.

A final caveat is that one needs to keep in mind the third of the troika—potassium. Over a period of time, IV magnesium may deplete potassium; the danger is that one may be tempted to increase the dose of magnesium, only to aggravate the low potassium picture. Always keep in mind that a potassium deficit may prevent magnesium repletion and vice-versa.

It is also, of course, possible to create a calcium deficit by the MP. However, potassium depletion, in my experience, is clinically more frequent and more symptom-provoking, and at times alarming. (If needed, give the potassium by mouth—**not** IV. **IV push potassium is FATAL**. I use Micro K Extendtabs, 10 MEQ, 1 to 2 times a day if potassium levels are under 4.0.) ■

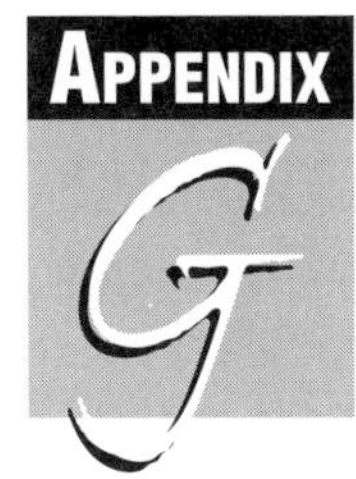

# Footnotes/References


## Introduction—From Pain to Pain Free!

1. Sipkoff, M. "Training Needed for Pain Treatment." The Quality Indicator, November 2003 pp 8 – 12.
2. David L. Caraway, M.D., Ph.D. Medscape—American Academy of Pain Medicine. Highlights of the American Academy of Pain Medicine CME http://www.medscape.com/viewarticle/472404.
3. Stewart W.F., et al. "Lost Productive Time and Cost due to Common Pain Conditions in the US Workforce." *Journal of the American Medical Association*, 2003; 290: 2443 – 2454.

## Chapter 1: Getting Started—Why We Have Pain

1. *Alternative Medicine*, February 2004 pp 84 – 85.

## Chapter 2: Optimizing Nutritional Support Easily

1. R.M. Marston and B.B. Peterkin. "Nutrient Content of the National Food Supply," *National Food Review*, Winter 1980, pp 21 – 25.
2. ibid and J.H. Nelson. "Wheat: Its Processing and Utilization." *American Journal of Clinical Nutrition*, 41, supplement (May 1985): 1070 – 1076.
3. H.A. Schroeder. "Losses of Vitamins and Trace Minerals Resulting from Processing and Preservation of Foods." *American Journal of Clinical Nutrition*, 24 (5) (May 1971): 562 – 573.
4. S.B. Eaton and N. Konner. "Paleolithic Nutrition. A Consideration of Its Nature and Current Implications." *The New England Journal of Medicine*, 312 (5) (31 January 1985): 283 – 289.
5. H.C. Trowell, ed. *Western Diseases: Their Emergence and Prevention* Cambridge, MA: Harvard University Press, 1981.
6. J.G. Travell and D.G. Simons. *Myofascial Pain and Dysfunction: The Trigger Point Manual*, Vol. I (Baltimore, MD: Williams & Wilkins, 1983), pp 103 – 164.
7. B. Kennes, I. Dumont, D. Brohee, et al. "Effect of Vitamin C Supplements on Cell-Mediated Immunity in Old People." *Gerontology*, 29 (1983): 305 – 310.
8. R.K. Chandra. "Effect of Macro and Micro Nutrient Deficiencies and Excess on Immune Response." *Food Technology*, February 1985, pp 91 – 93.
9. S. Chandra, et al. "Undernutrition Impairs Immunity." *Internal Medicine*, 5 (December 1984): 85 – 99.

10. R.K. Chandra, et al. "NIH Workshop on Trace Element Regulation of Immunity and Infection." *Nutrition Research*, 2 (1982): 721 – 733.

11. M.C. Talbott, L.T. Miller, and N.I. Kerkvliet. "Pyridoxine Supplementation: Effect on Lymphocyte Responses in Elderly Persons." *American Journal of Clinical Nutrition*, 46 (4) (October 1987): 659 – 664.

12. S.N. Meydani, M.P. Barklund, S. Liu, et al. "Vitamin E Supplementation Enhances Cell-Mediated Immunity in Healthy Elderly Subjects." *American Journal of Clinical Nutrition*, 52 (3) (September 1990): 557 – 563.

13. W. Mertz, ed. "Beltsville 1 Year Dietary Intake Survey." *American Journal of Clinical Nutrition*, 40, supplement (December 1984): 1323 – 1403.

14. E. Braunwald, ed. *Harrison's Principles of Internal Medicine,* 11th ed. (New York: McGraw Hill, 1987), p 1496.

15. S. Chandra, et al. "Undernutrition Impairs Immunity." op. cit.

16. R.K. Chandra, et al. "NIH Workshop on Trace Element Regulation of Immunity and Infection." op.cit.

17. T. Walter, S. Arredondo, M. Arevalo, et al. "Effect of Iron Therapy on Phagocytosis and Bactericidal Activity in Neutrophils of Iron-Deficient Infants." *American Journal of Clinical Nutrition*, 44 (6) (December 1986): 877 – 882.

18. T.F. Kirn. "Do Low Levels of Iron Affect Body's Ability to Regulate Temperature, Experience Cold?" *Journal of the American Medical Association*, 260 (5 August 1988): 607.

19. L.S. Darnell. "Abstract 21." *American Journal of Clinical Nutrition*, supplement.

20. D.C. Rushton, I.D. Ramsay, J.J. Gilkes, et al. "Ferritin and Fertility," Letter to the editor. *The Lancet*, 337 (8757) (22 June 1991): 1554.
J. Lindenbaum, E.B. Healton, D.G. Savage, et al. "Neuropsychiatric Disorders Caused by Cobalamin Deficiency in the Absence of Anemia or Macrocytosis." *The New England Journal of Medicine*, 318 (26) (30 June 1988): 1720 – 1728.

21. W.S. Beck. "Cobalamin and the Nervous System." Editorial. *The New England Journal of Medicine*, 318 (1988): 1752 – 1754.

22. J. Lindenbaum, I.H. Rosenberg, P.W. Wilson, et al. "Prevalence of Cobalamin Deficiency in the Framingham Elderly Population." *American Journal of Clinical Nutrition*, 60 (1) (July 1994): 2 – 11.

23. *The Health Resource Newsletter*. Volume 20 (1), 2004, p 2.

24. M.S. Seelig. "The Requirement of Magnesium by the Normal Adult." *American Journal of Clinical Nutrition*, 14 (June 1964) 342 – 390.

25. L. Lakshmanad, et al. "Magnesium Intakes and Balances." *American Journal of Clinical Nutrition*, 60 (6 Supplement) (December 1984): 1380 – 1389.

26. Prien EL, et al. "Magnesium oxide – pyridoxine therapy for recurring calcium oxalate urinary calculi." *Journal of Urology*, 112: 509 – 12, 1974
Wright JV. "Given IV, magnesium can help acute kidney stones to pass." *Nutrition and Healing*, Volume 10, issue 5 May 2003.

27. Presentation at the American College of Rheumatology annual meeting 2003. *Pain Medicine News*, January/February 2004. p15.

28. Plotnikoff G.A. Mayo Clinic Proceedings, December 2003; Volume 78: pp 1463 – 1470.

29. Web MD Medical News. Salynn Boyles. December 10, 2003.

30. InteliHealth. "High intake of vitamin D linked to reduced risk of multiple sclerosis" Jan 12 2004.

31. *Neurology*, 2004; 62: 275 – 280.

## Chapter 3: Getting 8 to 9 Hours of Sleep a Night—The Foundation of Pain Relief


1. Julia Sommerfeld. www.MSNBC.com/news/732683. April 3, 2002.
2. C.A. Everson. "Sustained Sleep Deprivation Impairs Host Defense." *The American Journal of Physiology*, 265 (5 Part 2) (November 1993): R1148 – R1154.
3. S. Pillemer, L.A. Bradley, L.J. Crofford, et al. "The Neuroscience and Endocrinology of FMS–[An NIH] Conference Summary." *Arthritis and Rheumatism*, 40 (11) (November 1997): 1928 – 939.
4. H. Moldofsky and P. Scarisbrick. "Induction of Neuresthenic Musculoskeletal Pain Syndrome by Selective Sleep Stage Deprivation." *Psychosomatic Medicine*, 38 (1) (January-February 1976): 35 – 44.
5. A.M. Drewes, K.D. Nielson, S.J. Taagholt, et al. "Slow Wave Sleep in FMS," Abstract. *Journal of Musculoskeletal Pain*, 3 (Supplement 1) (1995): 29.
6. Agargun, M.Y., et al. "Sleep Quality and Pain Threshold in Patients with Fibromyalgia." *Comprehensive Psychiatry*, 40(3): 226-228,1999.
7. Ursin, R., et al. "Relations among Muscle Pain, Sleep Variables, and Depression." *The Journal of Musculoskeletal Pain*, 7(3) 1999. p59 – 72.
8. Moldofsky H. "Sleep and Pain." *Sleep Med Rev*, 2001. Oct: 5(5): 385 – 396.
9. Moran N. [in the Doctors guide Review] "The Contribution of Pain: Report of Sleep Quality and Depressive Symptoms to Fatigue and Fibromyalgia." *Pain*, 2002 December;100(3): 271 – 9.
10. "Melatonin Use in Older Patients." *Family Practice News*, October 1, 2000: 16.
11. R. Cluydt. "Insomnia Treatment—A Postgraduate Medicine Special Report." 114 – 123.
12. Fibromyalgia Network. April 2004. p 6 – 7.
13. Todorov, A.B., et al. "Tiagabine and gabapentin in the management of chronic pain and sleep disturbances." Poster presentation. 22nd annual meeting of the American Pain Society, Chicago, Illinois, March 20 2 – 23, 2003.
14. Mathias, S., et al. The "GABA uptake inhibitor Gabitril promotes slow wave sleep in normal elderly subjects." *Neurobiology of Aging*, 22: 247 – 253, 2001.


## Chapter 4: Treating Hormonal Deficiencies


1. G.R. Skinner, R. Thomas, M. Taylor, et al. "Thyroxine Should be Tried in Clinically Hypothyroid but Biochemically Euthyroid Patients." *British Medical Journal*, 314 (7096) (14 June 1997): 1764.
2. G.R.B. Skinner, D. Holmes, A. Ahmad, et al. "Clinical Response to Thyroxine Sodium in Clinically Hypothyroid but Biochemically Euthyroid Patients." *Journal of Nutritional and Environmental Medicine*, 10 (2) (June 2000): 115 – 125.
3. R.A. Nordyke, T.S. Reppun, L.D. Madanay, et al. "Alternative Sequences of Thyrotropin and Free Thyroxine Assays for Routine Thyroid Function Testing Quality and Cost." *Archives of Internal Medicine*, 158 (3) (9 February 1998): 266 – 272.
4. J.G. Travell and D.G. Simons. *Myofascial Pain and Dysfunction: The Trigger Point Manual*, Vol. 1 (Baltimore, MD: Williams & Wilkins, 1983), pp 103 – 164.
5. J.G. Travell. "Identification of Myofascial Trigger Point Syndromes: A Case of Atypical Facial Neuralgia." *Archives of Physical Medicine and Rehabilitation*, 62 (1981): 100 – 106.

6. D.G. Simons. "Myofascial Pain Syndrome Due to Trigger Points." *International Rehabilitation Medicine Association Monograph Series*, 1 (November 1987).

7. J.C. Lowe, R.L. Garrison, A.J. Reichman, et al. "Effectiveness and Safety of $T_3$ Therapy for Euthyroid Fibromyalgia: A Double-Blind, Placebo-Controlled Response Driven Crossover Study." *Clinical Bulletin of Myofascial Therapy*, 2 (2/3) (1997): 31 – 58.

8. J.C. Lowe, A.J. Reichman, and J. Yellin. "The Process of Change During T3 Treatment for Euthyroid Fibromyalgia: A Double-Blind, Placebo-Controlled, Crossover Study." *Clinical Bulletin of Myofascial Therapy*, 2 (2/3) (1997): 91 – 124.

9. J. Teitelbaum and B. Bird. "Effective Treatment of Severe Chronic Fatigue: A Report of a Series of 64 Patients." *Journal of Musculoskeletal Pain*, 3 (4) (1995): 91 – 110.

10. McLean R. "Thyroid Hormone Therapy Reduces Chronic Pain and Fatigue." *Pain Medicine News*. p 20 – 21. Based on a Presentation at the 2003 Annual Meeting of the American College of Obstetricians and Gynecologists.

11. Press release on AACE web site: http://www.aace.com/pub/tam2003/press.php.

12. Canaris G.J., et al. "The Colorado Thyroid Disease Prevalence Study." *Archives of Internal Medicine*, Feb 28, 2000 p 526 – 534.

13. National Assn of Clinical Biochemistry web site. http://www.nacb.org/lmpg/thyroid_LMPG_PDF.stm.

14. Hak, A.S. "Subclinical Hypothyroidism is an independent Risk Factor for Atherosclerosis and MI in Elderly Women." *Annals of Internal Medicine*, 2000; 132: p270 – 278.

15. Allan, W.C, et al. "Maternal Thyroid Deficiency and Pregnancy Complications: Implications for Population Screening." *Journal of Medical Screening*, 2000 p 127 – 130.

16. Haddow, J.E., et al. "Maternal Thyroid Deficiency During Pregnancy and Subsequent Neuropsychological Development of the Child." *New England Journal of Medicine*, 1999: p 549 – 555.

17. J. Teitelbaum and B. Bird. "Effective Treatment of Severe Chronic Fatigue: A Report of a Series of 64 Patients." *Journal of Musculoskeletal Pain*, 3 (4) (1995): 91 – 110.

18. M. Jefferies, *Safe Uses of Cortisol*, 2nd edition, monograph (Springfield, IL: Charles C. Thomas, 1996).

19. R.A. Anderson, et al. "Chromium and Hypoglycemia." abstract, *American Journal of Clinical Nutrition*, 41 (4) (April 1985): 841.

20. W.M. Jefferies. "Low-Dosage Glucocorticoid Therapy. An Appraisal of Its Safety and Mode of Action in Clinical Disorders, Including Rheumatoid Arthritis." *Archives of Internal Medicine*, 119 (3) (March 1967): 265 – 278.

21. J.E. Teitelbaum, B. Bird, R.M. Greenfield, et al. "Effective Treatment of CFS and FMS: A Randomized, Double-Blind Placebo Controlled Study." *Journal of Chronic Fatigue Syndrome*, 8 (2) (2001).

22. W.M. Jefferies, *Safe Uses of Cortisol*, 2nd edition, monograph (Springfield, IL: Charles C. Thomas, 1996).

23. Tennant F. *Practical Pain Management*, July/August 2004, p 60.

24. Edwards E, et al. "Testosterone Propianate As a Therapeutic Agent in Patients with Organic Disease of the Peripheral Vessels." *New England Journal of Medicine*, 1939; 220 – 865.

25. Jaffee, M. "Effect of Testosterone Cypionate on Post Exercise ST Segment Depression." *British Heart Journal*, 1977: 39: 1217 – 1222.

26. Lesser, M. Testosterone Propionate Therapy in 100 Cases of Angina Pectoris. *Journal of Clinical Endocrinology*, 1946; 6: 549 – 557.

27. Reuters Medical News. June 22, 2000. "Testosterone Patches Improve Exercise Capacity in Men with Angina."

28. Winkler, U. *Effects of Androgens on Hemostasis.* Maturitas. 1996; 24: 147 – 155.

29. Wright, J.V., Lenard, L. *Maximize Your Vitality and Potency, for Men over 40.* Smart Publications; 1999 (an excellent reference for those who would like to explore the topic further).

## Chapter 5: Infections

1. William G. Crook. *The Yeast Connection and the Woman.* (Jackson, TN: Professional Books, 1995).

2. G. Reid, K. Millsap, and A.P. Bruce. "Implantation of Lactobacillus casei var. Rhamnosus into Vagina." *The Lancet*, 344 (8931): 1229.

3. G.P. Holmes, J.E. Kaplan, N.M. Gantz, et al. "Chronic Fatigue Syndrome: A Working Case Definition." *Annals of Internal Medicine*, 108 (1988): 387 – 389.

4. L. Galland, M. Lee, H. Bueno, et al. "Giardia as a Cause of Chronic Fatigue." *Journal of Nutritional Medicine*, 1 (1990): 27 – 32.

5. Ann Louise Gittleman. *Guess What Came to Dinner: Parasites and Your Health* (Garden City Park, NY: Avery Publishing Group, 1993).

6. D.G. Simons. "Myofascial Pain Syndrome Due to Trigger Points." *International Rehabilitation Medicine Association Monograph Series, I* (November 1987).

7. J.G. Travell and D.G. Simons. *Myofascial Pain and Dysfunction: The Trigger Point Manual*, Vol. I (Baltimore, MD: Williams & Wilkins, 1983), pp 103 – 164.

## Chapter 7: The Biochemistry of Pain

1. *Journal of the American Geriatrics Society.* 1998; 46: 635 – 651.

## Chapter 8: Neuropathic (Nerve) Pain and Reflex Sympathetic Dystrophy (RSD)

1. Grond S., et al. *Pain*, 1999: 79: 15 – 20.

2. Berger, A., Dukes, E.M, Oster, G. "Clinical characteristics and economic costs of patients with painful neuropathic disorders." *Journal of Pain*, 2004 Apr; 5 (3): 143 – 9.

3. Backonja, M. "Pathogenesis and treatment of neuropathic pain in older adults." *American Journal of Pain Management*, 14(2) April 2004. p 9S – 18S.

4. Ayres, S., et al. "Post herpes zoster neuralgia: response to vitamin E therapy." *Archives of Dermatology*, 108: 855 – 56, 1973).

5. Cochrane, T. Letter, *Archives of Dermatology*. 111: 396, 1975.

6. Furtado, D., et al. *Rev Clin Espan*, Madrid 5: 416, 1942.

7. Borsook, H., et al. "The relief of symptoms of major trigeminal neuralgia following the use of vitamin B 1 and concentrated liver extract." *Journal of the American Medical Association*, April 13, 1940, p 1421.

8. Schulz, J.B., et al. "Involvement of free radicals in excitotoxicity in vivo." *Journal of Neurochemistry*, 1995; 64: pp 2239 – 2247.

9. Backonja, M.M., et al. "Gabapentin for the symptomatic treatment of painful neuropathy in patients with diabetes colitis: a randomized controlled trial." *Journal of the American Medical Association*, 1998; 280: 1831 – 1836.

10. Backonja, M.M. "Anticonvulsants for neuropathic pain syndromes." *Clinical Journal of Pain*, 2000; 16 (2 suppl): s67 – s72.

11. Backonja, M.M. "Gabapentin monotherapy for symptomatic treatment of painful neuropathy: a multicenter, double-blind, placebo-controlled trial in patients with diabetes mellitus." *Epilepsia*, 1999; (40 suppl): s57 – s59.

12. *Neurology* 2003;60: 1391 – 2.
*International Journal of Pharmaceutical Compounding* 1998; 2: 122 – 7.

13. Meier, T., et al. "Efficacy of lidocaine patch 5 percent in the treatment of focal peripheral neuropathic pain syndromes: a randomized double-blind, placebo-controlled study." *Pain*, 2003; 106: 151 – 158.

14. *The Pain Clinic*, October 2003, p 27.

15. *Wounds*, 2003; 15 (eight): 272 – 276.
*The Pain Clinic*, 2000; 12 (1): 47 – 50.

16. *British Journal of Clinical Pharmacology*, 2000; 49: 574 – 9.

17. Reifg, Anesth. *Pain Med*, 2003 July – August; 28 (4): 289 – 93.

18. Davis, J.L., Smith, R.L. "Painful peripheral diabetic neuropathy treated with Venlafaxine extended-release capsules." *Diabetes Care*, 1999; 11: 1909 – 1910.

19. *Primary Psychiatry*, July 2003, Psychopharmacology Reviews, "Venlafaxine Effective for Painful Polyneuropathy." p 41.

20. Sindrup, S.H., et al. "Tramadol relieves pain and allodynia in polyneuropathy: a randomized, double-blind, controlled trial." *Pain*, 1999; 1: 85 – 90.

21. Vinik, A., et al. "Topiramate in the treatment of painful diabetic neuropathy: results from a multicenter randomized double-blind placebo-controlled trial," Abstract. *Neurology*, 2003; 60 (supplement 1): A154 – A155.

22. Zakrzewska, J.M., et al. "Lamictal in refractory trigeminal neuralgia: results from a double-blind placebo-controlled crossover trial." *Pain*, 1997; 2: 223 – 230.

23. Simpson, D.M., et al. "Lamictal for HIV associated painful sensory neuropathies: a placebo-controlled trial." *Neurology*, 2003; 9: 1508 – 1514.

24. Krusz, J. "Lamotrigine in the treatment of Neuropathic Pain" [abstract 758] *Journal of Pain*, 3(2, Suppl.1): 40, 2002.

25. Semenchuk, M.R. *Journal of Pain*, 1 (4) 2000. p 285 – 292.

26. Todorov, A.B., et al. "Tiagabine and gabapentin in the management of chronic pain and sleep disturbances," Poster presentation. 22nd annual meeting of the American pain Society, Chicago, Illinois, March 22 – 23, 2003.

27. Strickland, J., et al. "Use of Gabitril in the Management of Cancer Related Neuropathic Pain," Poster presentation. 22nd annual meeting of the American pain Society, Chicago, Illinois, March 22 – 23, 2003.

28. Hamza, M. "Initial experience with oxcarbazepine in the treatment of idiopathic neuropathic pain," [abstract 756] *Journal of Pain*, 3(2, Suppl.1): 40, 2002.

29. Ahmad, M., et al. "NMDA receptor antagonists – recent advances in chronic pain." *The Pain Clinic*, April 2001 p 25 – 31.

29A. *Journal of Pain Symptom Management*, 2001 Aug; 22(2): 699 – 703.

30. lson, B.D. *Primary Psychiatry*, November 2003; 49 – 52.

31. McMenamy, C., et al. "Treatment of CRPS in a multidisciplinary chronic pain program." *American Journal of Pain Management*, Via 14.(2). April 2004. p 56 – 62.

32. Gaby, A.R. "Literature Review and Commentary." *Townsend Letter for Doctors*, July 2000. p 32.

33. Crowley, K.L. "Clinical Application of Ketamine Ointment in the Treatment of Sympathetically Maintain Pain." *International Journal of Pharmaceutical Compounding*, Volume 2, #2, March/April 1998, pp 122 – 127.

34. Harbut, R.E., et al. "Successful Treatment of a Nine-year Case of Reflex Sympathetic Dystrophy with IV Ketamine Infusion in a warfarin anti-coagulated adult female patient." *Pain Medicine*, Vol 3 (2) 2002 p 147 – 155.

35. Jancin, B. "Adjunctive Therapies in Difficult Pain Patients." *International Medicine News*, May 1, 1999, p 16.

## Chapter 9: Myofascial (Muscles/Ligament/Tendon) and Fibromyalgia Pain

1. Teitelbaum, J., et al. "Effective Treatment of Fibromyalgia and Chronic Fatigue Syndrome; a Randomized Double-blind, Placebo-controlled Study." *Journal of Chronic Fatigue Syndrome*, 8(2) 2001. p 3 – 28.

2. McLain, D. "An open labeled dose finding trial of Zanaflex for treatment of fibromyalgia." *Journal of Musculoskeletal Pain*, 10(4) 2002. p 7 – 18.

3. Holman, A.J. "Safety and efficacy of the dopamine agonist, Pramipexole, on pain score for refractory fibromyalgia." Abstract presented at the American College of Rheumatology National Meeting. Philadelphia, November, 2000.

## Chapter 10: Arthritis Pain

1. Adam, O., Beringer, C., et al. *Rheumatol Int*, 2003; 23: 27 – 36.

2. Leventhal, L.J., et al. "Treatment of rheumatoid arthritis with gamma linolenic acid." *Annals of Internal Medicine,* 1993; 119: 867 – 873.

3. Gibson, T., et al. "A controlled study of diet in patients with gout." *Annals of Rheumatic Disease*, 42 (2): 123 – 27, 1983.

4. www.temple.edu/news_media/ej0312_462.html reporting on Tallarida, R., et al. "Anti-nociceptive synergy with combinations of Oral glucosamine plus non-opioid analgesics in mice." *Journal of Pharmacology and Experimental Therapeutics*, November 2003.

5. Lawrence, R.M. "MSM: a double-blind study of its use in degenerative arthritis." *International Journal of Antiaging Medicine*, 1998; and 1(1): 50 abstract.

5A. http://www.reutershealth.com/en/index.html.

6. Reginister. J., et al. "Glucosamine sulfate slows down osteoarthritis progression in postmenopausal woman: pooled analysis of two large independent, randomized, placebo-controlled, double-blind, prospective, three year trials." ULAR 2002 European Congress of Rheumatology; June 12-15, 2002; Stockholm, Sweden. Abstract 196.

7. Deal see, et al. "Nutriceuticals as therapeutic agents in osteoarthritis. The role of Glucosamine, Chondroitin sulfate, and collagen hydrolysate." Rheumatic Disease Clinics of North America 1999; 25: 379 – 95.

8. McAlindon, T., et al. "Nutrition: risk factors for osteo arthritis." *Annals of Rheumatic Disease*, 1997; 56: 397 – 402.

9. Konig, B. "A long-term [two year] clinical trial with SAM-e for the treatment of osteoarthritis." *American Journal of Medicine*, 1987; 835A: 89 – 94.

10. Lean, M., et al. "Impairment of health and quality-of-life using new US federal guidelines for the identification of obesity." *Archives of Internal Medicine*, 1999; 159: 837 – 843.

11. Felson, D., et al. "Weight loss reduces the risk for symptomatic knee osteoarthritis in women." The Framingham Study. *Annals of Internal Medicine*, 1992; 116: 535 – 9.

12. Miller, G., et al. "The Arthritis, Diet, and Activity Promotion Trial (ADAPT)." Control Clinical Trials 2003; 24: 462 – 80.

13. Walker, W.R., et al. "An investigation of the therapeutic value of the copper bracelet: dermal assimilation of copper in arthritic/rheumatoid conditions." Agents Actions 6: 454, 1976.

14. McLean, R. *Pain Medicine News* – based on the study presented at 2003 American Academy of physical medicine and Rehabilitation. January/February 2004. P 14.

## Chapter 11: Inflammatory Pain

1. Buskila, D., et al. "Fibromyalgia and systemic lupus erythematosus: prevalence and clinical implications." *Clinical Review of Allergy and Immunology*, 2003 August; 25 (1): 25 – 8.

2. Huisman, A.M., et al. "Vitamin D Levels in Women with Systemic Lupus Erythematosus and Fibromyalgia." *Journal of Rheumatology*, 2001; 28: 2535 – 9.

3. *Arthritis and Rheumatism*. 2002; 46 (7): 1820 – 1829.

4. Church, T.S., et al. "Reduction of C reactive protein levels through the use of a multivitamin." *American Journal of Medicine*, 2003 December 15; 115 (9): 702 – 7.

## Chapter 12: Other Pains—Osteoporosis and Cancer Pain

1. Meunier, P.J., et al. "Strontium ranelate: dose-dependent effects on established postmenopausal vertebral osteoporosis—a two-year randomized placebo-controlled trial." *Journal of Clinical Endocrinology and Metabolism*, May 2002; 87 (5): 2060 –6.

2. Meunier, P.J., et al. "The effects of strontium on the risk of vertebral fracture in women with postmenopausal osteoporosis." *New England Journal of Medicine*, 2004, January 29; 350 (5): 459 – 68.

3. McCaslin, F.E., et al. "The effect of strontium lactate in the treatment of osteoporosis." Proceedings of the Staff Meetings of the Mayo Clinic 34: 329-34, 1959.

4. *Inflammation and Aging*. Ronald E. Hunninghake, M.D. (Tape) The Center For the Improvement of Human Functioning International (run by Hugh Riorden, M.D.).

5. Skoryna, S.C. *Canadian Medical Association Journal*, 125: 703 – 712. 1981.

6. Aun, N.C. "Myofascial Pain Syndrome in Cancer Pain Management." *Chinese Journal of Pain*, 1996; 6: 111 – 118.
7. Crosby, V., et al. "The safety and efficacy of a single dose of intravenous magnesium sulfate in neuropathic pain poorly responsive to strong opioids analgesics in patients with cancer." *Journal of Pain Symptom Management*, 19: 2000: 35 – 39.

## Chapter 13: Headaches and Facial Pain

1. Educational resources: National Headache Foundation; headache fact sheet page. www.headaches.org/consumer/general info/factsheet.html.
2. Fox, R. "Natural Agents Offer Relief from the Misery of Migraines." *Life Extension*, February 2004 p 72 – 78.
3. *Pain Medicine News*, November/December 2003. p 6.
4. Martin Araguz, A., et al. "Treatment of Chronic Tension Type Headaches with Mirtazapine and Amitriptyline." *Rev Neurol*, 2003; 37: 101 – 105.
5. Holroyd, K.A., et al. *Headache*, 2003; 43: pp 999 – 1004.
6. Marcus, D.A. *Headache and Pain*, Nov 2003: p 180 – 185.
7. Oliver, R.L. "Choosing the right triptan." *Practical Pain Management*, January/February 2003; pp 15 – 18.
8. *Headache*, 2003 Sep; 43(8): 835 – 844.
9. *Lancet*, 1995; 346: 923 – 926.
10. *Functional Neurology*, 2000; 15 supplement 3: 196 – 201.
11. Wilner, A.N. *Pain Medicine News*. Vol 1 #4 p 1 and 5, 2003.
12. Wilner, A.N. *Pain Medicine News*. Vol 1 #4 p 1 and 5, 2003.
13. Demirkaya, S., et al. "Efficacy of Intravenous Magnesium Sulfate in the Treatment of Acute Migraine Attacks." *Headache*, 2001; 41: 171 – 177.
14. *Clinical Science*, 1995; 89: 633 – 6.
15. Dora, B. "Migraine Headache and Magnesium Sulfate." *Clinical Pearls News*, April 2002.
16. Singer, R.S., et al. "Oral Transmucosal Fentanyl Citrate in the Outpatient Treatment of Severe Pain from Migraine Headache." *The Pain Clinic*, Jan/Feb 2004; p 10 – 13.
17. Singer, R.S., et al. *The Pain Clinic*, Jan/Feb 2004; p 10 – 13.
18. Dora, B. *The Journal of Headache and Pain*, 2000; 1: 179 – 186.
19. *Clin Sci* [lond], 1995 December; 89 (6): 633 – 6.
20. *Headache*, 1996 March; 36 (3): 154 – 60.
21. Peikert, A., et al. "Prophylaxis of migraine with oral magnesium: results from a prospective, multi-center, placebo-controlled and double-blind randomized study." *Cephalgia*, 1996 June; 16 (4): 257 – 63.
22. Facchinetti, F., et al. "Magnesium prophylaxis of mention migraine: effects on intracellular magnesium." *Headache*, 1991 May; 31 (5): 298 – 301.
23. Schoenen, J., et al. "High-dose riboflavin as a prophylactic treatment of migraine: results of an open pilot study." *Cephalgia*, 1994 October; 14 (5): 328 – 9.
Schoenen, J., et al. "Effectiveness of high-dose riboflavin in migraine prophylaxis. A randomized controlled trial." *Neurology*, 1998 February; 50 (2): 466 – 70.
24. Van Der Kuy, P.H.M., et al. "Hydroxycobalamin, a nitric oxide scavenger, in the prophylaxis of migraine: an open, pilot study." *Cephalgia*, 2002; 22: 513 – 519.

25. Murphy, J.J., et al. "Randomized double-blind placebo-controlled trial of feverfew in migraine prevention." *Lancet*, 1988 July 23; 2May (8604); 189 – 92.

26. Prusinski, A., et al. "Feverfew as prophylactic treatment of migraine." *Neurol Neurochir Pol*, 1999; 33 supplement 5: 89 – 95.

27. Brown, D.J. "Standardized butterbur extract Petadolex – herbal approach to migraine prophylaxis." *Townsend Letter for Doctors and Patients*, October 2002.

28. Glueck, C.J., et al. "Amelioration of severe migraine with omega-3 fatty acids: a double-blind placebo-controlled clinical trial," Abstract. *American Journal of Clinical Nutrition*, 43: 710, 1986.

29. McCarren, T., et al. "Amelioration of severe migraine by fish oils," Abstract. *American Journal of Clinical Nutrition*, 41: 874 a, 1985.

30. Rozen, T.D., et al. "Open label trial of coenzyme Q10 as a migraine preventive." *Cephalgia*, 2002. March; 22 (2): 137 – 41.

31. British Medical Journal Online 2004: 10.1136/bmj.38029.421863.EB.

32. Mansfield, L.E., "Food allergy and migraine." *Postgraduate Medicine*, 83 (7): 46 – 55, 1988.

33. Mansfield, L.E., et al. "Food allergy and adult migraine." *Annals of Allergy*, 55: 126, 1985.

34. Monroe, J., et al. "Migraine is a food allergic disease." *Lancet*, 2: 719 – 21, 1984.

35. Egger, J., et al. "Is migraine food allergy?" *Lancet*, 2: 865-9, 1983.

36. Lipton, R., et al. "Aspartame as a dietary trigger of headache." *Headache*, 29: 90 – 92, 1989.

37. Koehler, S.M., et al. "The effect of aspartame on migraine headaches." *Headache*, 28 (1): 10 – 14, 1988.

38. Grant, E.C.G. "Food Allergies and Migraines." *Lancet*, May 5, 1979; 966 – 969.

39. Freitag, F.G. *Headache and Pain*, Nov 2003. p 151 – 2.

40. Manfredini, D., Romagnoli, M., Cantini, E., Bosco, M. "Efficacy of tizanidine hydrochloride in the treatment of myofascial face pain." *Minerva Med*, 2004 Apr; 95(2): 165 – 71.

41. Femiano, F., Scully, C. "Burning mouth syndrome: a double-blind controlled study of alpha lipoic acid therapy." *Journal of Oral Pathol Medicine*, 2002: 31: 267 – 269.

## Chapter: 14 Back Pain

1. *Practical Pain Management*, July/August 2003, p 36.

2. Kovacs, F.M., et al. *Lancet*, November 15, 2003; 362: pp 1599 – 1604.

3. *USA Weekend*, May 28, 2004 p 16.

4. Rask, M.R. "Colchicine use in 3000 patients with diskal and other spinal disorders." *Journal of Neurological and Orthopedic Surgery*, Vol 6, Issue 3, 1985. p 1 – 8.

5. Meek, J.B., et al. "Colchicine confirmed effective in disk disorders. Final results of a double blind study." *Journal of Neurologic and Orthopedic Medicine and Surgery*, Vol 6, Issue 3, 1985. p 211 – 218.

6. *USA Weekend*, May 28, 2004 p 16.

7. Krusz, J. "Lamotrigine in the treatment of Neuropathic Pain" [abstract 758] *Journal of Pain*, 3(2, Suppl.1): 40, 2002.

## Chapter 16: Spastic Colon


1. Teitelbaum, J., et al. "Effective treatment of chronic fatigue syndrome and fibromyalgia—a randomized double-blind placebo-controlled study." *Journal of Chronic Fatigue Syndrome*, p 3 – 24, 8(2), 2001.


## Chapter 17: Noncardiac Chest Pain


1. Jenson, M., et al. "Use of the lidocaine patch in the treatment of Costochondritis." *The Pain Clinic*, December 2003 pp 15 – 17.


## Chapter 18: Pelvic Pain Syndromes—Menstrual Cramps, Vulvadynia, Interstitial Cystitis, Endometriosis, and Prostadynia


1. Mulkey, V.H. "Interstitial Cystitis." *Continuing Education Topics and Issues*, Jan 2001. p 11 – 14.
2. *Journal of Urology*, 2002;167: 1338 – 1343.
3. Korting, G.E. et al. "A randomized double-blind trial of Oral L – arginine for treatment of interstitial cystitis." *Journal of Urology*, 1999; 161: 558 – 565.
4. Gutierrez, M., et al. "Mechanisms involved in the spasmolytic effect of extracts from Sabal serrulata fruit on smooth muscle." *Gen Pharmac*, 27: 171 – 176, 1996.
5. Stewart, E.G. "Diagnosis and management of generalized vulvodynia." *Practical Pain Management*, May/June 2004. p 38 – 41.
6. *Urology*, 63: 13 – 16. 2004.
7. Shoskes, D.A., et al. "Quercetin in men with category 3 chronic prostatitis: a preliminary prospective, double-blind, placebo-controlled trial." *Urology*, 1999; 54: 960 – 963.


## Chapter 19: Wrist, Hand, Shoulder, Leg, and Foot Pains


1. Hoffberg, H,J. "Carpal Tunnel Syndrome." *Practical Pain Management*, 2002; November/December. p 10 – 15.
2. Rep̀ice, R.M., et al. "Wrist Traction As a New Method for Treatment of Carpal Tunnel Syndrome." *American Journal of Pain Management*, 2003: 14; 31 – 36.
3. Drug Therapy Bulletin 34: 7, 1996 and Postgraduate Medicine 99 (2): 177, 1996.


## Chapter 20: Natural Therapies


1. "Money Colors Drug Research," *Journal of the American Medical Association*, 1/22/03 reported in <u>USA Today</u>,1/22/03 P 6.
2. Chrubasik, S., et al. "Treatment of low back pain exacerbations with willow bark extract: a randomized double-blind study." *American Journal of Medicine*, 2000 Jul; 109 (1): 9 – 14.

3. Chrubasik, S., Kunzel, O., et al. "Potential economic impact of using a proprietary willow bark extract in outpatient treatment of low back pain: an open non-randomized study." *Phytomedicine*, 2001 Jul; 8(4): 241 – 51.
4. Marz, R.W., Kemper, F. "Willow bark extract—effects and effectiveness. Status of current knowledge regarding pharmacology, toxicology and clinical aspects>" [Article in German] *Wien Med Wochenschr*, 2002; 152(15-16): 354 – 9.
5. Schmid, B., et al. "Efficacy and tolerability of a standardized willow bark extract in patients with osteoarthritis: randomized placebo-controlled, double blind clinical trial." *Phytother Res*, 2001 Jun; 15(4): 344 – 50.
6. Highfield, E.S., Kemper, K.J. "White willow monograph." Longwood Herbal Task Force. Accessed on June 7, 2004. Available at: http://www.mcp.edu/herbal/willowbark/willow.pdf.
7. Hedner, T., Everts, B. "The early clinical history of salicylates in rheumatology and pain." *Clinical Rheumatology*, 1998; 17: 17 – 25.
8. Chrubasik, S., Eisenberg, E. "Treatment of rheumatic pain with herbal medicine in Europe." *Pain Digest*, 1998; 8: 231 – 6.
9. Meier, B., Sticher, O., Julkunen-Tiitto, R. "Pharmaceutical aspects of the use of willows in herbal remedies." *Planta Medica* 1988: 559 – 60.
10. Singh, G.B., Atal, C.K. *Agents and Actions* 1986; 18: 407.
11. Sharma, M.L., et al. *Agents and Actions* 1988; 24: 161.
12. Sharma, M.L., et al. *International Journal Immunopharm*, 1989; 11: 647.
13. Kar, A., Menon, M.K. *Life Sciences* 1969; 8: 1023.
14. Menon, M.K., Kar, A. *Planta Medica* 1971; 19: 333.
15. Sander, O., Herborn, G., Rau, R. [Is H15 (Resin extract of Boswellia serrata, "incense") a useful supplement to established drug therapy of chronic polyarthritis? Results of a double-blind pilot study] *Z Rheumatol*, 1998; 57: 11 – 6. German.
16. Sharma, M.L., et al. *Agents and Actions* 1988; 24: 161.
17. Etzel, R. *Phytomedicine* 1996; 3(1): 91 – 94.
18. Kimmatkar, N., Thawani, V., Hingorani, L., et al. *Phytomedicine* 2003; 10(1): 3 – 7.
19. Safayhi, H., et al. "Inhibition by Boswellic acids of human leukocyte elastase." *Journal of Pharmacological Experimental Therory*, 1997 Apr; 281(1): 460 – 3.
20. Gupta, I., et al. "Effects of a Boswellia resin in patients with bronchial asthma: results of a double-blind, placebo-controlled, six week clinical study." *European Journal of Medical Research*, 1998; 3: 511 – 514.
21. Gupta, I., et al. "Effects of gum resin of Boswellia serrata in patients with chronic colitis." *Planta Medica* 2001 Jul; 67(5): 391 – 5.
22. Hostanska, K., et al. "Cytostatic and apoptosis-inducing activity of boswellic acids toward malignant cell lines in vitro." *Anticancer Res*, 2002 Sep-Oct;22(5): 2853 – 62.
23. Huang, M.T., et al. "Anti-tumor and anti-carcinogenic activities of triterpenoid, beta-boswellic acid." *Biofactors*, 2000; 13(1-4): 225 – 30.
24. Seeram, N.P., et al. "Cyclooxygenase inhibitory and antioxidant cyanidin glycosides in cherries and berries." *Phytomedicine*, 2001 Sep; 8(5): 362 – 9.
25. Kang, S.Y., et al. "Tart cherry anthocyanins inhibit tumor development in Apc(Min) mice and reduce proliferation of human colon cancer cells." *Cancer Letter*, 2003 May 8; 194(1): 13 – 9.
26. Blau, L.W. "Cherry diet control for gout and arthritis." *Tex Report on Biol Medicine*, 1950; 8: 309 – 11.

27. Gabor, M. "Pharmacologic effects of flavonoids on blood vessels." *Angiologica.* 1972; 9: 355 – 74.

28. Havsteen, B. "Flavonoids, a class of natural products of high pharmacological potency." *Biochem Pharm*, 1983; 32: 1141 – 1148.

29. Lawrence, R.M. "MSM: a double-blind study of its use in degenerative arthritis." *International Journal of Antiaging Medicine*, 1998; and1(1): 50 abstract.

30. Reginister, J., et al. "Glucosamine sulfate slows down osteoarthritis progression in postmenopausal woman: pooled analysis of two large independent, randomized, placebo-controlled, double-blind, prospective, three year trials." ULAR 2002 European Congress of Rheumatology; June 12-15, 2002; Stockholm, Sweden. Abstract 196.

31. Deal see, et al. "Nutriceuticals as therapeutic agents in osteoarthritis. The role of Glucosamine, Chondroitin sulfate, and collagen hydrolysate." Rheumatic Disease Clinics of North America 1999; 25: 379 – 95.

32. Femiano, F., Scully, C. "Burning mouth syndrome: a double-blind controlled study of alpha lipoic acid therapy." *Journal of Oral Pathol Medicine*, 2002: 31: 267 – 269.

33. Konig, B. "A long-term (two years) clinical trial with SAM-e for the treatment of osteoarthritis." *American Journal of Medicine*, 1987; 835A: 89 – 94.

34. Fleming, T., ED. "Jamaica Dogwood" PDR for herbal medicines. 1998 pp 428 – 9.

35. ."Humulus Lupus," Monograph. *Alternative Medicine Review*, 8(2)2003.190 – 192.

36. Cronin, J.R. "Passionflower—Reigniting Male Libido and Other Potential Uses." *Alternative and Complementary Therapies*, April 2003. pp 89 – 92.

37. Dhawan, K., et al. "Reversal of Morphine Tolerance and Dependence by Passiflora Incarnata." *Pharmaceutical Biology*, 2002; 40 (8): 576 – 580.

38. Hadley, S., et al. "Valerian." *American Family Physician*, 2003; 67 (8): 1755 – 1758.

39. Blonstein, J.L. "Control of Swelling in Boxing Injuries." *Practitioner*, 1969; 203: 206.

40. Donath, F., et al. "Dose related bioavailability of Bromelain and trypsin after repeated oral administration." *Clin Pharm Therapy*, 61, 157 1997.

41. Bailey, S.P. "Effects of protease supplementation on muscle soreness following downhill running." *Medicine and Science in Sports and Exercise*, May 1999; 31 (Five): a 214, S. 76.

42. Ramirez-Bosca, A., et al. "Antioxidant curcuma extracts decrease the blood lipid peroxide levels of human subjects." *Age*, 18: 167-9, 1995.

43. Arjun, R., et al. "Curcumin attenuates allergen induced airway hyper responsiveness in sensitized guinea pigs." *Biol Pharm Bulletin*, 26(7)1021 – 1024 (2003).

44. Joe, B., et al. "Biological properties of curcumin-cellular and molecular mechanisms of action." *Crit Rev Food Sci Nutr*, 2004; 44(2): 97 – 111.

45. Cronin, J.R. "Old spice is a new medicine." *The Biochemistry of Alternative Medicine in Alternative and Complementary Therapies*, February 2003: 34 – 38.

46. *Chem Pharm Bulletin* 1992; 40: 187 – 91.

47. Brown, D.J. "Standardized butterburr extract for migraine treatment: a clinical overview." *HerbalGram* # 58, 2003 p 19.

48. Sindrup, S.H., et al. "St. John's wort has no [statistically significant] effect on pain in polyneuropathy." *Pain*, 2001; 91: 361 – 365.

## Chapter 21: Structural Therapies—Chiropractic and Osteopathic Medicine


1. E Basch, M.D. and C Ulbricht Pharm D. "Chiropractic Discipline Addresses Multitude of Health Concerns." *Alternative Medicine Research Report*, October 2003 pp 109 – 116.


## Chapter 22: Prescription Therapies—We're Way Past Aspirin!


1. Trnavsky, K., et al. "Efficacy and safety of 5 percent ibuprofen cream treatment in knee Osteoarthritis: Results of randomized, double-blind, placebo-controlled study." *Journal of Rheumatology*, 2004; 31: 565 – 572.
2. Backonja, M. "Pathogenesis and treatment of neuropathic pain in older adults." *American Journal of Pain Management*, 14(2) April 2004. p9S – 18S.
3. *Mortar and Pestle*, May 2000.
4. Chase, M. "The race to make a gentler painkiller faces high standards." *Wall Street Journal*, May 30, 1998.
5. Scheman, J., et al. "Fibromyalgia—A special Indication for Chronic Pain." Rehabilitation Highlights of the American Academy of Pain Medicine Meeting, March 3 – 7, 2004: Orlando Florida. Abstract 113.
6. Singh, G. "Recent considerations in nonsteroidal anti-inflammatory drug gastropathy." *American Journal of Medicine*, 1998; 105 31S – 38S.
7. Goldenberg, D.L., et al. "A randomized, controlled trial of amitriptyline and Naprosyn in the treatment of patients with fibromyalgia." *Arthritis and Rheumatism*, volume 29, 11, November 1986, 1371 – 1377.
8. Laine, L., et al. *Gastroenterology*, 116: a229, April 1999.
9. *Journal of Rheumatology*, June 2004.
10. "Beware of Overdosing of Over-the-counter Analgesic Containing Medicines." *Pain Medicine News*, March/April 2004. p 1.
11. Pembrook, L. "NSAIDs Superior to Acetaminophen in Treating Osteoarthritis Pain," Based on a presentation at the 2003 annual meeting of the American College of Rheumatology. *Pain Medicine News*, March/April 2004. p 13.
12. *Primary Psychiatry*, November 2003. p 17.
13. Todorov., A.B., et al. "Tiagabine and gabapentin in the management of chronic pain and sleep disturbances." Poster presentation. 22nd annual meeting of the American Pain Society, Chicago, Illinois, March 22 – 23, 2003.
14. Mathias, S., et al. "The GABA uptake inhibitor Gabitril promotes slow wave sleep in normal elderly subjects." *Neurobiology of Aging*, 22: 247 – 253, 2001.
15. Jung, A.C., et al. "Selective Serotonin Reuptake Inhibitors Are Effective for Mixed Chronic Pain." *The Journal of General Internal Medicine*, June 1997; 384 – 389.
16. Goldenberg, D.L. "A Review of the Role of Tricyclic Medications in the Treatment of Fibromyalgia Syndrome." *Journal of Rheumatology*, 1989; (Supplement 19) 16: 137 – 9.
17. O Malley, P.G., et al. "Treatment of fibromyalgia with antidepressants. A metaanalysis." *Journal of General Internal Medicine*, 2000 Sep; 15; 659 – 66.

18. Jancin, B. "Adjunctive Therapies in Difficult Pain Patients." *Internal Medicine News*, May 1, 1999, p 16.

19. Bennett, R.M., et al. "A Comparison of Cyclobenzaprine and Placebo in the Management of Fibrositis." *Arthritis and Rheumatism Primary Care Review*, Volume 2, 4 July 1990, pp 16 – 24.

20. Quimby, L.G., et al. "A randomized trial of Cyclobenzaprine for the treatment of fibromyalgia." *Journal of Rheumatology*, 1989: supplement 19; 16. p 140 – 3.

21. *Practical Pain Management*, Nov/Dec 2003, p 36.

22. Grothe, D.R., et al. "Treatment of pain syndromes with Effexor." *Pharmacotherapy*, 2004 May: 24 (5): 621 – 9.

23. Jancin, B. "Adjunctive Therapies in Difficult Pain Patients." *Internal Medicine News*, May 1, 1999, p 16.

24. "Treatment of Sexual Side Effects [of Antidepressants]." Report and references available at www.Medscape.com/reviewarticle/430614_5.

25. Hoffmann, V., et al. "Successful Treatment of Post herpetic Neuralgia with Oral Ketamine." *The Clinical Journal of Pain*, 10: 240 – 242. 1994.

26. Furuhashi-Yonaha, A., et al. "Short and long-term efficacy of Oral ketamine in 8 chronic pain patients." *Canadian Journal of Anesthesiology*, 2002; 49: 886 – 887.

27. "Successful Use of Gabapentin for Benzodiazepine Detoxification." *Primary Psychiatry*, July 2001. p 18.

28. *Pain* 1994 Dec; 59(3)361 – 8.

29. Nelson. *Neurology* 48: 1212, 1997.

30. Clark, S.R., Bennett, R.M. *AFSA Update*, October 2000, p 5.

31. Chevlen, E.M. "Optimizing the use of opioids in the elderly population." *American Journal of Pain Management*, 14 (2) April 2004 P 19 S – 24S.

32. Slatkin, N.E. "Treatment of Opiate Related Sedation: Utility of the Cholinesterase Inhibitors." *Journal of Supportive Oncology*,1: p 53 – 63, 2003.

33. Alsager, D.E. "Oxycommon use associated with Perleche (B2 deficiency)." *Clinical Practice of Pain*, August 2001 pp 25 – 26.

34. Jancin, B. "Adjunctive Therapies in Difficult Pain Patients." *Internal Medicine News*, May 1, 1999, p 16.

35. *Pain* 1994 December; 59, 3; 361 – 368.
*The Mortar and Pestle*, January 1998.

36. Karst, M., et al. "Analgesic effect of the synthetic Cannabinoid CT-3 on chronic neuropathic pain-a RCT." *Journal of the American Medical Association*, 2003: 290: 1757 – 1762.

37. Campbell, F.A., et al. *British Medical Journal*,2001 July 7, 323: 1 – 6.

38. "Open Label Study for Oral Cannabinoids for Neuropathic Pain." *Pain Management*, May/June 2004.

39. Russo, E.B. "Clinical endocannabinoid deficiency (CECD): Can this concept explain the therapeutic benefits of cannabis in migraine, fibromyalgia, irritable bowel syndrome and other treatment resistant conditions?" *Neuroendocrinology Letter*, February – April 2004; 25 (1 – 2): 31 – 9.

40. Reed, J.C. "Magnesium Therapy in Musculoskeletal Pain Syndromes—Retrospective Review of Clinical Results." Magnesium Trace Elements 1990; 9: 330.

41. J.H. Raphael, et al. "Efficacy and adverse effects of intravenous lignocaine therapy in fibromyalgia syndrome." *BMC Musculoskeletal Disorders*, 2002, 3: 21.

42. Sorensen, J., et al. *Journal of Rheumatology*, 1997; 24: 1615 – 1621.

43. Bennett, M.I., Tai, M.A. *International Journal of Clinical Pharmacology*, Res XV(3) 115 – 119 (1995).

44. Graven-Nielsen, T., et al. “Ketamine reduces muscle pain, temporal summation, and referred pain in fibromyalgia patients.” *Pain*, 85 (2000) p 483 – 491.

45. *Pain Medicine News*, March/April 2003 p 10 (based on a poster presentation at the 2002 annual meeting of the New York State Society of Anesthesiologists).

## Chapter 23:Prolotherapy

1. Banks, A.R. “A Rationale for Prolotherapy.” Journal of Orthopaedic Medicine 1991; Vol 13, No 3.

2. Hackett, G.S., Hemwall, G.A. Montgomery GA. *Ligament and Tendon Relaxation Treated by Prolotherapy*. 1993, 5th Edition, 2nd Printing, Oak Park Illinois.

3. Klein, R.G. “Proliferant Injectionas for Low Back Pain: Histologic Changes of Injected Ligaments and Objective Measures of Lumbar Spine Mobility before and After Treatment.” *Journal of Neurology, Orthopedic Medicine and Surgery* 1989; 10: 141 – 144.

4. Klein, R.G., Eek, B.C., DeLong, W.B., Mooney. V. “A Randomized Double-Blind Trial of Dextrose-Glycerine-Phenol Injections for Chronic Low Back Pain.” *Journal of Spinal Disorders*, 1993; Vol 6, No 1: 23-33.

5. Liu YK, Tipton CM, Matthes RD, Bedford TG, Maynard JA, Walmer HC. “An In Situ Study of the Influence of a Sclerosing Solution in Rabbit Medial Collateral Ligaments and Its Junction Strength.” Connective Tissue Research 1983; Vol 11: 95-102.

6. Maynard J, et al. “Morphological and Biochemical Effects of Sodium Morrhuate on Tendons.” Journal of Orthopaedic Research 1985; 3: 234-248.

7. Mooney, V. “Prolotherapy in the Spine and Pelvis: An Introduction.” *SPINE: State of the Art Reviews*, 1995; Vol 9, No 2: 309 – 311.

8. Mooney, V. “Prolotherapy at the fringe of medical care, or is it the frontier?” *The Spine Journal*, 3 (2003) 253 – 254.

9. Ongley, M.J., Dorman, T.A., Klein, R.G., Eek, B.C., Hubert, L.J. “A New Approach to the Treatment of Chronic Low Back Pain.” *The Lancet*, July 18, 1987: 143 – 146.

10. Ongley, M.J., Dorman, T.A., Eek, B.C., Lundgren, D., Klein, R.G. “Ligament instability of knees: a new approach to treatment.” *Manual Medicine*, 1988; 3: 152 – 154.

11. Reeves, K.D. “Treatment of Consecutive Severe Fibromyalgia Patients with Prolotherapy.” *Journal of Orthopaedic Medicine*, 1994; Vol 16, No 3.

12. Reeves, K.D. “Prolotherapy: Present and Future Applications in Soft-Tissue Pain and Disability.” Physical Medicine and Rehabilitation Clinics of North America, November 1995; Vol 6, No 4: 917 – 926.

13. Reeves, K.D., Hassanein, K. “Randomized Prospective Double-Blind Placebo-Controlled Study of Dextrose Prolotherapy for Knee Osteoarthritis with or without ACL Laxity.” *Alternative Therapies Health Medicine*, March 2000; Vol 6, No 2: 68 – 80.

14. Reeves, K.D., Hassanein, K. “Randomized, Prospective, Placebo-Controlled Double-Blind Study of Dextrose Prolotherapy for Osteoarthritic Thumb and Finger (DIP, PIP, and Trapeziometacarpal) Joints: Evidence of Clinical Efficacy.” *The Journal of Alternative and Complementary Medicine*, 2000; Vol 6, No 4: 311 – 320.

15. Reeves, K.D. "Prolotherapy: Basic Science, Clinical Studies, and Technique." In: Lennard, T.A., ed. *Pain Procedures in Clinical Practice.* 2[nd] ed. Philadelphia, PA: Hanley and Belfus; 2000: 172 – 190.

16. Reeves, K.D., Hassanein, K.M. "Long Term Effects of Dextrose Prolotherapy for Anterior Cruciate Ligament Laxity." *Alternative Therapies*, May/June 2003, Vol. 9, No. 3.

17. Schultz, L.W. "A Treatment for Suluxation of the Temporomandibular Joint." *Journal of the American Medical Association*, Sept 25, 1937; Vol 109, No 13: 1032 – 1035.

18. Schultz, L. "Twenty years experience in treating hypermobility of the temporomandibular joints" *American Journal of Surgery*, Vol 92, Dec, 1956, pp 925 – 928.

19. Schwartz, R.G., Sagedy, N. "Prolotherapy: A Literature Review and Retrospective Study," *The Journal of Neurological and Orthopaedic Medicine and Surgery*, 1991; Vol 12, No 3.

20. Wilkinson, H.A. *The Failed Back Syndrome: Etiology and Therapy.* New York, Springer-Verlag, 1992: 147-169.

## Chapter 24: Traditional Chinese Medicine: Acupuncture for Coordinated Wellness-Care

1. Eisenberg, D.M., Davis, R.B., Ettner, S.L., Appel, S., Wilkey, S., Van Rompay, M., and Kessler, R.C. "Trends in Alternative Medicine Use in the United States, 1990-1997: Results of a Follow-Up National Survey." *Journal of the American Medical Association*, 1998. 280(18): 1569 – 75.

2. Culliton, P.D. "Current Utilization of Acupuncture by United States Patients." National Institutes of Health Consensus Development Conference on Acupuncture, Program & Abstracts (Bethesda, MD, November 3-5, 1997). Office of Alternative Medicine and Office of Medical Applications of Research. Bethesda: National Institutes of Health, 1997.

3. Beinfield, H. and Korngold, E.L. *Between Heaven and Earth: A Guide to Chinese Medicine. New York.* Ballantine Books, 1991.

4. Brown, D. "Three Generations of Alternative Medicine: Behavioral Medicine, Integrated Medicine, and Energy Medicine." Boston University School of Medicine Alumni Report. Fall 1996.

5. Senior, K. "Acupuncture: Can It Take the Pain Away?" *Molecular Medicine Today*, 1996. 2(4): 150 – 3.

6. Raso, J. *Alternative Health Care: A Comprehensive Guide. Buffalo.* Prometheus Books, 1994.

7. National Institutes of Health Consensus Panel. Acupuncture. National Institutes of Health Consensus Development Statement (Bethesda, MD, November 3-5, 1997). Office of Alternative Medicine and Office of Medical Applications of Research. Bethesda: National Institutes of Health, 1997.

8. Dale, R.A. "Demythologizing Acupuncture. Part 1. The Scientific Mechanisms and the Clinical Uses." *Alternative and Complementary Therapies Journal*, April 1997. 3(2): 125 – 31.

9. Takeshige, C. "Mechanism of Acupuncture Analgesia Based on Animal Experiments." *Scientific Bases of Acupuncture.* Berlin: Springer-Verlag, 1989.

10. Han, J.S. "Acupuncture Activates Endogenous Systems of Analgesia." National Insti-

tutes of Health Consensus Conference on Acupuncture, Program & Abstracts (Bethesda, MD, November 3-5, 1997). Office of Alternative Medicine and Office of Medical Applications of Research. Bethesda: National Institutes of Health, 1997.

11. Wu, B., Zhou, R.X., and Zhou, M.S. "Effect of Acupuncture on Interleukin-2 Level and NK Cell Immunoactivity of Peripheral Blood of Malignant Tumor Patients." Chung Kuo Chung Hsi I Chieh Ho Tsa Chich. 1994. 14(9): 537 – 9.

12. Wu, B. "Effect of Acupuncture on the Regulation of Cell-Mediated Immunity in the Patients with Malignant Tumors." Chen Tzu Yen Chiu. 1995. 20(3): 67 – 71.

13. Eskinazi, D.P. "National Institutes of Health Technology Assessment Workshop on Alternative Medicine: Acupuncture." *Journal of Alternative and Complementary Medicine*, 1996. 2(1): 1 – 253.

14. Tang, N.M., Dong, H.W., Wang, X.M., Tsui, Z.C., and Han, J.S. "Cholecystokinin Antisense RNA Increases the Analgesic Effect Induced by Electroacupuncture or Low Dose Morphine: Conversion of Low Responder Rats into High Responders." *Pain*, 1997. 71(1): 71 – 80.

15. Cheng, X.D., Wu, G.C., He, Q.Z., and Cao, X.D. "Effect of Electroacupuncture on the Activities of Tyrosine Protein Kinase in Subcellular Fractions of Activated T Lymphocytes from the Traumatized Rats." *Acupuncture and Electro-Therapeutics Research*, 1998. 23(3-4): 161 – 170.

16. Chen, L.B. and Li, S.X. "The Effects of Electrical Acupuncture of Neiguan on the PO2 of the Border Zone between Ischemic and Non-Ischemic Myocardium in Dogs." *Journal of Traditional Chinese Medicine*, 1983. 3(2): 83 – 8.

17. Lee, H.S. and Kim, J.Y. "Effects of Acupuncture on Blood Pressure and Plasma Renin Activity in Two-Kidney One Clip Goldblatt Hypertensive Rats." *American Journal of Chinese Medicine*, 1994. 22(3-4): 215 – 9.

18. Okada, K., Oshima, M., and Kawakita, K. "Examination of the Afferent Fiber Responsible for the Suppression of Jaw-Opening Reflex in Heat, Cold and Manual Acupuncture Stimulation in Anesthetized Rats." *Brain Research*, 1996. 740(1-2): 201 – 7.

19. Lao, L., Bergman, S., Langenberg, P., Wong, R., and Berman, B. "Efficacy of Chinese Acupuncture on Postoperative Oral Surgery Pain." *Oral Surgery, Oral Medicine, Oral Pathology*. 1995. 79(4): 423 – 8.

20. Lewith, G.T. and Vincent, C. "On the Evaluation of the Clinical Effects of Acupuncture: A Problem Reassessed and a Framework for Future Research." *Journal of Alternative and Complementary Medicine*, 1996. 2(1): 79 – 90.

21. Tsibuliak, V.N., Alisov, A.P., and Shatrova, V.P. "Acupuncture Analgesia and Analgesic Transcutaneous Electroneurostimulation in the Early Postoperative Period." *Anesteziologiia i Reanimatologiia*, 1995. 2: 93 – 7.

22. Bullock, M.L., Pheley, A.M., Kiresuk, T.J., Lenz, S.K., and Culliton, P.D. "Characteristics and Complaints of Patients Seeking Therapy at a Hospital-Based Alternative Medicine Clinic." *Journal of Alternative and Complementary Medicine*, 1997. 3(1): 31 – 7.

23. Deihl, D.L., Kaplan, G., Coulter, I., Glik, D., and Hurwitz, E.L. "Use of Acupuncture by American Physicians." *Journal of Alternative and Complementary Medicine*, 1997. 3(2): 119 – 26.

24. Ter Reit, G., Kleijnen, J., and Knipschild, P. "Acupuncture and Chronic Pain: A Criteria-Based Meta-Analysis." *Clinical Epidemiology*, 1990. 43: 1191 – 9.

25. "Acupuncture Needles No Longer Investigational." U.S. *Food and Drug Administration. FDA Consumer Magazine*, June 1996. 30(5).

26. Lytle, C.D. "An Overview of Acupuncture." 1993. Washington: U.S. Department of Health and Human Services, Health Sciences Branch, Division of Life Sciences, Office of Science and Technology, Center for Devices and Radiological Health, Food and Drug Administration.

27. Berman, B., Lao, L., Bergman, S., Langenberg, P., Wong, R., Loangenberg, P., and Hochberg, M. "Efficacy of Traditional Chinese Acupuncture in the Treatment of Osteoarthritis: A Pilot Study." *Osteoarthritis and Cartilage*. 1995. (3): 139 – 42.

28. Allen, John J.B. "An Acupuncture Treatment Study for Unipolar Depression." *Psychological Science*, 1998. 9: 397 – 401.

29. Sonenklar, N. "Acupuncture and Attention Deficit Hyperactivity Disorder." National Institutes of Health, Office of Alternative Medicine Research grant R21 RR09463. 1993.

30. Milligan, R. Breech Version by Acumoxa. National Institutes of Health, Office of Alternative Medicine Research grant R21 RR09527. 1993.

31. Cardini, F. and Weixin, H. "Moxibustion for Correction of Breech Presentation: A Randomized Controlled Trial." *Journal of the American Medical Association*, 1998. 280: 1580 – 4.

32. White House Commission on Complementary and Alternative Medicine Policy. Interim Progress Report: White House Commission on Complementary and Alternative Medicine Policy. Washington: White House Commission on Complementary and Alternative Medicine Policy, 2001.

33. "Doctor, What's This Acupuncture All About? A Brief Explanation for Patients." American Academy of Medical Acupuncture. Los Angeles: American Academy of Medical Acupuncture, 1996.

34. Lao, L. "Safety Issues in Acupuncture." *Journal of Alternative and Complementary Medicine*, 1996. 2(1): 27 – 9

## Chapter 25: Sexual Dysfunction, Depression, and Mind-Body Aspects of Pain

1. Teitelbaum, J., et al. Unpublished data.

2. *Pain Medicine News*, March/April 2004 p 1.

3. Jonathan V. Wright, M.D. and Lane Lenard. Ph.D. *Maximize Your Vitality and Potency for Men Over 40*. Smart Publications, 1999. (contains multiple references) The study's findings were presented at the 2004 52nd Annual Clinical Meeting of the American College of Obstetricians and Gynecologists (ACOG).

4. Elliott, T. "Chronic pain, depression, and quality of life: correlations with gender, age, and number of pain types." Program and abstracts of the American Academy of Pain Medicine 20th Annual Meeting; March 3 – 7, 2004; Orlando, Florida. Abstract 115.

5. Pinzon, E.G., "Persistent Spine Centered Chronic Pain Scenarios and Treatment Options" *Practical Pain Management*, March/April 2004 pp 17 – 22.

6. Bressa, G.M. "SAM-e as an antidepressant: meta analysis of clinical studies." *Acta Neurol Scand*, Suppl 1994;154: 7 – 14.

7. Peet, M., et al. "A dose ranging study of the effects of eicosapentaenoate in patients with ongoing depression despite apparently adequate treatment with standard drugs." *Archives of General Psychiatry*, 2002; 59 (10): 913 – 919.

8. Su, K., et al. "Omega-3 fatty acids and major depressive disorders: a preliminary double-blind placebo-controlled trial." *Eur Neuropsychopharmacal*, 2003;13(4): 267 – 261.

9. Lake, J. "The Integrative Management of Depressed Mood." *Integrative Medicine*, 3(3)June/July 2004. p 34 – 43.

10. Birdsall, T.C. "5HTP: a clinically effective serotonin precursor." *Alternative Medicine Review*, 1998; 3 (4): 271 – 280.

11. Fieve, R., et al. "Rubidium: Biochemical, behavioral, and metabolic studies in humans." *Am Journal of Psychiatry*,1973; 130: 55 – 61.

12. Carolei, A., et al. "Azione farmacologica del cluorodi rubidio—effeto antidepressivo: confronts con l'imipramina." *Clin Ter*, 1975; 75: 469 – 478.

13. Calandra, C., Nicolisi, M. "Confronts fra due farmaci ad azione antidepressiva: rubidio cluoro a chlorimipramina." Proc 34th Congress Italian Society of Psychiatry, Catania, Italy, 1980.

14. Placidi, G., et al. "Exploration of the clinical profile of rubidium chloride in depression: a systemic open trial." *Journal of Clinical Psychopharmacology*,1988; 8(3): 184 – 188.

15. Torta, R., et al. "Rubidium chloride in the treatment of major depression." *Minerva Psichiatr*, 1993; 34(2): 101 – 110.

16. Brundisino, A., Cairoli, S. "The pharmacological action of rubidium chloride in depression." *Minerva Psichiatr*, 1996; 37(1): 45 – 49.

17. Williams, R., Maturen, A., Sky-Peck, H. "Pharmacologic role of rubidium in psychiatric research." *Comprehensive Therapy*, 1987; 13(9): 46 – 54.

18. Torta, R., et al. "Rubidium chloride in the treatment of major depression." *Minerva Psichiatr*,1993; 34(2): 101 – 110.

19. Pippa, Wysong. *Medscape Orthopaedics and Sports Medicine*. 8(1), 2004. © 2004 Medscape.

## Chapter 26: Eliminating Weight Gain

1. Teitelbaum, J., et al. unpublished data.

## Appendix E: Why Physicians Do Not Focus on Pain Medicine

1. "Just 335 Physicians Treat Pain of 2.3 Million Patients in Ohio." *Pain Medicine News*, March/April 2004, p 5.

2. "Worried Pain Doctors Decry Prosecutions." *Washington Post*, p 1 and 4, December 29, 2003.

3. Gupta, S. "Knowledge and comfort level in opioid management amongst physicians." Program and abstracts of the American Academy of Pain Medicine 20th Annual Meeting; March 3 – 7, 2004; Orlando, Florida. Abstract 124.

4. *USA Today*, Wednesday, January 22, 2003. p 6D. ■

# Index

## B



## C

## D



## E



## F

## G



## H



## I

## J



## K



## L



## M

## N



## O

## P

## X



## Y



## Z

## Promises, Promises

While walking down the street one day a U.S. senator is tragically hit by a truck and dies. His soul arrives in heaven and is met by St. Peter at the entrance.

"Welcome to heaven," says St. Peter. "Before you settle in, it seems there is a problem. We seldom see a high official around these parts, you see, so we're not sure what to do with you."

"No problem, just let me in," says the man.

"Well, I'd like to but I have orders from higher up. What we'll do is have you spend one day in hell and one in heaven. Then you can choose where to spend eternity."

"Really, I've made up my mind. I want to be in heaven," says the senator.

"I'm sorry but we have our rules."

And with that, St. Peter escorts him to the elevator and he goes down, down, down to hell. The doors open and he finds himself in the middle of a green golf course. In the distance is a club and standing in front of it are all his friends and other politicians who had worked with him. Everyone is very happy and in evening dress.

They run to greet him, shake his hand, and reminisce about the good times they had while getting rich at expense of the people.

They play a friendly game of golf and then dine on lobster, caviar and champagne.

Also present is the devil, who really is a very friendly guy and who has a good time dancing and telling jokes. They are having such a good time that, before he realizes it, it is time to go.

Everyone gives him a hearty farewell and waves while the elevator rises.

The elevator goes up, up, up, and the door reopens on heaven, where St. Peter is waiting for him.

"Now it's time to visit heaven."

So, 24 hours pass with the head of state joining a group of contented souls moving from cloud to cloud, playing the harp and singing. They have a good time and, before he realizes it, the 24 hours have gone by and St. Peter returns.

"Well then, you've spent a day in hell and another in heaven. Now choose your eternity."

*Continued on next page*

*(continued)*

The senator reflects for a minute, then the senator answers: "Well, I would never have said it before, I mean heaven has been delightful, but I think I would be better off in hell."

So St. Peter escorts him to the elevator and he goes down, down, down to hell.

Now the doors of the elevator open and he's in the middle of a barren land covered with waste and garbage.

He sees all his friends, dressed in rags, picking up the trash and putting it in black bags.

The devil comes over to him and puts his arm around his shoulder.

"I don't understand," stammers the senator. "Yesterday I was here and there was a golf course and club, and we ate lobster and caviar, drank champagne, and danced and had a great time. Now all there is, is a wasteland full of garbage and my friends look miserable. What happened?"

The devil looks at him, smiles and says,

"Yesterday we were campaigning. Today you voted for us.

# Notes

# Notes